EXPOSURE THERAPY FOR ANXIETY

Exposure Therapy for Anxiety

Principles and Practice

Jonathan S. Abramowitz
Brett J. Deacon
Stephen P. H. Whiteside

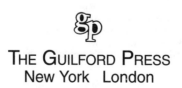

THE GUILFORD PRESS
New York   London

© 2011 The Guilford Press
A Division of Guilford Publications, Inc.
72 Spring Street, New York, NY 10012
www.guilford.com

Printed in the United States of America

This book is printed on acid-free paper.

Last digit is print number: 9 8 7 6 5 4 3

The authors have checked with sources believed to be reliable in their efforts to provide
information that is complete and generally in accord with the standards of practice that
are accepted at the time of publication. However, in view of the possibility of human error
or changes in behavioral, mental health, or medical sciences, neither the authors, nor
the editor and publisher, nor any other party who has been involved in the preparation
or publication of this work warrants that the information contained herein is in every
respect accurate or complete, and they are not responsible for any errors or omissions or
the results obtained from the use of such information. Readers are encouraged to confirm
the information contained in this book with other sources.

Library of Congress Cataloging-in-Publication Data

Abramowitz, Jonathan S.
  Exposure therapy for anxiety : principles and practice / by Jonathan S. Abramowitz,
Brett J. Deacon, and Stephen P. H. Whiteside.
     p. ; cm.
  Includes bibliographical references and index.
  ISBN 978-1-60918-016-4 (hardcover : alk. paper)
  ISBN 978-1-4625-0969-0 (paperback: alk. paper)
  1. Anxiety disorders—Treatment. 2. Exposure therapy. I. Deacon, Brett J.
II. Whiteside, Stephen P. H. III. Title.
  [DNLM: 1. Anxiety Disorders—therapy. 2. Implosive Therapy—methods. WM 172]
  RC531.A27 2011
  616.85′22—dc22
                                                                    2010037386

*To the many patients we have treated
and therapists we have supervised; you have taught
us much about the nature and treatment of anxiety*

*To Stacy, Emily, and Miriam Abramowitz
with all my love*
—J. S. A.

*To my parents, Robert and Sharon Deacon,
with love and gratitude*
—B. J. D.

*To my wife, Catherine, and my parents, Jim and Mary;
thank you for all your patience and support*
—S. P. H. W.

About the Authors

Jonathan S. Abramowitz, PhD, ABPP, is Professor and Associate Chair of the Department of Psychology and Research Associate Professor in the Department of Psychiatry at the University of North Carolina (UNC) at Chapel Hill. He is also Director of the UNC Anxiety and Stress Disorders Clinic. Dr. Abramowitz conducts research on anxiety disorders and has published 10 books and over 150 peer-reviewed research articles and book chapters. He currently serves as Associate Editor of the journals *Behaviour Research and Therapy* and *Journal of Cognitive Psychotherapy* and on the editorial boards of several other scientific journals. He is a member of the board of directors of the Anxiety Disorders Association of America and the Scientific Advisory Board of the International OCD Foundation. Dr. Abramowitz received the Outstanding Contributions to Research Award from the Mayo Clinic Department of Psychiatry and Psychology in 2003 and the David Shakow Early Career Award for Distinguished Scientific Contributions to Clinical Psychology from Division 12 of the American Psychological Association in 2004. He regularly presents papers and workshops on anxiety disorders and their treatment at regional, national, and international professional conferences.

Brett J. Deacon, PhD, is Associate Professor in the Department of Psychology at the University of Wyoming and Director of the University of Wyoming Anxiety Disorders Clinic in Laramie. Dr. Deacon has published over 50 peer-reviewed research articles on the nature and treatment of anxiety disorders. He serves on the editorial boards of numerous scientific journals and is a member of the Clinical Advisory Board of the Anxiety Disorders Association of America. He is the recipient of numerous teaching and research awards from the University of Wyoming as well as the Northern Illinois University College of Liberal Arts and Sciences Golden Anniversary Alumni Award in 2009. Dr. Deacon regularly presents workshops on cognitive-behavioral therapy for anxiety disorders at regional and national conferences.

Stephen P. H. Whiteside, PhD, ABPP, is Associate Professor of Psychology and Director of the Child Anxiety Disorders Program at the Mayo Clinic in Rochester, Minnesota. He conducts research on the assessment and treatment of childhood anxiety disorders, including the use of neuroimaging to examine the effects of cognitive behavioral therapy. He has received research funding from the International OCD Foundation and has published 35 articles and book chapters. Dr. Whiteside serves on the editorial board of the *Journal of Anxiety Disorders* and on the Education and Training Committee of the Minnesota Psychological Association.

Acknowledgments

This book reflects how we understand and treat clinical anxiety problems. The conceptual model and intervention strategies elucidated herein are based on a firm foundation of scientific literature that we are at once students of and contributors to. We wish to thank all of those who have helped us learn from and add to this knowledge, including the countless patients with whom we have worked (some successfully and some unsuccessfully) and therapists we have supervised, as well as the many outstanding teachers who have been instrumental in our growth and learning. Several individuals who have served as our teachers and mentors deserve specific mention: Edna Foa, Martin Franklin, Arthur Houts, Paul Kettlewell, Michael Kozak, Don Lynam, and David Valenteiner. We thank these individuals for their insights and hope they will see their influence reflected in this book. We are also enormously fortunate to have an outstanding network of collaborative relationships with fine clinicians and scholars in the field of anxiety disorders. We are especially grateful to Julie Dammann, Sarah Kalsy, Dean McKay, Bunmi Olatunji, Brad Riemann, Steven Taylor, Mike Tiede, and David Tolin, who have helped us refine our thinking about the concepts and techniques discussed in this book. And, most of all, we would like to thank our families, who have been very patient with us while we labored over this project. We hope you are as proud of us as we are of you.

Preface

Over the last 30 years, empirically supported treatment manuals for specific anxiety disorders have become extremely popular. Although these manuals serve an important purpose, they are sometimes criticized as being written with an assumption that "one size fits all," that every patient with a particular anxiety disorder has similar "classic" symptoms, and that every patient with a given problem requires (and will respond to) the same treatment procedures, delivered according to the same schedule. Finally, disorder-focused manuals sometimes assume that patients with one anxiety disorder do not have symptoms of other anxiety disorders or that all patients will fit neatly into our diagnostic boxes. Research and clinical experience, however, question all of these assumptions. Thus, while treatment manuals are critical for conducting research to establish whether a therapy is effective (which involves the use of homogeneous patient samples), manuals for particular disorders may be of less value for clinicians in typical mental health settings, where anxiety symptoms are often manifested in diverse and complex forms (e.g., many people with social phobia also have panic attacks and abuse alcohol or drugs).

A cursory inspection of treatment manuals for various anxiety disorders, however, reveals that despite some variability, the centerpiece of each manual is essentially the same technique, *therapeutic exposure*, which involves helping the patient confront his or her fears. Repeated and prolonged confrontation with situations and stimuli that are associated with excessive fear weakens clinical anxiety, because it teaches the person that such situations and stimuli are not as dangerous as was previously thought and that anxiety and fear themselves are not harmful. Accordingly, the main difference across the disorder-specific treatment manuals is the way in which exposure must be engineered to help the individual confront the feared situations, stimuli, contexts, and cues that are characteristic of each anxiety disorder. Manuals for treating social phobia, for example, discuss how best the clinician can arrange for individuals with this disorder to confront social performance or evaluative situations. Manuals for treating obsessive–compulsive disorder help the clinician arrange patients' exposure to items or places that provoke obsessional fear, such as knives, bathrooms, or cemeteries, outside the context of any reassurance-seeking compulsive rituals.

With this brief overview in mind, our aim in writing *Exposure Therapy for Anxiety: Principles and Practice* was to put under one cover a comprehensive and practical guide to using exposure therapy for the treatment of a wide range of anxiety problems. Because of its broad scope and relevance to clinical and research activity, this book will appeal to practicing clinicians, researchers, and students. An important recurring theme is that exposure is an effective (i.e., empirically supported or "evidence-based") treatment method for overcoming excessive (clinical) fear and anxiety *regardless of the patient's diagnostic category or status*. Instead of focusing on implementing exposure for different anxiety *disorders*, we focus on how clinicians can use the principles of exposure therapy to help patients overcome different types of *fears* that may occur in one or more anxiety disorders or even among individuals not meeting formal diagnostic criteria.

The successful application of exposure therapy requires a mastery of multiple skills. Sometimes, exposure is relatively straightforward to implement, such as in the treatment of many animal phobias. At other times, it is fraught with conceptual challenges, as in the treatment of obsessional fears about going to hell, getting cancer 40 years in the future, and hitting pedestrians with one's car. Treating trauma survivors (i.e., patients with posttraumatic stress disorder), who experience fear when they remember or encounter reminders of horrific events, presents additional practical challenges. Regardless, clinicians need to be able to convey confidence and engage patients in an emotionally demanding treatment. To this end, we share our extensive knowledge and clinical expertise with exposure-based therapy to provide the reader with a resource for planning and conducting challenging exposures. This book will increase the reader's confidence in exposure through user-friendly reviews of the history and science behind exposure, through easy-to-follow guides to assessing anxiety symptoms, and through setting up and conducting the therapy itself. Its copious case examples and ideas for exposure exercises further enhance readers' ability to design their own exposures for even the most unique of patients.

We have divided the book into three parts. Part I comprises six chapters covering topics that are fundamental to the practice of exposure therapy. Chapter 1 provides a definition and historical perspective on exposure, and Chapter 2 reviews the research attesting to its efficacy for anxiety-related problems. Chapter 3 provides the conceptual basis for the use of exposure therapy and discusses the nature of clinical anxiety and its treatment. Chapters 4 and 5 are highly practical and cover specialized assessment techniques, as well as how to develop a treatment plan and ascertain that the client is ready to engage in treatment. Chapter 6 then presents a general overview of how to implement the various exposure techniques.

Part II contains nine chapters, each pertaining to a particular domain of situations and stimuli that can evoke clinical fear and anxiety and for which therapeutic exposure has demonstrated efficacy. In the relatively brief, yet highly practical, Chapters 7 through 15, we describe how to apply the material in Chapters 4, 5, and 6 to each type of fear. These chapters adhere to a consistent format for presenting examples of treatment plans and illustrative case examples to facilitate readability and comparisons across chapters.

Part III consists of six chapters on important ancillary topics that clinicians routinely face, such as managing common complexities (Chapter 16), adapting exposure therapy for children (Chapter 17), working within the context of family or couple therapy (Chapter 18), the use of exposure when a patient is taking medication for anxiety (Chapter 19), and maintaining treatment gains even after exposure therapy has ended (Chapter 20). Last, Chapter 21 addresses the risks and benefits of exposure, as well as other ethical considerations in the use of this technique.

Optimally, books on psychological treatment techniques should delineate the essential principles of assessment and treatment and provide the clinician with procedural guidelines for their implementation. The challenge in writing such a book is to specify abstract principles of treatment with enough detail that they can be applied to a variety of patients, but not in so much detail that the text becomes unwieldy and cumbersome. Striking this balance is never more relevant than in the case of anxiety, since the manifestation of clinical anxiety is exceptionally broad and patient-specific. Indeed, there is no book that could adequately address the implementation of exposure therapy (or any other treatment procedure) across the countless possible personal variations of clinical anxiety and fear. Therefore, our solution is to present reasonably standardized guidelines for case formulation and treatment for the most common presentations of anxiety, noting the need for ongoing assessment, flexibility, and creativity in dealing with the more idiosyncratic symptoms likely to be encountered in clinical practice. For the most part, unanticipated obstacles can be managed by adhering to the conceptual principles that form the basis of successful exposure therapy.

Contents

PART III. SPECIAL CONSIDERATIONS
IN THE USE OF EXPOSURE TECHNIQUES

EXPOSURE THERAPY FOR ANXIETY

Part I

The Fundamentals of Exposure Therapy

The first part of this book contains six chapters that cover topics that are fundamental to the practice of exposure therapy. In Chapter 1, we provide a definition and historical perspective on exposure. Chapter 2 then reviews research attesting to the efficacy of this intervention in the treatment of anxiety-related problems. The nature of clinical anxiety and the conceptual basis for the use of exposure therapy are discussed in Chapter 3. Chapters 4 and 5 are highly practical and cover assessment techniques that are specific to exposure therapy, as well as how to develop an exposure treatment plan and ensure that the client is ready to engage in treatment. In Chapter 6, we present a general overview of how to implement the various exposure techniques. As we note throughout the chapters in this part of the book, clinical anxiety is tremendously heterogeneous and patients' complaints are highly idiosyncratic. Therefore, this part of the book (specifically, Chapters 3, 4, 5, and 6) is intended to provide the reader with a general framework for conceptualizing and assessing clinical anxiety problems and for implementing exposure techniques. Specific material for conceptualization, assessment, and use of exposure techniques as applied to particular presentations of clinical anxiety appear in the chapters in Part II.

1
Overview and History of Exposure Therapy for Anxiety

The range of human fears is immeasurable. While some people break out in a cold sweat at the thought of riding in an elevator or driving over a bridge, others fear animals (large and small), loss of control, speaking to strangers, or experiencing sexual arousal. Still others are afraid of eternal damnation, "immoral" thoughts and "unlucky" numbers, acting on unwanted impulses to harm loved ones, and using public restrooms. There are even those who become immobilized at the sight of a hospital, a cemetery, or their own navel.

In order to help people overcome distressing and disabling anxiety, mental health professionals face the daunting task of selecting an effective treatment strategy from the myriad of available options. Some of these strategies are purportedly effective for a wide range of psychological problems. Some are designed for individual therapy and others for group settings. Some are touted as short term or "brief," while others work over a longer period. Although proponents of most of these therapies claim that they are effective, acceptable and convincing scientific evidence to support these claims is lacking in the majority of cases.

With so many possibilities, it is inevitable that many interventions that seem plausible are in the end ineffective, or even harmful. Indeed, the treatment of anxiety has a long and colorful history dating back well past the fifth century B.C. Dimopoulos, Robinson, and Fountas (2008) recount instructive examples of "treatment" for panic attacks by trephination as described by contemporaries of Hippocrates. Essentially, "physicians" of the day—who had little knowledge of human anatomy—bored holes into the sufferer's skull, presumably to coax out from the brain demons that were thought to cause "insanity." While we may snicker at this practice now, variations of this approach have endured and are still in use in some parts of the world today. Practitioners used trephination because it "worked," by which we mean it was occasionally followed by the cessation of panic attacks. However, one can achieve this same *spontaneous remission* of symptoms in about a third of panic sufferers without intervening (Swobota, Amering, Windhaber, & Katschnig, 2001), thus saving patients a hole in their head. Given the complexity and subtlety of clinical fear and anxiety, it is no surprise that so many different treatments have been tried, and so many have persisted despite a lack of evidence supporting their effectiveness.

This somewhat unruly state of the field demands not only that treatments prove their muster in carefully conducted research trials, but also that we gain knowledge about the process by which they produce their outcomes. Accomplishing this task requires demarcating potentially useful and valid principles of therapeutic change. Several candidates common to most, if not all, psychological treatments for pathological fear and anxiety include the therapeutic relationship, the milieu in which the patient is treated, and the patient's (and therapist's) expectations of improvement (Frank, 1989). Yet another common principle of change—that which we concern ourselves with in this book—derives from the observation that alterations in thoughts, feelings, and behavior appear to occur following a strong emotional response to material presented within the context of therapy. Psychodynamically oriented therapists, for example, confront patients with information about so-called unconscious conflicts and unacceptable wishes through *free association* and the interpretation of dreams (Freud, 1949/1989). Likewise, gestalt therapists use imagery, role enactment, and group interactions to coax the patient into confronting information that he or she has avoided (Perls, 1969). In this volume, we focus on a cognitive-behaviorally oriented approach—namely, exposure therapy—that involves a more direct sort of confrontation with fearful events.

Exposure therapy refers to the process of helping a patient engage in repeated and prolonged contact with a feared stimulus. Anxiety-evoking stimuli can be alive (e.g., snakes, clowns), inanimate (e.g., balloons, toilets), situational (e.g., funeral homes, bridges), cognitive (e.g., thoughts of harming a loved one, memories of a traumatic event), or physiological (e.g., racing heart, dizziness). Exposure to the objectively safe (or "low-risk") fear-eliciting stimulus typically precipitates a response ranging from mild apprehension to intense panic, the basis for which is the patient's exaggerated expectation of danger. It is thought that learning of one form or another takes place when a person repeatedly confronts a feared stimulus in the absence of an actual threat or dreaded consequence. Although debate continues regarding what exactly happens in the brain during therapeutic exposure, a new behavioral repertoire seems to be cultivated and strengthened each time an individual effectively handles a previously feared situation.

However, before we discuss the implementation of exposure therapy, let us explore the concepts of normal and abnormal anxiety and the history of exposure treatment.

ANXIETY: NORMAL AND ABNORMAL

While a complete definition of anxiety is outside the scope of the present volume (entire books have been written on the subject; e.g., Barlow, 2002), *anxiety* is, broadly speaking, an organism's response to the *perception* of threat.[1] This implies that actual threat need not be present in order to experience anxiety. The reader will surely recall instances of intense fear and apprehension that turned out to be baseless. Similarly, one might actually be in danger, yet not become anxious if one does not perceive a significant threat. We have probably all had experiences in which it was only later that we realized how potentially dangerous a particular situation was. Either way, everyone is familiar with the psychological experience of feeling threatened, whether we label it as *anxiety, apprehension, fear, panic, worry, stress*, or something else. Moreover, we are all familiar with the physiological arousal that accompanies this emotion.

Normal Anxiety

At a neurophysiological level, the anxiety response appears to be implemented in various brain structures, including the visual thalamus, visual cortex, and the amygdala. The brain stimulates the release of adrenaline from the adrenal glands, which activates the sympathetic nervous system and initiates the *fight-or-flight response*, the body's built-in way of priming the organism for reacting to a perceived threat by attacking (fighting for one's life) or running (fleeing to safety).

The fight-or-flight response occurs simultaneously on three levels. First, at a physiological level, the body prepares for physical exertion by enriching the blood with oxygen, which is converted to energy for use by the body's

---

[1]In this book we use the terms *anxiety* and *fear* somewhat interchangeably, although these concepts can be differentiated from one another. Anxiety is a future-oriented mood state associated with preparation for possible, upcoming negative events, and fear is an alarm response to present or imminent danger (real or perceived) (Barlow, 2002).

muscles. This change involves abrupt and noticeable increases in the intensity of the heart rate and depth of breathing. In addition, feelings of nausea are also common since digestion is not typically involved in fleeing for one's life, and thus resources are diverted to other areas of the body. Second, at a cognitive level, attention automatically shifts toward the perceived threat so that it might seem difficult to concentrate on any extraneous matters. This focus serves as a constant reminder of the potential for harm and allows for early detection of threats. Finally, at a behavioral level, the individual takes actions that are geared toward avoiding or escaping the feared stimulus, such as by running away, thereby increasing the odds of survival. The urge to act aggressively (fight) is also part of this response.

The fight-or-flight response is critical to the survival of humankind (and most other species in the animal kingdom). Just imagine what would happen if you were crossing a busy street in a large city—cars bearing down on you—and you felt absolutely no stress or anxiety. Most of us can recall a time where spontaneous actions motivated by the fight-or-flight response probably saved our life, or at least helped us avoid serious injury. As more than one author has put it, "in times of danger, anxiety can be a person's best friend" (e.g., Rosqvist, 2005, p. 1).

Abnormal Anxiety

Unfortunately, sometimes the fight-or-flight response is the kind of friend that relieves us of the need for enemies. This happens when anxiety occurs in the absence of danger or when it is out of proportion relative to the actual threat. In these situations, such as giving a speech, having your body prepared to run for safety probably won't keep you safe, but may make you sweaty. Such excessive and pathological anxiety—stemming from the misperception of a safe situation as dangerous—appears to form the basis of most clinical anxiety problems (i.e., anxiety disorders; Barlow, 2002; Beck, Emery, & Greenberg, 1985). In such instances, the fight-or-flight response is triggered unnecessarily and may even worsen the situation by leading to more negative thoughts, such as "I'm *feeling* anxious, therefore I must *be* in danger." This sort of emotional reasoning bias serves to increase the perception of threat (Arntz, Rauner, & van den Hout, 1995) and maintain physiological responding, thereby creating a vicious cycle in which threat perception leads to anxious responding, which leads to more threat perception, and so on.

Another unfortunate consequence of habitually misperceiving objectively safe stimuli as dangerous is the development of strategies for avoiding these fear cues. These strategies may include "passive avoidance," such as a student with social phobia who refrains from raising her hand in class because she fears her peers will laugh at her if she gives an incorrect answer.

Other feared stimuli, including germs and traumatic memories, cannot be completely avoided. In such instances, the anxious individual will often develop strategies that serve as an "escape" from the feelings of anxiety that accompany exposure to these triggers (Barlow, 2002). Such "active avoidance" strategies include compulsive washing and cleaning to prevent illness after handling money and remaining close to a "safe person" for protection in a circumstance reminiscent of a traumatic event. By minimizing exposure to stimuli associated with pathological (unrealistic) anxiety, regardless of the form of avoidance, the person never has the opportunity to learn that such stimuli really are objectively safe (i.e., low risk; Clark, 1999). That is, the person cannot correct his or her misperception of the fear trigger, and he or she goes on believing (erroneously) that it is very dangerous.

Not only do efforts to escape and avoid perceived threats prevent pathological anxiety from self-correcting over time, they may actually *worsen* the very problems they are intended to alleviate. Accordingly, much of the devastating effects of pathological anxiety result from the extreme lengths people go to in trying to keep themselves safe by avoiding and escaping from (largely nonthreatening) fear cues. For example, we know of one man with a fear of AIDS who couldn't leave his bedroom for 5 years after someone with HIV had visited his home. A woman drove 45 miles out of her way to work each day to avoid having to cross a certain bridge. Another woman relocated from the West Coast to Rochester, Minnesota, just so she could be near the Mayo Clinic in case she suffered a serious medical emergency. Although she was medically healthy, she restricted herself to traveling no more than a few miles from the hospital, and at all times carried with her various medical devices, self-test kits, and medicines. More detailed information regarding the development and maintenance of abnormal anxiety is presented in Chapter 3.

Anxiety Disorders

The *Diagnostic and Statistical Manual of Mental Disorders* (DSM; e.g., American Psychiatric Association, 2000) assumes a categorical stance and defines *anxiety disorders* based on observable signs and symptoms. These disorders are intended to inform the clinician about the likely course of the problem and what treatments would be appropriate. In the fourth edition of the DSM (American Psychiatric Association, 2000), the major anxiety disorders, as listed in Table 1.1, are characterized by pathological anxiety associated with different feared stimuli. For example, social phobia is marked by fear and avoidance of social situations, while in obsessive–compulsive disorder anxiety is triggered by unwanted thoughts and images (i.e., obsessions). Research has established the reliability and construct validity of these

TABLE 1.1. Anxiety Disorders in DSM-IV

Major anxiety disorders

    Panic disorder with or without agoraphobia

    Specific phobia

    Social phobia

    Obsessive–compulsive disorder

    Posttraumatic stress disorder

    Generalized anxiety disorder

    Separation anxiety disorder

Other anxiety disorders

    Acute stress disorder

    Anxiety disorder due to a general medical condition

    Substance-induced anxiety disorder

diagnoses. Moreover, treatment manuals for almost all of the anxiety disorders have been developed and evaluated.

Despite the general acceptance of the current system, the DSM diagnostic approach has a number of limitations that encumber its use for treatment planning. To begin with, the neat and distinct categories of disorders outlined in the DSM cannot fully capture the breadth and depth of human emotional experience. As far as the major anxiety disorders are concerned, the DSM diagnostic labels merely reflect topographical and superficial differences among problems that have essentially the same fundamental psychological mechanism (e.g., Abramowitz & Deacon, 2005). That is, all the major anxiety disorders can be conceptualized using the framework outlined above in which relatively safe stimuli are misperceived as dangerous, leading to anxiety, and what amount to unnecessary avoidance or escape behaviors that perpetuate the problem. Each diagnostic entity, however, has a somewhat unique set of fear cues, ways in which these cues are misperceived, and maladaptive coping responses. Table 1.2 shows these phenomena across the seven major anxiety disorders in DSM-IV.

The DSM also makes an arbitrary distinction regarding the level of symptomatology that constitutes an anxiety disorder (Widiger & Miller, 2008). In this system anxiety disorders are treated like a medical disease, such as diabetes, which you either have or (preferably) do not have. However, as can be seen from the discussion of normal versus pathological anxiety, fears and worries are more like blood pressure; everyone has it, but having too high (or too low) levels can be problematic. A categorical-based

TABLE 1.2. Fear Cues, Misperceptions, and Maladaptive Coping Responses in the Major Anxiety Disorders

Anxiety disorder	Fear cue(s)	Misperception(s)	Maladaptive coping responses
Obsessive–compulsive disorder	Intrusive thoughts, situational cues	Thoughts are highly significant and equivalent to actions; inflated responsibility for preventing harm	Avoidance, compulsive rituals (e.g., checking, washing, covert neutralizing), reassurance seeking
Specific phobia	Snakes, heights, injections, etc.	Overestimation of the likelihood or severity of danger	Avoidance, use of drugs (alcohol, benzodiazepines), distraction
Social phobia	Social situations	Other people are highly judgmental; negative evaluation is intolerable	Avoidance, in-situation safety behaviors (e.g., using alcohol at a party)
Panic disorder and agoraphobia	Arousal-related body sensations; situational cues	Misinterpretation of arousal-related body sensations as dangerous (e.g., racing heart means a heart attack)	Agoraphobic avoidance, in-situation safety behaviors (e.g., going to emergency room), and safety signals (e.g., have safe person nearby, carry cell phone)
Posttraumatic stress disorder	Intrusive memories of traumatic events	Nowhere is safe	Avoidance of reminders, distraction, safety signals (e.g., carrying a gun)
Generalized anxiety disorder	Thoughts/images of low probability negative events	Intolerance of uncertainty; overestimation of the likelihood and severity of negative outcomes	Reassurance seeking, worrying as a form of problem solving
Separation anxiety disorder	Physical separation from parents or other caregivers	Overestimation of the likelihood of threat of harm or permanent separation	Clinging to parents, crying, avoiding situations in which separation is required

diagnostic system does not provide treatment recommendations for individuals whose symptoms do not fall into a specific category or who have subthreshold symptoms.

An alternative approach to diagnosis is to view psychopathology as a "dyscontrolled organismic impairment in psychological functioning" that falls along a continuum of severity (Widiger & Miller, 2008). In other words some *mechanism* within the individual, such as how he or she is responding to certain fear cues, is not functioning optimally. This operationalization is compatible with the view that effective psychological therapies don't treat "disorders" as much as they change (or reverse) maladaptive psychological mechanisms that are present in these "disorders" (Abramowitz & Deacon, 2005). As the reader will find, we approach exposure therapy as targeting the processes underlying the persistence of pathological anxiety—regardless of the specific fear triggers and cues—rather than as a treatment for a specific "disorder" (see Chapter 3).

Although exposure therapy must be modified depending on the particular fear trigger (see the chapters in Part II), this is not the same as using a different *treatment* or *treatment manual* for each different anxiety disorder. As we argue in this book, the same basic principles of utilizing exposure therapy can be applied to any patient's anxiety problem, regardless of which DSM diagnostic category best describes it. This *transdiagnostic approach* frees the therapist from the arduous task of learning to use a bookshelf full of treatment manuals for all the anxiety-related DSM disorders and instead emphasizes understanding and treating the common psychological mechanisms that underlie the maintenance of anxiety-related problems in general.

Etiology versus Maintenance

The reader will also note that exposure therapy and its conceptual framework for understanding pathological anxiety are focused on the psychological processes that *maintain* the problem rather than those that lead to its development or *etiology*. One reason for this is that whereas the maintenance factors in anxiety are well understood based on careful clinical observation and empirical research (e.g., Clark, 1999), we understand much less about the factors that dictate why some people are more vulnerable to developing such problems than are others. Recently, Mineka and Zinbarg (2006) proposed a comprehensive etiological model of anxiety disorders that incorporates early learning experiences, the occurrence and context of stressful events, and genetic or temperamental vulnerability. In other words, the tendency to respond in excessively fearful ways—on a physiological, emotional, and behavioral level—appears to be mediated by environmental and biological variables.

Psychological treatments, however, cannot "undo" historical events or change genetic and temperamental predispositions. That is, they can't directly address the initial causes of anxiety problems. In fact, therapists cannot even reliably determine the precise ways in which learning experiences and vulnerability factors interact to cause a particular individual's anxiety problem to develop. Yet, treatment can address the *maintenance factors*, phenomena that interfere with the natural process of overcoming a fear. If we view excessive anxious responding as learned *patterns* of maladaptive thinking, feeling, and acting, we can help the patient learn healthier patterns to replace his or her maladaptive ones. From this perspective, two elements are necessary for the treatment of clinical fear and anxiety: first, information must be presented that is incompatible with the patient's threat-related beliefs and misperceptions: second, behaviors that interfere with the incorporation of this new information must be eliminated. If these criteria are met, then emotional change will occur (Foa & Kozak, 1986). This idea provides the theoretical basis for the use of exposure therapy to treat most problems with excessive fear and anxiety. The remainder of this chapter provides an overview and a history of the development of this treatment technique.

CONTEMPORARY EXPOSURE THERAPY: AN OVERVIEW

As we detail in the pages of this volume, exposure therapy is both a science and an art. While there is more than adequate empirical support for its conceptual basis and efficacy (see Chapter 2), implementing exposure still requires careful artistry and therapeutic know-how. No two anxious individuals present with precisely the same fears and avoidance patterns, and therefore no two exposure therapy programs will be exactly the same. This need for a patient-specific, or *idiosyncratic*, approach is one important challenge and a key characteristic of exposure therapy. In Chapter 4, we describe how to conduct a careful assessment that allows the clinician to tailor the treatment to the needs of the patient. The need to persuade anxious individuals to confront their greatest fears also represents a hurdle to successful exposure therapy. In Chapter 5, we present suggestions for conveying a clear and coherent rationale for treatment. What follows next is a general overview of contemporary exposure therapy procedures as commonly implemented. Further below, we step back and take a historical perspective.

Assessment and Treatment Planning

In general, exposure therapy begins with a thorough assessment of the patient's problem with anxiety. This "functional (or *behavioral*) assessment" (as we discuss in detail in Chapter 4) focuses on understanding (1) the contexts in which fear and anxiety are triggered, (2) the anticipated feared consequences of encountering fear triggers, and (3) the strategies used to reduce anxiety by avoiding and escaping from these triggers. The therapist next thoroughly explains the exposure procedures and why they are expected to be helpful. Providing a clear rationale helps to motivate the patient to tolerate the distress that typically accompanies the actual exposure exercises. As we describe in Chapter 5, a good rationale includes not only a clear and coherent explanation of the problem in terms that are readily understandable to the patient, but also information about how exposure therapy is commonly experienced, including the provocation and diminution of distress during prolonged exposure. The information gleaned from the functional assessment is then used to plan the exposure exercises that will be pursued.

The preparatory stage of therapy also introduces the patient to the importance of reducing (if not completely eliminating) subtle and not-so-subtle avoidance and escape strategies that prevent the natural extinction of fear, that is, response prevention. Depending on the nature of the patient's anxiety problem and the type of anxiety-reduction strategies he or she uses, response prevention may take different forms. For example, individuals with compulsive rituals are taught to abstain from such ritualizing. Those who use benzodiazepine medication or alcohol to cope with anxious feelings are helped to safely reduce the use of these agents. Those who use safety cues such as not leaving home without a "safe person," cell phone, or water bottle are helped to complete exposure exercises without these safety signals.

Practicing Exposure

How exposure therapy is carried out depends on the nature of the individual's fear. Patients typically begin by confronting moderately distressing stimuli and gradually work up to more difficult situations. For instance, a person with acrophobia (fear of heights) can be helped to visit increasingly higher floors of a building, ending with the observation deck of a skyscraper or the top floor of a parking garage. Exposure might occur in imagination when it is not possible to confront the actual feared situation—such as for someone with fears of impulsively attacking a child. Here, mentally visualizing this event (i.e., exposure in imagination) would be the technique of choice. In cases where physiological states, such as anxious arousal itself, are the feared stimuli, the preferred method is interoceptive exposure in which the patient purposely elicits such internal stimuli (e.g., by engaging in physical activity or using caffeine). In any case, successful confrontation with the feared situation, thought, or internal sensation eventually brings about a decrease in the person's anxiety response to this stimulus.

Each individual exposure exercise lasts until anxiety has subsided to a mild level, and exposure to each stimulus is repeated until it no longer induces significant distress. In general, it seems that the more intense or pervasive the fear, the more exposure time is required to achieve anxiety reduction within a treatment session and between sessions. As alluded to above, exposure therapy has been rigorously evaluated with thousands of anxious patients, treated by hundreds of therapists in a variety of clinics located around the world. This literature, which we review in Chapter 2, consistently demonstrates the efficacy and effectiveness of therapeutic exposure.

A HISTORY OF EXPOSURE THERAPY

Exposure, as a therapy procedure for reducing pathological fear, has its roots in the behavior therapy movement of the 1950s. The first behavior therapists emerged from multiple schools of psychotherapy, including the then dominant psychoanalytic view in the United States and the United Kingdom (Krasner, 1971; Krasner & Houts, 1984). Some of the earliest efforts to treat phobias and other anxiety-related problems came from research-oriented psychologists and psychiatrists in South Africa, many of whom eventually made their way to England and the Maudsley Hospital training program directed by Hans Eysenck (Houts, 2005).

As a psychiatrist with enthusiasm for learning theory and experimental psychology, Joseph Wolpe (1915–1997) turned to his psychologist colleagues to find like-minded individuals with whom to discuss clinical problems from a behavioral point of view. Among those he consulted was James G. Taylor (1897–1973) in the psychology department of the University of Cape Town, South Africa. In the 1950s Taylor had used behavioral therapy procedures for the treatment of anxiety. Unfortunately, he did not publish most of his case studies and only hints of his work survive in published form. In an interview with Leonard Krasner, Taylor described treating several anxiety cases using techniques we would today call situational exposure with response prevention (Krasner, 1971). For example, in a case of driving phobia, he accompanied the patient on drives designed to evoke anxiety. He also exposed compulsive hand washers to more and more anxiety-provoking circumstances and blocked their washing behavior. Although Taylor might have been the first behavior therapist to use systematic exposure techniques, investigators who published more prolifically usually receive credit for bringing this form of therapy to the forefront of anxiety treatment.

Systematic Desensitization

One of the first forms of exposure to emerge in the era of behavior therapy was *systematic desensitization* (SD). Initially described by Salter (1949), but later elaborated by Wolpe (1958), SD involves weakening the association between anxiety and an objectively nondangerous phobic stimulus by pairing the phobic stimulus with a physiological state that is incompatible with anxiety. Procedurally, the patient and the therapist first develop a *fear hierarchy*, a list of the patient's phobic situations and objects ordered from the least to the most fear-provoking. Next, the therapist helps the patient become relaxed. Then, the anxiety-provoking stimuli are either gradually visualized or actually presented to the patient while he or she is in the relaxed state. Stimuli are confronted in order from the least to the most distressing. If the patient becomes anxious, the feared stimulus may be withdrawn until the patient can once more become relaxed.

The goal of SD is for the patient to be completely relaxed while in the presence of his or her phobic stimuli. Wolpe adopted Jacobson's (1938) progressive muscle relaxation technique as the primary anxiety-inhibiting procedure. Once mastered by the patient, Wolpe believed, this technique could be employed at almost any time and in various circumstances both in and outside of the therapist's office. Wolpe also found that the use of imagined, rather than actual, exposure to feared stimuli expanded the range of phobic stimuli that could be addressed by SD. Therefore, although presentation of actual phobic material was occasionally used, SD usually involved exposure to thoughts and images of feared situations and stimuli.

Wolpe derived his techniques for SD largely from his earlier laboratory research (Wolpe, 1958) and from that of Mary Cover Jones (1924), which demonstrated that phobic responses (in animals and humans) could be weakened if a response that was the opposite of anxiety (and incompatible with it) occurred in the presence of the phobic stimulus. Wolpe, for example, conditioned cats to become afraid of their cage through the administration of electric shocks to the floor of the cage. He then found that he could weaken this phobic response by giving the cats food at locations progressively closer to the cage. Eating was viewed as a pleasant response antagonistic to phobic anxiety. Wolpe hypothesized that the cats were undergoing a process he called *reciprocal inhibition* (i.e., anxiety inhibits feeding and feeding inhibits anxiety) which became the theoretical basis of SD.

A large body of clinical and experimental research amply demonstrates the efficacy (success in the laboratory) and effectiveness (success in non-laboratory clinical settings) of SD, particularly for problems such as specific phobias, social phobia, and agoraphobia. In a classic study of patients with fears of public speaking, Paul (1966) found that SD was more effective than insight-oriented therapy. After only five treatment sessions, 100% of patients receiving SD were improved or much improved compared to 47% who received insight-oriented treatment. Moreover, the therapists in this study had not been schooled in behavior therapy, suggesting that SD did not require intensive behaviorally oriented training. However, as other behavioral therapies, such as flooding and implosive therapy, emerged in the 1970s and 1980s research and clinical interest in SD began to decline (McGlynn, Smitherman, & Gothard, 2002).

Flooding and Implosive Therapy

Other precursors to contemporary exposure include *flooding* and *implosive therapy (implosion)*. Flooding refers to a nongraduated approach in which the patient rapidly confronts his or her most feared stimuli, either in imagination or in real life, while minimizing escape from the fear-provoking context (i.e., response prevention). For example, a child with a phobia of large dogs might be placed in a room with such a dog and prevented from leaving until his anxiety subsides. Alternatively, the child might imagine strongly anxiety-eliciting scenes involving a large dog for a prolonged period of time. The assumption is that flooding results in the activation of anxiety, which then subsides over time in the absence of avoidance patterns and results in the extinction of the fear.

Implosive therapy was considered a variation of flooding (Stampfl & Levis, 1967) with the following differences: First, all presentations of fear-evoking situations were done in imagination. Second, the imagined scenes were often exaggerated or impossible situations designed to provoke as much anxiety as possible. Third, although derived from learning theory (Stampfl, 1966) and considered a behavioral technique, implosive therapy contained psychodynamic elements. Specifically, the scenes were often based on dynamic sources of anxiety such as hostility toward parental figures, rejection, sex, death wishes, and concepts such as the Oedipus complex. In illustrating implosive therapy for a person with snake phobia, Hogan (1968) described scenes including images of a snake crawling in the patient's lap, the snake biting the patient's fingers off and blood dripping from the fingers, the snake biting the patient's face and pulling the eyes out and eating them, and the snake crawling into the eye socket and nose. Another scene involved falling into a pit filled with thousands of snakes. Assuming the snake is a symbol of male sexuality, a female patient might imagine a large snake sexually violating her and mutilating her sexual organs.

As fear reduction strategies, flooding and implosive therapy derive from the well-established laboratory principle of *extinction* in which the repetition of the feared stimulus in the absence of the feared consequence and any escape or avoidance behaviors will result in the reduction of the fear. The use of these strategies to successfully treat phobias, posttraumatic stress reactions, and obsessive–compulsive problems proliferated in the 1960s and 1970s. Soon, influential behavior therapists and researchers such as Victor Meyer (1966), Jack Rachman (Rachman, Marks, & Hodgson, 1971, 1973), and Issac Marks (1973) realized that flooding, implosion, and SD all involved exposure to fear-provoking stimuli and abstinence from fear-reducing escape and avoidance responses. This recognition led in the 1970s and 1980s to the development and testing of contemporary gradual (hierarchy-driven) exposure therapy that is devoid of the relaxation component of SD and the psychodynamic element of implosive therapy.

CONCLUSIONS

This chapter provides a historical and theoretical framework for using exposure therapy to treat clinical anxiety and fear-based problems. Although the idea that facing one's fears will lead to a reduction in fear responses has probably been recognized for millennia, it is only within the last century that research has been applied to understanding the reasons this approach works and the extent to which it does so. In the next chapter, we review the treatment outcome literature that speaks to the efficacy and effectiveness of this form of therapy.

2

How Well Does
Exposure Therapy Work?

As mentioned in the previous chapter, some interventions for anxiety disorders, such as trephination, have been ineffective if not counterproductive. Even if a treatment itself is not iatrogenic, pursuing an intervention that is unlikely to be beneficial can place an undue burden on a patient in terms of time and money and may reduce his or her willingness to seek further help. Thus, the clinician has a responsibility to select the treatment with the greatest likelihood of safely and efficiently alleviating symptoms. The scientific method provides an excellent, although not infallible, tool for sorting through the plethora of potential interventions. However, some professionals feel uncomfortable with research and prefer to rely on their clinical judgment when making treatment decisions. Thus before we review the empirical literature supporting exposure therapy, we briefly discuss some of the reasons why it is important to base clinical wisdom on a solid research foundation.

BARRIERS TO IDENTIFYING
EFFECTIVE TREATMENTS

At first glance, the task of identifying effective treatments appears fairly unambiguous. If you intervene to help someone with distressing symptoms and he or she gets better, then it stands to reason that your intervention was effective. Repeat that process with a few hundred patients with similar problems and you can be confident that you have discovered a good treatment. Unfortunately, given the ambiguity and fluctuating nature of emotional problems, identifying the components that lead to change is rarely this straightforward. Even in everyday life, determining how we affect other people's behavior involves a complicated interaction among our actions, the other person's characteristics, the environment we are in, and our perception of the entire process. If we considered all of that information in every decision we made, we would be paralyzed with information overload and never get anything accomplished.

In order to efficiently handle such complex decisions, people naturally develop *heuristics*, informal decision-making rules that prune down the available information to a less unwieldy size. In general, these strategies help us cut corners by applying previous experiences to new situations. For example, our heuristics tend to work to make the world seem more controllable by exaggerating our own effect on our surroundings and by giving added weight to information that seems to confirm what we already believe (sometimes called *confirmatory bias*; Turk & Salovey, 1985). Although heuristics make the world seem more manageable, they can interfere with our ability to make accurate decisions in complex situations. Clinicians and researchers alike have been interested in how such cognitive shortcuts affect one's clinical decision making (Beutler, 2004; Dawes, 1986; Meehl, 1996; Morton & Torgeson, 2003; Turk & Salovey, 1985).

It turns out that the impossibility of knowing what would have happened if we had done something else or even nothing at all provides a fundamental barrier to evaluating the effectiveness of the treatment that we deliver. To manage these situations we use heuristics to fill in the information void. For instance, when a patient's phobic symptoms abate, we naturally tend to attribute that therapeutic success to our specific intervention. Yet in doing so, we overlook a number of other factors that might also have contributed to the patient's improvement including regression to the mean (Morton & Torgerson, 2003), the natural course of the problem (i.e., spontaneous remission), support from a friend or parent, other life changes, or the beneficial effects of a warm, therapeutic relationship. Once we believe in the effectiveness of an intervention, we bolster this belief with recollections of other successful patients, as well as with similar experiences described by colleagues. Conversely, we closely scrutinize treatment failures and dissenting opinions to discover the extenuating circumstances, such as lack of motivation or noncompliance, which explain the negative outcome. In other words, we tend to welcome agreement and dismiss discrepancies.

These cognitive shortcuts can present a formidable obstacle to using exposure therapy with anxious patients. Specifically, therapists are understandably reticent to adopt a treatment plan that deliberately (if only temporarily) increases a patient's already distressing anxiety. Consequently, a therapist would only select this treatment if she believed that it was the best method for helping her patients in the long run. However, when other approaches seem equally effective, many reasonable therapists would choose one that seems less aversive, especially if they have previous experience with an alternative treatment. This is precisely where the heuristics just described come in to play. It is almost impossible for even the brightest and most observant among us to objectively evaluate the success of an intervention with its inherent complexity and variation. Thus, to make sense of our professional experience, we fall back on our cognitive shortcuts. Unfortunately, these shortcuts often lead to inaccurate decisions.

In the abstract such heuristics may seem unlikely to occur among trained professionals with good "clinical judgment" (we have found that many educated professionals tend to deny that they could be affected by any such mental foibles). But examples abound in the psychological and medical literature. One concrete illustration of the pitfalls of relying on clinical judgment alone can be found in medicine (for further examples, see Friedman, Furbeg, & DeMets, 1998). For many years high-concentration oxygen was administered to premature babies to prevent brain damage. However, it was later discovered that this intervention raised the infant's risk of blindness (Silverman, 1977). Similar, less dramatic, examples can be found in the field of mental health. For instance, many treatments that achieved passing popularity, such as facilitated communication and critical incident stress debriefing, later were discredited as ineffective and, at times, harmful (Jacobson, Mulick, & Schwartz, 1996). These examples stand as reminders that relying primarily on one's own judgment when making decisions about interventions can be problematic.

STRATEGIES FOR IDENTIFYING EFFECTIVE TREATMENTS

On what basis, then, should a clinician make decisions about treating a patient or client that minimizes interference from the heuristics described earlier? Although not infallible itself, the scientific (experimental) method provides a procedure for making these decisions by setting out strict procedures for evaluating the effects of treatments and requiring that these findings be scrutinized and replicated by other investigators. In experimental research, the ways in which patients are selected and assigned to treatments, as well as how data are collected and analyzed, decrease the extent to which our natural cognitive shortcuts interfere with the evaluation of a treatment's effects.

The "gold standard" type of investigation for determining whether a given treatment is more effective than another treatment, or than receiving no treatment at all, is the randomized controlled trial (RCT). An RCT is a prospective study comparing the effect of an intervention provided to one group against a control group in which every participant has an equal chance of being in each group based on random assignment (Friedman et al., 1998). Since the experience of each group is the same, except for the intervention, any differences in improvement are attributable to the treatment. This paradigm controls for the effects of regression to the mean, natural disease course, and, if a placebo is employed, the nonspecific effects of treatment such as warmth, attention, and expectations of improvement.

Although RCTs control for many factors, differences between studies, such as patient population, therapist characteristics, and random variations, can affect their outcome. Often, after multiple trials have been completed, there will be a range of outcomes providing varying degrees of support for a given treatment. To make sense of multiple, at times conflicting, studies, meta-analyses are conducted to quantitatively synthesize the results and characterize the general effectiveness of various treatments. The outcomes of meta-analyses are generally expressed as *effect sizes* (ESs) which standardize the difference between the average scores of two groups—perhaps scores from a treatment group and a control group. The ES is statistically computed by subtracting the mean (average) of one group from the mean of the second group and dividing this difference by the pooled standard deviation from both groups, and can be used to examine two types of comparisons. For our purposes, the "within-group" or "pre–post" ES refers to those calculated from a treatment group's average scores before and after treatment. A "between-group" ES refers to the standardized difference between a treated group and a control group (or a second treated group) following treatment. As a rule, within-group ESs are greater than between-group ESs as the former reflect change caused by both specific and nonspecific factors that occur during treatment. Cohen (1977) suggested that an ES of 0.2, 0.5, and 0.8 represents a small, medium, and large effect, respectively.

Despite the potential benefits of using the scientific method to inform clinical practice, RCTs have been met with skepticism from some quarters of psychology (e.g., Levant, 2004). These arguments typically question the relevance of RCTs to real-world practice by claiming that study patients are more likely to be middle-class white individuals with less severe and less complicated psychopathology than patients treated in typical clinical settings. In addition, it has been argued that RCTs focus solely on a relatively unimportant aspect of therapy, that is, technique, to the exclusion of other factors such as the therapeutic relationship. Finally, critics argue that the focus on RCTs leads to the dismissing of treatments that have not been tested even though the fact that a treatment has not been studied does not equate to it being ineffective. These arguments typically conclude with a call for placing clinical judgment on par with research findings in guidelines for evidence-based practice (e.g., Levant, 2004).

Responses to these criticisms often reference research investigating the relevance of RCTs (e.g., Beutler, 2004). To begin with, empirical efforts to compare patients in research studies with clinical populations generally indicate that the samples in research studies are similar to those treated in clinical practice and often tend to be *more* severe and complex. Moreover, relationship and technique appear to be similarly important, each accounting for approximately 10% of variance in treatment outcome, and so methods to improve each of them should be pursued. Alas, as much as we would like to think that our "clinical judgment" is accurate, it is important to acknowledge that the combination of incomplete information and normal human cognitive processes render even the most thoughtful and careful clinical decisions and predictions subject to error. Although further progress needs to be made, RCTs and meta-analyses provide the best evidence currently available for determining which treatments are most effective.

EXPOSURE THERAPY FOR ANXIETY: A REVIEW OF THE EVIDENCE

The decision to use exposure-based therapy for treating problems with anxiety and fear is supported by a vast research literature. In fact, behavioral and cognitive therapies are the most widely studied psychological interventions for anxiety disorders (Barlow, 2002). Numerous RCTs indicate that these methods can be highly effective in reducing these symptoms. Because of the enormous volume of research, our review focuses primarily on meta-analyses of RCTs, highlighting clinically relevant aspects of the research for each type of problem.

Although the intent of this chapter is to review the evidence supporting the use of exposure specifically, the bulk of the research involves treatment packages that incorporate multiple techniques. Specifically, much of the research focuses on cognitive-behavioral treatment (CBT) that combines exposure therapy with cognitive approaches, such as verbally challenging inaccurate beliefs thought to lead to anxiety. In some areas, with a long history of treatment research, behavioral interventions (exposure) have been evaluated independently from cognitive interventions. In other areas, these two approaches have not been separated.

As we will see in later chapters, disentangling cognitive and exposure techniques can be difficult given that their delivery is often intertwined. The fact that similar treatments are sometimes labeled differently further complicates this endeavor. For instance, in the panic disorder literature, highly similar treatment packages that utilize both cognitive therapy and exposure components have been variously termed *cognitive therapy* (e.g., Beck, Sokol, Clark, Berchick, & Wright, 1992), *behavioral therapy* (e.g., Barlow, Craske,

Cerny, & Klosko, 1989), and *cognitive-behavioral therapy* (e.g., Telch et al., 1993). Similarly, some treatments described as "cognitive therapy" include exposure techniques in the form of "behavioral experiments" (McLean et al., 2001). Thus, for the current review, we focus on any treatment protocol that contains exposure to anxiety-provoking stimuli as a central component of the treatment package. We anticipate that most clinicians will use exposure therapy along with other techniques, rather than in isolation. In the remainder of this chapter we review the empirical evidence supporting the use of exposure-based treatments for the anxiety (and related) disorders. Mean effect sizes from meta-analyses of exposure-based treatments for different forms of anxiety are presented in Figure 2.1.

Specific Phobias

Basic exposure paradigms have been used to treat specific phobias for decades. Although the administration of exposure therapy to specific phobias is fairly straightforward, variations in the provision of treatment, such as the frequency of sessions, augmentation with cognitive techniques, and method of confronting the feared stimuli (*in vivo*, imaginal, or virtual reality exposure) may affect outcome. Recently, Wolitzky-Taylor, Horowitz, Powers, and Telch (2008) conducted a meta-analysis of 33 treatment outcome studies with adults conducted between 1977 and 2004. Overall, they found exposure-based treatment to be more effective than no treatment, with a between-group ES of 1.05. As explained earlier in this chapter, an ES greater than 0.8 is considered large. In addition, exposure-based treatments outperformed placebo and non-exposure-based interventions at posttreatment (ESs = 0.48 and 0.44), and follow-up (ESs = 0.80 and 0.35). Moreover, the authors found exposure to be more effective when administered across multiple sessions as opposed to within a single session. In addition, situational (*in vivo*) exposures were more effective than alternative methods (e.g., imaginal exposure) at posttreatment, although not at follow-up. Adding cognitive techniques did not enhance the impact of exposure therapy (Wolitzky-Taylor et al., 2008).

Panic Disorder

Interventions utilizing behavioral techniques have consistently demonstrated efficacy in the treatment of panic disorder with or without agoraphobia (Gould, Otto, & Pollack, 1995). Exposures to feared locations and bodily sensations (i.e., interoceptive exposure) are often combined with (1) education about the nature and physiology of anxiety and panic, (2) cognitive techniques designed to modify the tendency to catastrophically misinterpret bodily sensations, and (3) coping skills for managing bodily symptoms. Unfortunately, many outcome studies were conducted prior to the advent of modern cognitive-behavioral approaches (e.g., Barlow et al., 1989; Clark et al., 1994), and utilized primarily situational exposure to agoraphobic situations. As a result, meta-analyses often do not include the more contemporary interoceptive exposure techniques that we describe in later chapters of this book.

Multiple meta-analyses support the effectiveness of exposure-based therapy for panic disorder. For instance, Chambless and Gillis (1993) found that CBT led to 72% of patients being panic-free compared to 25% in waitlist and placebo conditions. In a more recent meta-analysis, Westen and Morrison (2001) found that exposure-based treatments led to a large improvement at posttreatment (ES = 1.55), which was greater than the change in the control conditions, resulting in a median between-group ES of 0.80. Earlier studies focusing on situational exposures found larger effects on agoraphobia symptoms than on panic attacks (e.g., agoraphobia ES = 1.38; panic

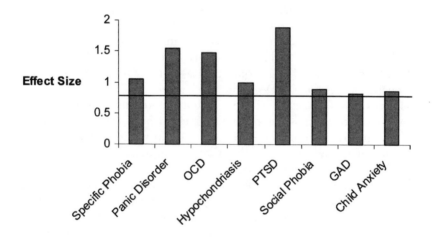

FIGURE 2.1. Mean ESs for exposure-based therapy of anxiety disorders. The horizontal line indicates an ES of 0.80, which is considered a large treatment effect. ESs reflect examinations of exposures as a stand-alone treatment or combined with other interventions (e.g., CBT). Comparisons are pre–post or to no treatment. References: Specific phobia, Wolitzky-Taylor, Horowitz, Powers, and Telch (2008); panic disorder, Westen and Morrison (2001); OCD, Van Balkom and colleagues (1994); HC, Taylor, Asmundson, and Coons (2005); PTSD, van Etten and Taylor (1998); social phobia, Gould, Buckminster, Pollack, Otto, and Yap (1997); GAD, Mitte (2005); childhood anxiety, In-Albon and Schneider (2007.

ES = 0.79; Bakker, van Balkom, Spinhoven, Blaauw, & van Dyck, 1998). However, studies that have examined contemporary behavioral approaches have found that interoceptive exposure with cognitive restructuring is more powerful than wait-list or supportive therapy for panic symptoms (ES = 0.66; Gould et al., 1995).

Overall, at least seven meta-analytic reviews of the panic disorder treatment literature support the efficacy of cognitive-behavioral interventions that include exposure therapy. In addition, these analyses indicate that exposure therapy alone is an effective treatment for panic disorder in general, and the agoraphobic avoidance component in particular (e.g., Clum, Clum, & Surls, 1993).

Obsessive–Compulsive Disorder

Until the 1960s, obsessive–compulsive disorder (OCD) was generally considered unresponsive to psychotherapy, which at the time typically included psychoanalytic and supportive approaches. However, with the introduction of exposure and response prevention (ERP) in the 1960s (Meyer, 1966), the prognosis for this problem improved substantially. Numerous studies conducted in various centers around the world have established ERP as a highly efficacious therapy for OCD (Foa et al., 2005). Abramowitz (1996) conducted a meta-analysis of 24 exposure treatment studies for OCD conducted between 1975 and 1995 encompassing over 800 patients. He found that this treatment produced large pre–post treatment ESs for outcome assessed by patient self-report (ES = 1.16) and by an interviewer (ES = 1.31). In addition, these large ESs remained at follow-up, suggesting that the improvements persisted even after the treatment had been ended.

The unique effects of ERP in the alleviation of OCD symptoms, as opposed to effects common to therapy in general (i.e., imparting hope or therapeutic relationship), can be examined through studies comparing ERP to other interventions. A second meta-analysis by Abramowitz (1997) included only RCTs in which two treatments were compared; ES was calculated as the standardized comparison between two interventions at post-treatment. Comparisons between ERP and a relaxation control yielded a large ES in favor of ERP (ES = 1.18). Similarly, in the largest meta-analysis conducted (86 studies), Van Balkom and colleagues (1994) were able to examine treatments that were described as "behavioral," as opposed to "cognitive" or a combination. Their results supported the effectiveness of stand-alone exposure techniques with an ES of 1.46 for self-reported OCD symptoms and an ES of 1.47 for assessor-rated symptoms. Taken as a whole these studies provide strong support for the effectiveness of exposure alone or in combination with cognitive techniques for OCD.

Hypochondriasis and Health-Related Anxiety

Compared to other problems with anxiety, exposure-based treatments have only recently been applied to health anxiety, commonly known as hypochondriasis (HC). HC is characterized by a preoccupation with fears of having a serious disease based on misinterpretation of bodily sensations (American Psychiatric Association, 2000). Although HC is currently classified as a somatoform disorder under the DSM nomenclature, researchers have suggested that it may be more appropriately grouped with the anxiety disorders (Olatunji, Deacon, & Abramowitz, 2009). One such approach views HC as similar to OCD in that it consists of obsessive thoughts regarding the presence of disease and attempts to relieve distress through compulsively checking one's health, such as through doctor visits (Abramowitz & Moore, 2007). Based on this conceptualization, HC can be treated using ERP. Accordingly, exposure has also been incorporated into CBT packages along with psychoeducation, self-monitoring, and cognitive restructuring (Taylor, Asmundson, & Coons, 2005).

Although a limited number of clinical trials have examined the efficacy of treatments for HC, Taylor et al. (2005) conducted a meta-analysis of the controlled and uncontrolled trials. This study combined 15 studies, six of which included ERP or CBT. The results supported the use of CBT, with ESs of 2.05 at posttreatment and 1.54 at follow-up. The utility of exposure therapy was supported by ESs of 1.00 and 1.19 for posttreatment and follow-up, respectively. Although these results are promising, the authors cautioned that the small number of trials included in the meta-analysis limited the impact of the study.

Posttraumatic Stress Disorder

Many psychological treatment programs for posttraumatic stress disorder (PTSD) involve exposure, cognitive restructuring, and anxiety management skills. Exposure-based treatments emphasize confrontation with fear-evoking memories of the traumatic event (i.e., imaginal exposure) as well as situations or stimuli that have come to evoke avoidance or anxiety symptoms (i.e., situational exposure). Foa, Steketee, and Rothbaum (1989) asserted that the purpose of therapeutic exposure is twofold: first, to weaken conditioned fear responses associated with trauma cues; and second, to modify overestimates of the dangerousness of the world and threat to personal safety. Stress inoculation training (SIT; Veronen & Kilpatrick, 1983) and cognitive processing therapy (CPT; Calhoun & Resick, 1993) involve combinations of educational, exposure, relaxation, and cognitive interventions to help the patient manage anxiety symptoms and challenge maladaptive beliefs.

Eye movement desensitization and reprocessing (EMDR; Shapiro, 1991) is an effective, yet controversial, treatment involving a form of imaginal exposure to traumatic memories along with coping statements that are introduced during recall of the trauma. Simultaneously, patients engage in saccadic eye movements such as tracking the therapist's finger from side to side across the field of vision. Shapiro (1995) suggested that the eye movements specifically aid processing and integration of the traumatic memories, thus reversing neural pathology. Others have proposed that it is the imaginal exposure that accounts for the effectiveness of EMDR (e.g., Lilienfeld, 1996). In fact, a meta-analysis demonstrated that EMDR has similar efficacy with or without the eye movements and is no more effective than exposure therapy (Davidson & Parker, 2001).

Two recent meta-analyses have been published on the effects of CBT for PTSD. One review by van Etten and Taylor (1998) included 61 trials from 39 treatment studies. Psychotherapies were grouped as behavior therapy (13 trials), EMDR (11 trials), relaxation (1 trial), hypnosis (1 trial), and dynamic therapy (1 trial). Mean within-group ESs for "behavior therapies" were 1.27 and 1.89 for self-report and observer-rated measures of PTSD severity, respectively. For EMDR, which was also considered a form of CBT, self-report and observer-rated ESs were 1.24 and 0.69, respectively. Because the group of "behavior therapies" actually incorporated both cognitive and behavioral interventions (e.g., exposure-based treatments, SIT, and CPT) averaged together, estimation of the effect of exposure procedures alone could not be gleaned from this study. Nevertheless, van Etten and Taylor's (1998) results suggest that CBTs that include exposure exercises are highly effective in reducing PTSD symptoms.

The second meta-analytic review on PTSD, published by Sherman (1998), included only those treatment studies comparing an active treatment to a comparison group (e.g., wait-list control). Seventeen such studies were identified; the authors also attempted to locate unpublished findings by contacting prominent researchers in the field. The specific treatment interventions studied included exposure therapy, EMDR, SIT, CPT, hypnosis, and various inpatient treatment programs. Comparison group conditions included no treatment (waiting list), supportive counseling, and dynamic therapy. The average mean ES between treatment and control across all studies was 0.52 at posttreatment and 0.53 at follow-up. These findings indicate that overall, psychological treatments yield moderate positive effects on symptoms of PTSD.

Social Phobia

Psychological treatments for social phobia typically involve cognitive restructuring, various forms of exposure (imaginal, situational), social skills training, or combinations of these approaches. Behavioral approaches emphasize prolonged exposure to social stimuli both within and between sessions via homework assignments (e.g., Newman, Hofmann, Werner, Roth, & Taylor, 1994). Cognitive therapy relies on techniques aimed at correcting maladaptive beliefs about the self and others, particularly beliefs that exaggerate the probability and consequences of negative social evaluation (Rapee & Heimberg, 1997). CBTs typically utilize both cognitive restructuring and exposure to feared social situations as means of addressing negative cognitive appraisals and overestimations of negative consequences. CBT for social phobia is often delivered in a group format (e.g., Heimberg et al., 1990) since this setting constitutes a form of exposure and affords ample opportunity to confront feared social situations.

Recently, there have been four published meta-analytic reviews of CBTs for social phobia. Feske and Chambless (1995) examined 15 treatment outcome studies, 9 of which included exposure therapy alone and 12 of which examined the combination of exposure plus cognitive restructuring. Across studies, exposure alone and exposure plus cognitive restructuring were equally effective at both posttreatment and follow-up on most measures of social phobia, depression, and general anxiety. Similarly, Gould, Buckminster, Pollack, Otto, and Yap (1997) reviewed 16 studies that examined CBT. Although statistical tests of differences between these cognitive, behavioral, and combined treatments were not conducted, the results suggest that exposure therapy either alone or in combination with cognitive restructuring is somewhat more effective than cognitive restructuring alone. Specifically, within-group ESs at posttreatment, averaged across dependent variables, were 0.89 for exposure alone, 0.80 for exposure plus cognitive restructuring, and 0.60 for cognitive restructuring alone.

Taylor's (1996) meta-analysis reviewed 24 studies of exposure, cognitive therapy, cognitive therapy plus exposure, and social skills training for social phobia. Analysis of within-group ESs indicated that all psychological treatments were superior to control treatments. On measures of social phobia, mean ESs were 1.06 for cognitive therapy plus exposure, 0.82 for exposure alone, and 0.63 for cognitive therapy alone. In the most recent meta-analytic review of social phobia treatment, Fedoroff and Taylor (2001) computed within-group ESs for 7 trials of exposure therapy, 7 of cognitive therapy, and 21 of combined exposure and cognitive therapy. Although exposure alone had the largest ES, it was not significantly different from no effect due to high variability in results and lack of power from a small number of studies. At follow-up, behavioral, cognitive, and combination treatments were judged to be efficacious with no differences between them.

Overall, meta-analytic findings on psychological treatments for social phobia provide consistent support for the effectiveness of cognitive-behavioral interventions. Exposure therapy alone appears to be effective as well, yet results are equivocal regarding whether adding cognitive restructuring confers additional benefits.

Generalized Anxiety Disorder

Exposure methods have enjoyed long-standing acceptance as effective treatments for anxiety disorders in which specific fear-provoking stimuli can be identified. However, the diffuse nature of external triggers for anxiety found in generalized anxiety disorder (GAD) makes the applicability of exposure less intuitive (Borkovec & Whisman, 1996). Consequently, psychological treatments for GAD have been characterized by a variety of techniques including progressive muscle relaxation, self-monitoring and early cue detection, applied relaxation, self-control desensitization (Goldfried, 1971), cognitive restructuring, and combinations of the above (e.g., Borkovec & Costello, 1993). At least four meta-analytic studies have reviewed treatment outcome results for GAD.

Borkovec and Whisman (1996) summarized results from 11 controlled trials. Within-group ESs were calculated separately for each of five commonly used measures of anxiety and depression. At posttreatment, all psychological treatments reviewed (including "nonspecific" treatments) were superior to wait list. Although ESs varied somewhat across dependent variables, behavioral techniques (i.e., relaxation training, imaginal exposure) tended to produce stronger effects relative to cognitive therapy, while the highest ES was evidenced by treatments incorporating the combination of behavioral and cognitive procedures. For example, at posttreatment the ES on the State–Trait Anxiety Inventory—Trait version (STAI-T; Spielberger, Gorsuch, Lushene, Vagg, & Jacobs, 1983) was 0.24 for cognitive therapy, 0.90 for behavior therapy, and 1.01 for combined approaches. At followup, combined treatment demonstrated higher ESs than behavior therapy for each dependent measure. These findings provide support for the effectiveness of behavioral, particularly cognitive-behavioral, interventions for GAD.

Gould, Otto, Pollack, and Yap (1997) conducted a meta-analysis of GAD treatment studies, including 22 comparisons of CBTs. Combined treatment approaches and anxiety management training had the highest ESs (ES for both = 0.91), followed by relaxation (ES = 0.64), cognitive therapy (ES = 0.59), behavior therapy (ES = 0.51), and relaxation with biofeedback (ES = 0.34). Statistical comparisons among these conditions yielded only one significant finding: combined treatment was significantly more effective than relaxation with biofeedback. A subsequent meta-analysis focused on a relatively small number of studies reinforced previous conclusions supporting the effectiveness of CBTs for GAD with an overall ES of 2.09 at posttreatment (Weston & Morrison, 2001).

The most recent and extensive meta-analysis included a total of 65 studies examining CBT and pharmacotherapy (Mitte, 2005). Although the author of the studies differentiated between cognitive and behavioral approaches, most treatments combined both elements and included some form of exposure. CBT was found to be more effective than no treatment (ES = 0.82) and placebo controls (ES = 0.57). The study author did not compare cognitive to behavioral approaches and the relative effectiveness compared to medication varied depending on the meta-analytic methods applied. Finally, patients tolerated CBT well with an average dropout rate, 9%, that was significantly lower than the rate with pharmacotherapy.

Overall, the meta-analytic literature supports the effectiveness of CBT for GAD. Although exposure exercises appear to be an effective intervention, their combination with cognitive techniques leads to more effective treatment of GAD than either component in isolation.

Childhood Anxiety Disorders

The research summarized so far in this chapter has been conducted with adults. As is the case with many areas of psychological research, the investigation of treatment effects in children has lagged behind the adult literature. Treatment outcome studies of childhood anxiety disorders typically combine patients with GAD, social phobia, and separation anxiety disorder. CBT interventions, such as "The Coping Cat" manualized treatment for childhood anxiety disorders (Kendall, 2000), are the most extensively studied interventions (e.g., In-Albon & Schneider, 2007). Kendall's approach begins with eight sessions devoted to psychoeducation and development of an anxiety management plan. The remaining eight sessions consist of graduated exposures to anxiety-provoking situations and stimuli.

A recent meta-analysis including 10 studies of CBT for childhood anxiety disorders found that 56.5% of patients treated with CBT no longer met criteria for an anxiety disorder, compared to 34.8% of children who received no treatment (Cartwright-Hatton, Roberts, Chitsabesan, Fothergill, & Harrington, 2004). Moreover, these differences remained at follow-up. A more recent meta-analysis of 24 RCTs including 1,275 patients also supported the efficacy of CBT for childhood anxiety disorders, with a recovery rate of 68.9% compared to 12.9% for the waiting list (In-Albon & Schneider, 2007). Furthermore, the ES for the treatment group was 0.86 (1.36 at follow-up) compared to 0.13 for wait-list control and 0.58 for attention placebo control. Thus, exposure-based treatment appears to be appropriate for anxiety symptoms in children.

In addition to evidence regarding treatment of the three main childhood anxiety disorders, outcome studies have also been conducted for other anxiety symptoms. For instance, a meta-analysis of treatment for pediatric

OCD concluded that ERP was more effective then other treatment modalities (Abramowitz, Whiteside, & Deacon, 2005). In this review ERP, had a pre- to posttreatment ES of 1.98, compared to 1.13 for medication and 0.48 for placebo. Similarly, a review of treatments for specific phobias concluded that participant modeling and reinforced practice are well-supported treatments, while imaginal and *in vivo* desensitization, filmed and live modeling, and CBT are probably effective (Ollendick & King, 1998). Importantly, exposures have been singled out as the common element underlying all of these treatments (Davis & Ollendick, 2005). Finally, some anxiety problems, such as school phobia, occur predominately in children and do not have an extensive adult literature to consult. In a qualitative review of behavioral treatments, two uncontrolled trials supported the effectiveness of behavior therapy for school phobia (Thyer & Sowers-Hoag, 1988).

Although derived from a more limited research base than the adult literature, meta-analytic reviews support the effectiveness of treatments for childhood anxiety disorders. Overall, these studies have supported the efficacy of exposure-based treatments.

EXPERT CONSENSUS GUIDELINES

Based on the literature investigating treatment for anxiety disorders, a number of organizations have developed practice guidelines for clinicians. For example, the American Psychiatric Association has recommended that exposure-based CBT and serotonin reuptake inhibitors be considered first-line treatments for OCD, PTSD, and panic disorder depending on the patient's preference for therapy or medication. Moreover, the guidelines developed by the National Institute for Health and Clinical Excellence (NICE), an independent organization that provides treatment recommendations to the National Health Services in England and Wales, provide further support for CBT. These standards designate exposure-based CBT as *the* treatment with the most empirical support and recommend it as the most appropriate first line intervention for OCD, PTSD, panic disorder, and GAD. Unfortunately, guidelines have not yet been established for other disorders, for example, social phobia.

CONCLUSIONS

A large body of empirical evidence supports the efficacy of exposure-based therapy for the various anxiety disorders. Although studies comparing the impact of different components of CBT are less numerous than those investigating treatment packages as a whole, a strong case can be made that exposure procedures constitute a critical ingredient in therapy for these conditions. Accordingly, many exposure-based treatments have attained the designation of "well-established treatments" in the American Psychological Association's reviews of evidence-based treatments. To qualify for this label, a treatment (delivered according to a manual) must have two or more RCTs (by separate investigators) demonstrating its superiority to placebo (Chambless et al., 1998). Currently, exposure-based treatments have attained this level of support for panic/agoraphobia, GAD, OCD, and specific phobia (Chambless & Ollendick, 2001). In addition, exposure-based treatment for PTSD, social anxiety disorder, and childhood anxiety disorders have achieved the level of "probably efficacious." In fact, the majority of well-established treatments for anxiety and stress disorders include exposure exercises.

3

The Nature
and Treatment
of Clinical Anxiety

Now that we have reviewed normal and pathological anxiety, the history of exposure therapy, and the outcome literature demonstrating its effectiveness, we turn our attention to the theoretical model underlying the conceptualization and treatment of clinical anxiety problems using exposure techniques. We believe that a firm grasp of this theoretical framework is necessary for clinicians to be able to transcend the traditional disorder-specific treatment manual and appropriately apply exposure techniques across the countless presentations of clinical anxiety. A solid understanding of the assumptions underlying the use of exposure also enables the clinician to present to the anxious person a clear and convincing rationale for engaging in exposure therapy. Therefore, in this chapter, we address how problems with clinical anxiety and fear are acquired, what causes them to persist (often for many years), and how exposure therapy helps to ameliorate them.

THE DEVELOPMENT OF CLINICAL ANXIETY

Four pathways have been proposed to explain how excessive fears are developed: (1) traumatic experiences, (2) modeling, (3) transmission of misinformation, and (4) evolutionary preparedness. We begin with a discussion of each pathway.

Traumatic Experiences (Classical Conditioning)

Perhaps the most obvious means of acquiring a fear is through a direct, negative experience with an object or situation. Through *classical conditioning*, a previously neutral stimulus acquires the power to elicit fear by being paired with an inherently aversive stimulus. This phenomenon was demonstrated in a classic experiment by Watson and Rayner (1920). The unfortunate subject of their experiment, an infant known as "Little Albert," initially showed no fear in response to a harmless white rat. However, by repeatedly pairing the rat with an aversive stimulus (a loud noise), the researchers were able to turn Little Albert's idle curiosity into fear of rats, as well as other objects that resembled rats in some way (e.g., a furry mask).

The process of classical conditioning involves learning new associations between stimuli and their consequences. Objects and situations previously considered harmless may be reevaluated as dangerous following an aversive conditioning experience. For example, following a car crash, a fearful individual may come to expect that the previously nonthreatening activity of driving to work is now very likely to lead to bodily harm. Accordingly, conditioning is a cognitive process that shapes people's expectations and beliefs about feared stimuli.

Individuals with clinical anxiety often fear objects and places that elicit a relatively "neutral" emotional response from most people. Examples include meeting dogs, driving cars, riding in elevators, and sitting in classrooms. Classical conditioning in the form of traumatic experiences involving these objects or situations may account for the development of such fears in some individuals. Many people with social anxiety, for example, describe having been the victim of severe teasing in childhood (McCabe, Antony, Summerfeldt, Liss, & Swinson, 2003). Similarly, poor dental health in childhood and early adolescence, and the increased opportunities for unpleasant and painful dental visits it brings, is associated with the development of dental fear at age 18 (Poulton et al., 1997).

An experience recounted by a patient concisely illustrates the role of classical conditioning in fear acquisition. On a warm summer day, the patient was mowing her lawn barefoot when she stepped on a harmless garter snake. She immediately experienced a severe panic attack and ran inside her home as the snake slithered away. Following this event, she experienced intense situational anxiety when in the presence of previously neutral stimuli she now associated with snakes, including her lawn, walking barefoot, and even her lawnmower. She subsequently sold her lawnmower, hired a lawn care company, and stopped walking barefoot (even inside her home). Her fear of snakes persisted for years despite the absence of any additional aversive experiences with these animals.

Latent Inhibition

Despite the importance of conditioning in fear acquisition, many people have traumatic experiences but never develop excessive fears (Ollendick, King, & Muris, 2002). This fact was illustrated by DiNardo, Guzy, and Bak (1988), who found that approximately two-thirds of people with no fear of dogs had experienced a conditioning event such as a painful dog bite. Of interest, this was the same percentage of negative experiences reported by those with dog phobia, suggesting that negative (traumatic) personal experiences do not necessarily give rise to fear.

Why might a traumatic experience fail to produce an excessive fear? One possibility is that prior positive experiences with a stimulus can protect an individual from acquiring a fear following a negative conditioning experience. This phenomenon, known as *latent inhibition*, helps to explain why traumatic experiences fail to produce clinically significant fears in most people. To illustrate, being bitten by a dog is less likely to produce a dog phobia among those who have had prior contact with dogs (Doogan & Thomas, 1992). Prior experience with dogs helps people distinguish playful from threatening behavior in dogs and increases the likelihood that a negative experience will be considered the exception rather than the rule. Research on latent inhibition suggests that lack of familiarity with an object or situation increases the probability that a traumatic experience will lead to an excessive fear.

Modeling (Vicarious Conditioning)

Vicarious conditioning, also known as modeling, refers to learning that occurs through observing others. Specifically, we may learn to fear certain objects or situations simply by witnessing other people's traumatic experiences or by observing others act in a fearful manner. A great deal of research attests to the powerful effects of vicarious conditioning in the development of fear (Mineka & Zinbarg, 2006). People with severe anxiety often relate personal accounts of vicarious learning experiences that appear to have triggered the onset of their symptoms. One such individual was Jennifer, a 20-year-old woman with panic disorder. During high school she witnessed a friend suffer a fatal asthma attack during which she dramatically gasped for air before being taken away in an ambulance. Jennifer, who suffered from very mild asthma herself, became concerned that she might suffer a similar tragic fate. She began to avoid activities and substances that she believed might trigger sensations of shortness of breath, and she experienced panic attacks when she noticed herself having difficulty breathing.

Transmission of Misinformation

Information transmitted by parents, peers, the media, and other sources might also contribute to the development of fears. For example, the message that germs are ubiquitous, dangerous, and require diligent cleansing is often conveyed by well-meaning family members, television commercials for antibacterial products, and sensationalistic reports in the news media. Individuals who internalize this message may acquire a fear of contamination in the absence of any negative personal or vicarious experiences with contaminants. In the same manner, the concern that immoral thoughts are equivalent to immoral actions (e.g., thinking about adultery is the moral equivalent to committing adultery) might be acquired through familiarity with the notion, advanced in some religious traditions, that morality is characterized by purity in both thought and deed (Berman, Abramowitz, Pardue, & Wheaton, 2010). In fact, as we discuss in Chapter 10, some individuals with OCD describe having acquired a fear of blasphemous, sacrilegious, and sexual thoughts in this manner.

Evolutionary Preparedness

It has long been observed that the distribution of fears is not random and does not reflect the types of objects and situations that are most likely to pose an actual threat to our present-day survival. People are more likely to be killed by a gun or an automobile than by a snake or a spider, yet fears of the former are rare compared to phobias of the latter. It appears that humans have a predisposition to fear stimuli that posed a survival threat during our evolutionary past. As a result, it is easier for people to acquire a fear of heights, for example, than to something unrelated to our evolutionary past, such as guns.

Support for an evolutionary contribution to fear acquisition was demonstrated in a fascinating series of studies by Poulton and colleagues (reviewed in Poulton & Menzies, 2002). These researchers found that negative conditioning experiences lead to higher rates of phobia for evolutionary *irrelevant* fears such as dental phobia, but to lower rates of phobia for evolutionary *relevant* fears such as heights. Rachman (1978) anticipated the implications of such findings when he asserted that "the predisposition to develop the most common fears is innate and universal, or nearly so, and that what we learn is how to overcome our existing predispositions. In large part, we learn to stop responding fearfully to predisposed or prepared stimuli" (p. 225). In other words, most people learn *not to fear* things like snakes, spiders, contaminants, heights, and so on. Many individuals who fear these things have simply failed to learn, perhaps through a lack of relevant life experiences, that they are not dangerous.

In summary, there is no single theory that adequately explains the development of excessive fear and anxiety. In contrast, it is likely that the pathways to the acquisition of excessive fears are multiply determined and include conditioning, learning, and genetic processes (Ollendick et al., 2002). Fortunately, the manner in which problematic fears and anxiety are maintained over time is more relevant to treatment than are the origins of those fears. This important topic is discussed next.

WHY DO ANXIETY PROBLEMS PERSIST OVER TIME?

At some point, most people experience, witness, or hear about a traumatic incident with the potential to produce a clinically significant fear. For example, most people experience public humiliation, a bad encounter with a ferocious dog, or a car accident. Some may even survive a physical or violent assault. For most of us, these experiences do not lead to clinically severe anxiety problems (i.e., anxiety disorders). More likely, they cause only a temporary increase in anxiety, distress, and feelings of vulnerability. For example, shortly after a painful bee sting a hiker may feel a sense of apprehension while walking in the woods, watch and listen carefully for bees, and even choose a different location in which to hike. Assuming the individual continues to hike without experiencing additional bee stings, the emotional, attentional, and behavioral changes described above would most likely fade away. In this manner, the hiker's apprehension would naturally self-correct. Put another way, the hiker would soon recover and feel as safe in the woods as he felt prior to the bee sting.

Now, consider the case of another hiker, James (age 16), who suffered a bee sting and subsequently developed a phobia of bees. How did the same conditioning event that had little effect on the fictional hiker above result in the development of a severe and debilitating anxiety disorder in James, who required treatment for a bee phobia? To begin with, James interpreted the bee sting he received at age 12 as a sign that bees and forests are inherently dangerous. Rather than viewing the bee sting as a context-specific stroke of bad luck, he believed that all forests were unsafe because they harbored bees that would sting him at first sight. Not surprisingly, he avoided hiking in the woods, walking in natural settings, and being outside in any environment where he might encounter bees. His fear gradually worsened to the point that he was unable to venture outdoors for more than a few minutes at a time during the summer months.

Cognitive-behavioral theory (e.g., Beck et al., 1985) regards psychological problems as the product of dysfunctional patterns of thinking and behavior. In James's case, the belief that bees and forests are inherently dangerous led him to feel anxious in situations where he believed he might be stung by a bee. He overestimated the likelihood of encountering bees in the outdoors, exaggerated the probability that bees would sting him, and catastrophized about the unendurable pain of getting stung. To manage his anxiety and prevent another bee sting, James avoided the outdoors, fled indoors upon sighting a bee, and even wore heavy long-sleeved clothing to protect his skin. In the context of these dysfunctional cognitions and extreme and unnecessary behaviors, his fear of bees persisted for 4 years despite the absence of another bee sting.

Whatever the manner of its acquisition, a fear may develop into a clinical anxiety problem as a result of maladaptive thinking and behaviors that maintain fear and interrupt the natural process of recovery, which in behavioral terms is called *extinction*. Next we discuss the psychological processes responsible for the maintenance of pathological anxiety, which are briefly described in Table 3.1. Consistent with the scope of this book, we eschew the DSM diagnostic boundaries and focus instead on *transdiagnostic* processes (i.e., biases in cognition, maladaptive behavioral patterns) that contribute to the maintenance of pathological anxiety and fear regardless of the syndrome or "disorder" in which it is found (e.g., Harvey, Watkins, Mansell, & Shafran, 2004).

Maladaptive Beliefs

Anxiety disorders are, by definition, irrational to some degree. That is, as mentioned in Chapter 1, they involve exaggerated estimates of threat. Objectively harmless situations and stimuli (i.e., those posing no more than normal everyday [low] risk) are misinterpreted as highly threatening or very dangerous. We thus begin our discussion of key psychological processes by reviewing different types of dysfunctional beliefs that maintain pathological anxiety.

Probability Overestimation

Most clinically anxious individuals habitually overestimate the probability (likelihood) that exposure to their feared stimuli will result in negative consequences. Patients with panic attacks, for example, often believe that the experience of arousal-related body sensations will result in physical catastrophes such as a heart attack or suffocation (Clark, 1986). Similarly, individuals who fear contamination may exaggerate the likelihood that touching "dirty" objects, such as toilet seats, will cause them to contract a disease. Most clinically anxious persons fear negative outcomes that are objectively unlikely to occur (although not altogether *impossible*), and their exaggerated expectations of danger almost always involve an inflated sense of the probability of harm.

TABLE 3.1. Psychological Processes That Maintain Clinical Anxiety Problems

Maintenance factor	Description
Maladaptive beliefs	
Probability overestimation	Exaggerating the likelihood of a feared outcome
Cost overestimation	Exaggerating the severity (badness) of a feared outcome if it were to occur
Intolerance of uncertainty	Refusal to be comfortable with even the remote possibility that a feared outcome might occur
Low coping self-efficacy	Belief that one is unable to tolerate or cope with feared stimuli and one's reaction to them
Beliefs about experiencing anxiety	Exaggerating how frightened one will feel in feared situations; belief that the symptoms of anxiety will lead to physical harm, loss of mental control, or negative evaluation
Beliefs about safety behaviors	Belief that safety behaviors prevent feared outcomes from occurring; beliefs about the mechanisms through which safety behaviors prevent disaster; belief that safety behaviors are necessary to cope with feared situations
Biased information processing	
Selective attention	Paying close attention to stimuli relevant to anxious concerns
Selective memory	Tendency to selectively recall information consistent with one's maladaptive beliefs
Safety behaviors	Actions intended to prevent disaster that inadvertently prevent the disconfirmation of maladaptive threat beliefs

Cost Overestimation

Sometimes feared events do occur; people stumble over their words while giving speeches or commit social faux pas at dinner parties. Relative to others, however, anxious individuals tend to overestimate the perceived cost (badness) of such feared outcomes *if they were to occur*. This is particularly true for social fears where patients believe it would be horrible if someone responded to them with annoyance or rejection or inappropriately laughed at what they said. This process can also occur with other fears, such as contamination. For instance, although it would be unfortunate to get sick from touching doorknobs, the illness would most likely be a nuisance cold that lasts a few days to a week. In addition, even patients who fear objectively severe outcomes still experience excessive anxiety due to inflated cost estimates. For example, patients with panic attacks often mistakenly believe that a heart attack, if it were to occur, would certainly be fatal. Some individuals with health anxiety believe that after finally succumbing to a terminal disease their consciousness will somehow endure, leaving them frightened and alone in their graves for all eternity (Furer, Walker, & Stein, 2007).

Intolerance of Uncertainty

Some patients manifest extreme anxiety despite their awareness that the probability of a feared outcome is quite low. For example, many people with a fear of flying experience panic attacks on airplanes despite their knowledge that the odds of being in a fatal plane crash are less than one in a million. These patients are unwilling to accept even the remote possibility that a feared catastrophe might occur. This tendency has been referred to as the *intolerance of uncertainty* (Dugas, Buhr, & Ladouceur, 2004) and appears closely linked to anxiety problems in which the habitual experience of uncertainty and ambiguity are central features. For individuals concerned with, for example, whether or not they turned off the stove, locked the front door, or hit a pedestrian with their car, obsessional anxiety and compulsive checking behavior revolve around the distress associated with *not knowing* if these catastrophes have occurred. The situation is much the same for individuals who wonder if bodily signs and sensations (e.g., lumps, moles, headaches) signify cancer and for those who worry about future catastrophes such as the abduction of their children or their spouse suffering a fatal car accident. It is as if the very *possibility* of disaster is amplified and considered unacceptable.

Low Coping Self-Efficacy

The appraisal of a situation as dangerous will probably not cause undue anxiety for persons who feel confident in their ability to cope with or be rescued from the danger. Consider the example of someone we know who is allergic to bees and could experience a potentially life-threatening anaphylactic reaction upon being stung. This person might be expected to experience extreme anxiety in areas where bees are present and to avoid these situations at all cost. In reality, however, he enjoys hiking and is quite comfortable with the presence of bees. What is his secret? He always carries an epinephrine injection kit on his person which can be used to slow down a potentially harmful allergic reaction and buy time for him to seek emergency medical treatment.

Beliefs about one's coping abilities play a key role in the experience of anxiety (Bandura, 1988; Beck et al., 1985). Clinically anxious patients typically underestimate their capacity to control or cope with perceived threats, as well as their fear reaction to such threats. It is not unusual for patients with PTSD, for example, to habitually suppress traumatic memories based on the belief that they would be unable to cope with the high anxiety caused by recalling traumatic experiences. The frequent emergency room visits and reliance on as-needed benzodiazepine medication among individuals with panic disorder attests to the ubiquity of low coping self-efficacy associated with this anxiety problem.

Beliefs about Experiencing Anxiety

Clinically anxious individuals not only tend to overpredict how frightened they will feel when encountering feared stimuli (Rachman & Bichard, 1988), but they also fear anxiety itself, a phenomenon labeled *anxiety sensitivity* (Taylor, 1999). For example, patients who present with fears of amusement park rides, enclosed spaces, and public speaking are often concerned that their arousal-related body sensations could lead to a heart attack, loss of consciousness, stroke, or suffocation if they become too intense. Some individuals believe that prolonged exposure to highly distressing stimuli, such as being stuck in an elevator, would cause them to lose control, go crazy, or even become permanently psychotic. Patients with a social evaluative component to their fears often describe concerns that others will notice their anxiety symptoms (e.g., trembling, blushing, sweating) and judge them as weird, stupid, or mentally ill. In each of these examples, the primary fear is not the object or situation per se, but rather its capacity to produce an anxiety reaction.

Biased Information Processing

In addition to maladaptive beliefs, the normal psychological processes of attention and memory tend to operate in a manner that maintains fear and anxiety. In addition, these processes and the maladaptive beliefs described above tend to reinforce each other. We review these processes below and summarize them in Table 3.1.

Selective Attention

When people become anxious, they tend to pay particularly close attention to stimuli relevant to their concerns, a phenomenon known as *selective attention*. The tendency to selectively attend to potentially threatening stimuli is normal, logical, and adaptive. Hikers in the backcountry of Glacier National Park, for example, know that the difference between spotting a grizzly bear from a safe distance and stumbling upon a bear around a bend on the trail can be a matter of life and death. As a result, safety-conscious individuals, as they hike, continuously scan the surrounding environment for any signs indicating the presence of a grizzly. Doing so increases the probability of detecting a threat to one's survival and escaping to live another day.

Unfortunately, selective attention can maintain, and even worsen, anxiety symptoms for individuals whose fears are out of proportion to the actual degree of danger present. To illustrate, some individuals frequently scan and check their bodies to assess potential threats associated with heart palpitations, such as numbness, difficulty breathing, feelings of unreality, sweating, and blushing. This *body vigilance* increases the awareness of feared (but generally harmless) body sensations and amplifies concerns about their potential consequences (Schmidt, Lerew, & Trakowski, 1997). Many people with obsessional problems have a similar dilemma in that their fear and selective attention are focused on their own unwanted thoughts (e.g., doubts, images). Thus, they become hyperaware of unwanted mental intrusions (i.e., obsessions) that often seem ubiquitous and tormenting (Abramowitz, 2006). Selective attention also amplifies the fear that contact with "contaminated" objects will result in disease. To prevent illness, fearful individuals pay close attention to potentially threatening objects in their environment. Objects associated with germs and contamination (e.g., door handles, light switches) are of course ubiquitous and unavoidable, and individuals who pay close attention to them quickly realize this fact. This increased awareness of threat cues may lead such persons to view themselves as especially vulnerable to contamination and reinforce or even exacerbate the maladaptive beliefs associated with this fear. That is, when one selectively attends to threat stimuli, the world seems more threatening because threat-related information is receiving preferential processing and signs of safety receive less consideration.

Selective Memory

When anxious, people also tend to selectively remember information that is consistent with their fear-related beliefs. This type of *selective memory* is adaptive when applied to objectively dangerous stimuli. However, this tendency also contributes to a *confirmation bias* in which people with anxiety-related problems tend to recall information that confirms their fear-based preconceptions and to avoid information that challenges them. Thus, evidence that seems to back up their fears is strongly considered while disconfirmatory evidence is given less weight. As a result, feared negative consequences seem more likely.

For clinically anxious patients, memories of occasional failures and traumatic experiences are much more accessible than memories of uneventful experiences with feared stimuli. Patients with a fear of flying, for example, often describe vivid memories of a turbulent flight in which they were convinced that a fatal crash was imminent. However, it may take a concerted effort for them to bring to mind the memory of the many unremarkable flights they may have taken. For individuals with this fear, the tendency to preferentially recall information about the "dangers" of flying contributes to probability overestimates concerning plane crashes. More generally, selective memory causes impaired access to the full range of memories (Harvey et al., 2004), thereby inhibiting the ability to accurately evaluate information associated with maladaptive beliefs. Selective attention and selective memory work together by increasing the probability that fear cues will be noticed, encoded into memory, and subsequently retrieved, thereby reinforcing the misperception of threat and maintaining the anxiety disorder.

Safety Behaviors

Actions intended to detect, avoid, or escape a negative or feared outcome, known as *safety behaviors*, are normal, logical, and (usually) adaptive responses to the perception of threat. Everyday examples include wearing seatbelts, learning CPR, and locking the front door at night. Such judicious use of safety behaviors in the presence of actual threat is essential for survival. However, the tendency for people with irrational anxiety and fear to employ excessive safety behaviors in the absence of objective danger plays an important role in maintaining (and even worsening) anxiety-related problems (Salkovskis, 1991).

As we discussed in Chapter 1, and as is summarized in Table 3.2, safety behaviors may maintain and even worsen anxiety problems in several ways. Because they reduce the perception of threat, safety behaviors produce a short-term reduction in anxiety. In other words, they seem to work—at least temporarily. However, because of the reduction in anxiety that they engender, safety behaviors are negatively reinforced and therefore develop into patterns (habits) that are used to cope with anxiety-provoking situations. This reliance on safety behaviors prevents the natural eventual extinction of inappropriate anxiety and discourages the development of positive coping strategies.

Safety behaviors may also paradoxically cause a *misattribution* of safety (Salkovskis, 1991). In this manner, the nonoccurrence of a feared catastrophe (e.g., heart attack) may be erroneously attributed to a safety behavior (e.g., sitting down). Inaccurate threat beliefs may even be *strengthened* when individuals conclude that the nonoccurrence of disaster constitutes a "near-miss" that was achieved only through the use of safety behaviors. Some safety behaviors also divert attentional resources away from information

TABLE 3.2. How Safety Behaviors Maintain and Worsen Anxiety Problems

Mechanism	Description
Negative reinforcement	Because they temporarily reduce anxiety, safety behaviors develop into habitual anxiety management strategies
Misattribution of safety	Attributing the nonoccurrence of feared outcomes to the power of one's safety behaviors, rather than the possibility that the situation was not dangerous
Distraction from disconfirmatory information	The attention required to engage in safety behaviors prevents the individual from attending to information that might disconfirm threat appraisals
Prevents development of adaptive coping strategies	Reliance on safety behaviors prevents opportunities to develop and practice positive coping strategies
Directly worsens feared stimuli	Some safety behaviors magnify the intensity of fear cues or increase the probability that feared outcomes will occur
Increases awareness of feared stimuli	Some safety behaviors increase selective attention to fear cues, which elicits greater awareness of them
Inference of danger	Safety behaviors may transmit information about the threatening nature of feared stimuli; individuals may infer the presence of danger from their own behavior

that might disconfirm inaccurate threat appraisals (Sloan & Telch, 2002). To illustrate, a person with social phobia who concentrates on avoiding eye contact during a speech may not notice the audience's favorable reaction.

Safety behaviors may further reinforce beliefs about one's inability to tolerate or cope with feared stimuli. By habitually relying on safety behaviors, patients are prevented from learning that they are able to successfully navigate distressing situations by using adaptive coping strategies. In some cases, this leads anxious individuals to believe that safety behaviors are necessary to cope with threat. For example, some people with agoraphobia are able to venture into feared situations only if accompanied by a "safe person."

Another way safety behaviors may maintain or exacerbate the very anxiety problems they are intended to solve is by amplifying the intensity of feared stimuli. For example, someone with severe health anxiety who is worried about skin cancer might inspect a harmless mole by poking and prodding it many times a day. As a result, the mole may become red and inflamed, thereby exacerbating overestimates of the likelihood of cancer, which in turn leads to additional checking, poking, and prodding. Similarly, socially anxious individuals who attempt to prevent negative evaluation by avoiding eye contact and keeping their conversation to a minimum may increase the odds of being evaluated by others as awkward or unintelligent. As discussed earlier, some safety behaviors (e.g., checking for potential contaminants, body scanning) may also increase the awareness of feared stimuli.

Lastly, individuals may infer the presence of danger from their performance of safety behaviors or the mere presence of safety signals (e.g., antianxiety medications). For instance, a dog with a muzzle appears more dangerous than one without. Similarly, the sight of hand sanitizer dispensers, face masks, and rubber gloves implies the presence of harmful bacteria. When anxious individuals use safety behaviors or carry safety aids in a particular situation, they may inadvertently reinforce the message that the situation is dangerous and unmanageable. For example, the patient who takes benzodiazepine medication during an episode of high anxiety while grocery shopping may conclude on the basis of this behavior that grocery shopping is threatening—a conclusion that many people with panic attacks and agoraphobia do indeed reach.

Types of Safety Behaviors

Safety behaviors come in many different forms and are highly individualized. Perhaps the most obvious variety involves attempts to avoid confronting feared stimuli altogether. Anxious individuals may also excessively check feared stimuli (e.g., door locks, skin blemishes) to try to verify the presence, absence, or degree of threat. Similarly, checking can involve seeking reassurance from others regarding the probability or cost of feared outcomes (e.g., "Do you think I contaminated my daughter? What if she gets sick?"). Safety behaviors are often used in feared situations to directly neutralize or prevent a feared outcome from occurring, as in the case of the patient who takes antianxiety medication because she believes that it is necessary to prevent a panic-induced heart attack.

In some cases, safety behaviors have a repetitious, stereotyped, or ritualistic quality. Examples include the compulsive rituals exhibited by many people with OCD, such as repetitively counting, washing, praying, or repeating words in a specific manner. As these examples demonstrate, safety behaviors can be *covert* (i.e., mental events) and unobservable to others. Lastly, patients may rely on safety signals or aids, such as a cell phone, water bottle, good luck charm, antianxiety medication, a safe person, and so on. Patients are often comforted by simply having access to these objects (and people) regardless of whether they are actually used. Whatever their form, all safety behaviors are intended to avoid or prevent disaster and have the secondary effect of preventing the disconfirmation of maladaptive threat beliefs (Salkovskis, Clark, Hackmann, Wells, & Gelder, 1999). A more detailed account of the different types of safety behaviors and clinical assessment strategies appears in Chapter 4.

Beliefs about Safety Behaviors

How is it possible that someone who reported experiencing over 1,000 panic attacks still expected to die during her next attack? Most likely, she misattributed the nonoccurrence of any catastrophes to the power of her safety behaviors. In other words, she believed that actions such as taking Xanax, sitting down, drinking water, and breathing deeply during panic attacks had kept her alive for years by preventing the disaster that would surely have taken place had she not engaged in these behaviors. Frequently, these beliefs apply to the mechanisms by which safety behaviors prevent harm. For example, the woman with panic attacks believed that the antianxiety medicine, relaxation strategies, and presence of trusted helpers kept her heart rate below the threshold at which she would experience a fatal heart attack. In addition, she believed that her safety behaviors were necessary for her to be able to cope with the experience of panic. As a result, her worst attacks occurred when she was alone and unable to solicit reassurance from "safe persons"; in these cases she often visited the emergency room. This case example illustrates the manner in which anxiety problems may be maintained by beliefs about (1) the extent to which safety behaviors are useful or even necessary to prevent disaster, (2) the mechanisms through which safety behaviors are successful in this regard, and (3) the extent to which safety behaviors are necessary to cope with feared stimuli and high-risk situations.

A MODEL OF THE MAINTENANCE OF ANXIETY DISORDERS

In this section we present an integrative framework for understanding how the various cognitive-behavioral processes described in this chapter work together to maintain anxiety-related disorders. This framework is intended to apply to anxiety-related problems in general. In the chapters of Part II we illustrate the application of this framework to specific presentations of anxiety and fear.

Figure 3.1 presents a basic conceptual framework for understanding the maintenance of clinical anxiety and fear. The model begins by assuming

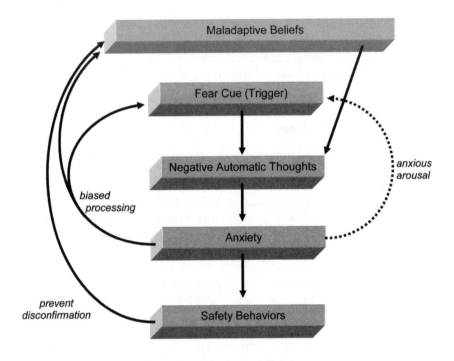

FIGURE 3.1. Cognitive-behavioral model of the maintenance of anxiety-related disorders.

that maladaptive beliefs (e.g., probability and cost overestimates) are the core maintenance factor that gives rise to the subsequent processes depicted in the diagram. The first ingredient in the experience of anxiety is the perception of a fear cue or "trigger" (i.e., a stimulus associated with a feared outcome). Depending on the individual, triggers may consist of external situations and stimuli, internal bodily signs and sensations, or mental events such as intrusive thoughts, impulses, doubts, images, and memories. The second ingredient is the appraisal of the fear cue as threatening or harmful (or for some anxiety problems, disgusting). In Figure 3.1, these appraisals are referred to as *automatic thoughts* because they often occur quickly and operate outside of the patient's conscious awareness. The appraisal of a situation or stimulus as harmful stems from the maladaptive probability and severity overestimates and naturally elicits anxiety.

As we have discussed, the anxiety response is accompanied by harmless but noticeable bodily signs and symptoms (e.g., pounding heart, shortness of breath, and dizziness). For individuals who believe these symptoms to be harmful, the experience of anxiety is a fear trigger in its own right. The dotted line leading from Anxiety to Triggers in Figure 3.1 depicts an additional maintenance process that affects those whose fear is triggered (and exacerbated) by their own anxiety reactions. Such individuals may experience a vicious circle in which threatening appraisals of arousal-related body sensations lead to more intense sensations, increasingly catastrophic appraisals, and so on, which may culminate in a full-blown panic attack (Clark, 1986). The experience of anxiety also naturally results in biased information processing in the form of selective attention and selective memory. By filtering out safety information and underscoring perceived threats, these cognitive processes make anxious persons especially likely to notice fear cues and to appraise them in a catastrophic manner consistent with their maladaptive beliefs. This biased information processing may in turn reinforce the maladaptive beliefs.

The natural reaction to the perception of danger is to seek safety. By engaging in safety behaviors, individuals can diminish or eliminate their aversive emotional state and seemingly prevent the occurrence of feared catastrophes. Thus, such behaviors become a habitual coping strategy. Unfortunately, safety behaviors have the paradoxical effect of maintaining and even strengthening the maladaptive beliefs responsible for the anxiety problem in the first place. This process becomes self-perpetuating in that as long as the maladaptive beliefs persist, so will the pathological anxiety and fear.

It is important to note that this cognitive-behavioral model does not assume that the psychological processes depicted in Figure 3.1 are part of a *disease* or *dysfunction*. By extension, individuals who experience anxiety problems are not thought to be suffering from an "illness" per se. It is indeed logical and adaptive to pay close attention to threats to one's safety in perceived high-risk situations, to feel afraid in the presence of danger, to experience noticeable body sensations when anxious, and to seek safety from harm. These responses are potentially lifesaving in the context of an actual threat to one's survival. The problem for anxious patients is that such individuals (mis)perceive a serious threat where the risk of true danger is actually low. In such instances, the responses described above are distinctly unhelpful and unfortunately (yet naturally) lead to the maintenance of their fear.

IMPLICATIONS FOR EXPOSURE THERAPY

The cognitive and behavioral processes that maintain anxiety comprise a vicious cycle that prevents the self-correction of pathological fear. In essence, anxious patients are "stuck" in this self-perpetuating cycle despite their best efforts to the contrary. The task for the exposure therapist is to help patients find their way out of this dysfunctional process. In this section, we discuss the mechanisms responsible for the effectiveness of exposure therapy and how this treatment targets the processes that maintain anxiety-related problems.

How Does Exposure Therapy Work?

Exposure therapy is generally thought to work by modifying pathological "fear structures" (Foa & Kozak, 1986), which contain associations between fearful emotions, cognitions, and behavior that maintain anxiety problems. Repeated and prolonged exposure modifies these associations by presenting patients with information that is incompatible with them. In other words, exposure disconfirms the following types of beliefs: maladaptive probability and cost overestimates, low coping self-efficacy, inaccurate beliefs about experiencing anxiety and uncertainty, and beliefs that safety behaviors are necessary to prevent feared catastrophes. Thus, the critical mechanism underlying successful exposure therapy is the correction of maladaptive beliefs, a phenomenon termed *emotional processing*.

Foa and Kozak (1986) proposed that the modification of maladaptive beliefs during exposure therapy is achieved by "activating" the fear structure and providing information that is incompatible with preexisting beliefs. From this perspective, exposure to corrective information should occur in the context of heightened arousal and subjective anxiety (e.g., through confronting feared situations). Information about the innocuous nature of feared stimuli can be presented to patients through psychoeducation, cognitive restructuring, modeling, and other therapeutic techniques. However, the most powerful corrective therapeutic experiences are those involving the repeated and prolonged direct confrontation with feared stimuli in the absence of the feared consequences. Accordingly, the exposure therapist's job is to thoughtfully design and implement exposure tasks in a manner that best corrects the patient's specific maladaptive beliefs.

Conventional wisdom holds that excessive fears are "unlearned" in exposure therapy. However, recent research suggests that older, fearful memories are not *weakened* or *erased*, but instead remain intact and actively compete with the new learning that occurs during exposures (Powers, Smits, Leyro, & Otto, 2007). Exposure therapy thus entails a process of "safety learning" in which patients *relearn* that they are safe in situations where they previously felt afraid. The new safety information acquired in exposure therapy competes with memories of previous experiences, with the winner determining the amount of anxiety experienced in a given situation.

Fear learning tends to readily generalize to multiple contexts. For example, a woman who was raped by an ex-boyfriend at a party subsequently feared being assaulted by men in general in a variety of situations. In contrast, safety learning is relatively context-dependent (a phenomenon that has obvious survival value). As a result, it took a month-long series of exposures involving attending parties, walking alone at night, and interacting with men in various contexts for this patient to believe that most men were unlikely to assault her. This context-dependent nature of safety learning has important implications for the practice of exposure therapy. Specifically, the degree of safety learning in every therapeutic exposure task is affected by the specific context, including the presence of the clinician, the therapeutic setting, safety behavior performance and access to safety signals (e.g., cell phone, defibrillator), the experience of a particular level of arousal, and the internal (and psychological) context created by a psychoactive substance or prescription medication. Each of these contexts can contribute to conditional safety learning during exposure (e.g., "I won't go crazy in enclosed spaces *as long as my therapist is there to keep me safe*").

The clinician's task is to engineer exposures that instill a broad sense of unconditional learned safety in their patients (e.g., "I won't go crazy in *any* enclosed spaces no matter what"). Clinicians can maximize the potency of exposure therapy and promote unconditional safety learning by paying close attention to *what is being learned from exposure* (Powers et al., 2007). Specifically, this involves ensuring that the patient conducts exposures in multiple contexts, at times without the therapist, and in the settings in which his or her symptoms tend to naturally occur. In addition, it is important for clinicians to monitor the patient's use of safety behaviors and ensure that they are discontinued.

Nonspecific Factors in Exposure Therapy

An honest discussion of why exposure therapy works needs also to acknowledge the benefits of what are often called *common* or *nonspecific* factors in psychological treatments. Variables such as motivation for change, the expectation of improvement, and a warm therapeutic relationship undoubtedly contribute to the effectiveness of exposure therapy, just as they do for other psychological treatments (Frank, 1989). Exposure probably benefits from a combination of common factors and the specific procedures for confronting fear triggers, and therapists need not feel threatened by the notion that nonspecific factors account for at least part of its potency. We believe that the scientifically grounded approach outlined in this book is uniquely capable of improving patients' lives through the combination of common factors, such as a strong therapeutic alliance and specific exposure techniques.

CONCLUSIONS

This chapter presents an overview of how fears are acquired, how they develop into anxiety disorders, and how exposure therapy works to correct them. A common theme throughout is the importance of maladaptive threat-related beliefs. Exaggerated threat beliefs set the stage for the development and maintenance of clinically significant anxiety symptoms. The information-processing biases and safety behaviors observed among anxious individuals are problematic primarily because they have the effect of maintaining maladaptive beliefs in the absence of evidence to support them. Exposure therapy works by providing experiences that correct these maladaptive beliefs, leading to reduced anxious feelings, thoughts, and more adaptive beliefs that reverse the vicious cycle that maintains irrational fear. In the next chapter we describe the nuts and bolts of assessing the anxiety-maintaining factors described above. Indeed, effective treatment of clinical anxiety begins with a thorough assessment.

4

Treatment Planning I

Functional Assessment

Exposure therapy is not administered by simply following a manual. The clinician first needs to develop an understanding of the patient's problems and then use this knowledge to plan a suitable treatment. This is the first of two chapters that describe and illustrate the information-gathering and treatment-planning strategies for exposure-based therapy for anxiety. In this chapter we cover *functional assessment*, which involves obtaining the information necessary for developing a treatment plan. Then, in Chapter 5, we discuss how to use this information to design a fear hierarchy and engage the patient in exposure therapy. The techniques presented in these two chapters are common to virtually all forms of exposure that the clinician will implement for any type of problem with anxiety or fear. To make these chapters as illustrative as possible, we have included case examples from across the various anxiety-related conditions. Forms and handouts are also included for use with patients. In Part II, we devote entire chapters to the specialized use of these techniques for different types of specific anxiety problems.

Functional assessment (a.k.a. "functional [behavioral] analysis") refers to the gathering of patient-specific information about the factors that control excessive anxiety or fear. These factors include the situations and stimuli that trigger anxiety (i.e., antecedents), the responses to anxiety (i.e., consequences), and the links between the two. Functional assessment is distinct from *diagnostic assessment* in that the former is theoretically driven and idiographic in its approach to understanding the individual's anxiety symptoms. Diagnostic assessment, on the other hand, is a nomothetic approach based more or less on atheoretical diagnostic criteria (usually the DSM). Although diagnostic assessment and classification have some important uses, the functional relations among the specific situations, stimuli, cognitions, and responses—over and above a diagnosis—are most critical when planning and implementing effective exposure therapy.

As readers familiar with anxiety disorders will recognize, the particular fears that patients have, and their maladaptive strategies for dealing with anxiety, are highly heterogeneous even within the various diagnostic categories. For example, whereas one person with a diagnosis of social phobia might be afraid of speaking to members of the *opposite* sex because of the fear of romantic rejection, another with the same diagnosis might be afraid of speaking to members of the *same* sex who are authority figures. Because exposure therapy targets the patient's specific fears, it is not enough to know that the individual has a diagnosis of "social phobia." Developing an effective exposure treatment plan requires the therapist to be cognizant of the particular situations and stimuli that trigger social fears, the feared consequences of facing these triggers, and the specific maladaptive strategies the individual uses to manage these fears. Functional assessment, relative to diagnostic assessment, provides a much more comprehensive and fine-grained analysis of these key clinical variables.

In the remainder of this chapter we delve into the details of conducting a functional assessment. The composition of this type of assessment for fear and anxiety problems is summarized in Table 4.1.

THE PROBLEM LIST

If they are not already apparent, the clinician might wish to begin assessment and treatment planning by assembling a list of the patient's major problems. To keep the list within manageable limits, up to 10 problems are included on the list, beginning with the chief problem. The following is the problem list for a 35-year-old married woman with the diagnosis of OCD:

1. Recurrent, intrusive thoughts of accidentally hitting pedestrians with my car.
2. Fear of actually hitting someone with my car.
3. Repeated checking of rearview mirrors, retracing driving routes, checking under the car, and seeking reassurance from others that I have not harmed anyone.
4. Avoidance of driving on certain roads and avoidance of driving at night.
5. Repeated doubts about having harmed my children by accident.
6. Fear and avoidance of knives and anything sharp that could be used to stab someone.

TABLE 4.1. Components of Functional Assessment of Anxiety

The problem list

Introduction of functional assessment

Background and medical history

Historical course of the problem and significant events or circumstances

    Personal and family history of anxiety

    Other events (e.g., media reports, illness outbreaks) that stand out as possible triggers of the current problem

Fear cues

    External situations and stimuli

    Internal cues: bodily signs and sensations

    Intrusive thoughts, ideas, doubts, images, and memories

Feared consequences of exposure to fear cues

    Overestimates of the likelihood and severity of danger

    Intolerance for uncertainty

    Beliefs about experiencing anxiety

Safety-seeking behaviors

    Passive avoidance

    Checking and reassurance seeking

    Compulsive rituals and covert, mini- (or mental) rituals

    Safety signals

    Beliefs about the power of safety behaviors to prevent feared consequences

Self-monitoring

7. Compulsions to ask my husband for assurance that I've never harmed the children.
8. Persistent depressed mood (without suicidal urges, plans, or intent).

The therapist need not attempt to remedy all the problems on the problem list using exposure therapy. As we have discussed, exposure is a set of procedures designed to help patients reduce excessive and inappropriate fear and anxiety. Thus, the therapist's first task is to decide which problems might best be conceptualized as such. This process involves formulating hypotheses about the nature of the problems in the problem list (e.g., that the rearview mirror checking is a response to the recurrent thoughts of hitting pedestrians) and then asking specific questions to further understand the nature of the patient's problem as described next.

INTRODUCING FUNCTIONAL ASSESSMENT TO THE PATIENT

Functional assessment of anxiety symptoms involves carefully identifying the idiosyncratic (patient-specific), circumstantial, cognitive, and behavioral features of the patient's presenting problem. The links between these features are then interpreted within the cognitive-behavioral theoretical framework as presented in Chapter 3. It is this patient-specific information that will guide the exposure therapy process. The clinician can expect to spend from 1 to 6 hours conducting the functional assessment depending on the complexity of the anxiety problem. This may mean setting aside multiple "information-gathering" sessions at the start of treatment. Not only are these sessions valuable because they provide critical information to the therapist, but they also serve to strengthen the therapeutic relationship and further reinforce the patient's understanding of the conceptual model and philosophy of treatment. Functional assessment, however, remains an ongoing process throughout therapy. The clinician should continuously be collecting information and incorporating this data into a conceptualization and treatment plan.

The process of functional assessment can be viewed as an exchange of information between the patient and the therapist: the patient provides information about his or her own problems with anxiety and the clinician draws on his or her expertise to fit these symptoms into the cognitive-behavioral framework. To this end, the therapist must ascertain the specific nuances of the patient's fears while the patient must learn how to understand these symptoms from a new perspective so that he or she can get the most out of treatment. We recommend informing the patient up front that the first few treatment sessions will be used to get to know one another and to develop a plan for therapy. Providing the patient with a clear expectation of what will occur during the initial sessions helps to reduce anticipatory anxiety. The following is a sample introduction to functional analysis for a patient with fears of embarrassment in social situations:

> "We have a lot to do today. In particular, we need to figure out how we can work together to help you reduce the problems you are having with social anxiety and the fear of being judged negatively. During our first few meetings together, we're going to spend time getting to know one another and exchanging important information. The way I like to think about this process is that we each bring our own expertise to the table: *I know a great deal about how to help people overcome their social anxi-*

ety. However, everyone with this problem is a little different and has his or her own specific issues that need to be addressed. So, I need to have a good understanding of *your* particular difficulties. That's where *your* expertise comes in. You're the expert on your own problems with social anxiety. You know best how it affects you and how you react to your feelings of fear. So, we need to put our heads together and use our combined expertise to figure out how best to help you."

To gain additional information about the patient's experience with anxiety symptoms, the clinician can ask for a description of a typical day in the patient's life. "Play-by-play" descriptions of a few recent episodes of anxiety are also helpful and can be used to focus the assessment on a particular symptom the clinician is having difficulty understanding. The clinician should listen carefully and begin to consider how the patient's symptoms can be conceptualized within the cognitive-behavioral framework as discussed in Chapter 3.

"For starters, could you walk me through a recent time when you experienced anxiety in a social situation? I'll probably stop you here and there to ask you some questions to make sure that I understand what you were thinking, feeling, and doing at various points. It's important that I understand every aspect of your problem. So, try to answer my questions in as much detail as you can. Sometimes you might think that certain details are not really important, possibly because some of these problems have become almost automatic for you. However, knowing this information will help me understand your difficulties better and that's what will allow me to help you. Okay?"

The clinician should help the patient go through one or more recent episodes of fear including his or her emotional, cognitive, and behavioral responses. Questions that can help elicit the necessary information include:

- "What was happening when the episode began?"
- "Was there a specific trigger? If so, what was it?"
- "How long did the anxiety last?"
- "What thoughts were going through your mind?"
- "What did you do?"
- "Did you attempt to reduce anxiety or escape from the feared situation?"
- "If used, what effect did these actions have on your anxiety? What happened next?"
- "How did the situation finally resolve itself and how did you feel afterward?"

The clinician can also use this dialogue to develop a common language and model for discussing and understanding the anxiety problem. This process begins with the therapist pointing out the relationships between thoughts and emotions, as well as the relationships between safety behaviors and anxiety reduction. For example:

> "We can think of social anxiety as involving a set of patterns of thinking, feeling, and acting, which are distressing, disabling, and difficult to get rid of by yourself. Specifically, the thinking patterns involve assuming that things will go badly in social situations. For example, if you assume that other people will find you boring, then naturally you will feel very anxious when you're around other people. Nobody likes being in situations that make them feel very anxious, so people with social anxiety try to avoid social interactions. They may also use strategies that minimize anxiety or embarrassment when a social interaction can't be avoided, such as using alcohol to take the edge off. These kinds of actions are called 'safety behaviors' because they make you feel safer. But safety behaviors don't work very well—although you might feel a little more relaxed for the moment, the next time you have to interact with other people, you're back to feeling anxious again.
>
> "Do you see how these patterns play out in your own problem with social anxiety? It sounds like when you started saying to yourself that other people at the holiday party wouldn't be interested in talking to you, that's what triggered your anxiety and made you decide not to go to the event after all. And by not going, you didn't get to find out whether or not your anxious predictions were correct. As a result, you continue to believe that going to parties would be an awful experience."

The information obtained through the patient's description of recent episodes provides the clinician with clues about the triggers that provoke anxiety, the thought processes that maintain it, and how the person tries to manage the associated distress using safety-seeking behaviors. The clinician should be prepared to ask detailed and sometimes uncomfortable personal questions to ensure that he or she obtains a full understanding of the symptoms. For instance, assessment may involve discussing sexual functioning, vulgar or horrific thoughts, and other very distressing situations to thoroughly understand the patient's fears, cognitions, and behavioral responses (e.g., "I go to the bathroom 10 times a day because I'm afraid I will pass gas in public"). Even aspects of the patient's life that seem relatively benign, such as hygiene, health maintenance behavior, diet, and sleep should be explored in depth to assess possible safety behaviors (e.g., excessively cleaning one's anus before social interactions). In the chapters of Part II, we discuss specific types of situations, triggers, cognitive factors, and behaviors to inquire about depending on the presentation of the anxiety problem.

MEDICAL EVALUATION

A medical evaluation from a qualified physician is generally recommended before beginning psychological treatment for anxiety since several medical conditions that can mimic anxiety should be ruled out. These include thyroid conditions, caffeine or amphetamine intoxication, drug withdrawal, or problems with the adrenal glands (e.g., pheochromocytoma, a tumor on the adrenal gland). Furthermore, some medical conditions can exacerbate anxiety problems, although anxiety and fear are likely to continue even if these conditions are successfully treated. Asthma, mitral valve prolapse (MVP), allergies, hyperhidrosis, and hypoglycemia (among others) fall into this category. These conditions can especially exacerbate panic and health anxiety since they produce physical sensations often feared by individuals with these problems. For example, MVP can produce heart murmurs, asthma can produce shortness of breath, hyperhidrosis can produce sweating, and hypoglycemia can produce dizziness and weak feelings. Finally, some medical conditions affect decisions about what exposures are appropriate. For example, interoceptive exposure to stimuli that might trigger seizures (e.g., flashing lights) is not appropriate for patients with epilepsy, and hyperventilation might not be used for those with severe asthma; exposures likely to provoke very intense anxiety responses would be avoided for patients who have cardiac diseases or are in advanced stages of pregnancy; and allergies might impinge on the use of situational exposure (e.g., to foods that might provoke allergic reactions).

HISTORICAL COURSE OF THE PROBLEM

The clinician should also assess the patient's history with the anxiety problem, including a family history of anxiety and related problems. When was the first episode and in what context did it occur? Were there any stressful events during the onset or first episode? What has the course of the problem been like? Although not essential to the use of exposure therapy, it can enhance therapist–patient rapport to briefly explore historical factors such as parental rearing practices and developmentally significant critical incidents that may impact the formation of dysfunctional attitudes and beliefs. The recollection of such information, of course, is likely to be affected by recall as well as by confirmation biases and should not be relied upon to draw firm conclusions about the causes of the current problems. Nevertheless, familiarity with the patient's understanding of the origin of his or her anxiety symptoms may provide insight into the beliefs that need to be challenged through exposure exercises. A general strategy for asking about these experiences is to use the following types of questions:

- "Why do you think you developed this problem?"
- "When was it that you first became anxious or fearful about _____?"
- "What was happening in your life at that time?"
- "Describe your physical health as you were growing up."
- "How did your parents [or caregivers] act when they became anxious?"
- "What has occurred in your life that could have influenced the way you think about ____?"

Very negative or painful experiences that occur in association with certain situations and stimuli can lead to connections between these stimuli and anxiety, fear, or other types of distress. In an obvious example, surviving a physical or sexual assault can lead to feeling afraid of the circumstances under which the assault took place. Patients can be asked if they can identify a very painful or frightening event to which they attribute the development of their fear. It can also be helpful to inquire whether patients can identify situations in which they witnessed a relative, close friend, or other important person become extremely fearful or severely injured.

Finally, it can be useful to ask patients whether their problems with anxiety were preceded by hearing particularly scary information or after receiving warnings about danger from authority figures (e.g., parents, teachers). One of the authors recently evaluated a woman with obsessive–compulsive fears of poisoning others by mistake whose symptoms escalated to clinical severity after hearing an actual news story in which a well-known restaurant cook mistakenly seasoned peoples' food with rust preventer instead of salt.

Anxious individuals *learn* to think and behave in maladaptive ways; thus the past may set the stage for the present difficulties they experience. However, because exposure therapy is aimed at reversing factors that *maintain* anxiety, rather than the *causes* of anxiety, one need not spend inordinate time or energy trying to identify the precise historical influences. Moreover, a patient's causal attributions may simply reflect an "effort after meaning," and may have little bearing on the true causes of his or her anxiety. It is also important not to place blame on particular people or situations since the extent to which such factors have actually played a role in the etiology of the anxiety problem cannot be determined for certain. That is, anxiety problems most likely arise as a consequence of numerous factors.

GATHERING INFORMATION
ON CURRENT SYMPTOMS

Generally, the clinician should aim to maximize the amount of information provided by the patient as long as it is relevant to the presenting problem. Providing a clear explanation of this task can be useful; the following example illustrates how we typically introduce the process:

> "I need to understand, as thoroughly as possible, what your experience of panic attacks and agoraphobia is like. The more you can teach me about what you struggle with, the better we'll be able to develop an effective treatment plan. Basically, I'd like to make a list of the situations you avoid, the physical symptoms you experience when you have a panic attack, and the precautions you take to try to prevent panic attacks. Why don't we begin by having you tell me about the situations you avoid because of your fear of having a panic attack?"

We have developed the form in Figure 4.1 for recording information obtained during the functional assessment. It is not essential to follow any specific order when collecting this information; clinicians often find themselves working back and forth across the various elements of the assessment. What matters most is that the therapist thoroughly understands the following:

- What are the situations in which fear and anxiety arise?
- What are the specific stimuli that trigger anxiety?
- What are the feared consequences of exposure to anxiety triggers?
- What situations are avoided because something frightening might occur if they were encountered?
- What safety behaviors are used to control anxiety or prevent feared consequences?
- What is the feared consequence of not performing a safety behavior?
- How do the safety behaviors prevent feared outcomes from occurring?

FEAR CUES: WHAT TRIGGERS ANXIETY?

Information about the context in which the patient's anxiety and fear occurs—the specific situations and stimuli that trigger anxiety—is crucial in developing an exposure treatment plan because it enables the therapist to design an exposure hierarchy that is tailored to the patient's particular fears.

FIGURE 4.1. Form for conducting a functional assessment of anxiety and fear.

Patient's name: _____

Age: _____

Duration of symptoms: _____

Educational level: _____

Occupation: _____

Relationship status: _____

Current living arrangement: _____

I. FEAR CUES

A. External/environmental situations and stimuli

B. Internal triggers: bodily signs, sensations

C. Intrusive thoughts, ideas, doubts, images, and memories

II. FEARED CONSEQUENCES OF EXPOSURE TO FEAR CUES

III. SAFETY-SEEKING BEHAVIORS

A. Passive avoidance

B. Checking and reassurance seeking

C. Compulsive rituals

D. Brief/covert (or mental) rituals

E. Safety signals

Triggers generally fall into three domains—external situations and stimuli, internal body sensations, and thoughts—as we describe next. It should be noted that many individuals with anxiety problems have triggers belonging to multiple domains.

External Triggers

Frequently, anxiety and fear are triggered by specific situations, objects, or other stimuli in the person's environment. The individual may try to avoid these triggers whenever possible. Sometimes, fears of specific stimuli generalize to related items, thereby increasing the number of situations and objects capable of provoking anxiety. For example, a fear of one particular dog might evolve into a fear of all dogs. As a result, the individual's life becomes more and more restricted. We find that some patients understand the relationship between their feared triggers and their avoidance or safety behaviors, whereas others need help to understand this association. The most straightforward way to identify situational anxiety cues is to ask directly using questions such as:

- "What specific things are you afraid of? What situations do you avoid?"
- "In what situations do you start to feel anxious or afraid? What are your triggers?"
- "In what situations do you have to use safety behaviors, such as _____?"

Internal Triggers: Bodily Signs and Sensations

For many anxious individuals, fear is triggered by internal stimuli such as bodily sensations (e.g., sudden stomach pain, feelings of fatigue) and physiological changes related to the stress and anxiety response (e.g., dizziness, increased heart rate). Changes in skin, hair, and the color, odor, or form of products that are expelled from the body may also trigger anxiety. These feared stimuli may be medically explained or unexplained, but are frequently misunderstood by the patient and often misinterpreted as very serious.

Questions to elicit information about feared bodily stimuli include:

- "What bodily symptoms are you concerned with?"
- "What happens to your body that makes you feel afraid?"
- "What kinds of symptoms set off concerns about your health?"

To ensure a comprehensive list of feared bodily stimuli, Warwick (1995) recommends asking the patient to record the incidence of each feared internal sensation, its severity, and the situation in which it occurred for 1 week. Some patients are easily able to describe their fear-evoking internal triggers. Patients with health anxiety, for example, can often point to specific body signs (e.g., lumps) and symptoms (e.g., numbness) as evidence of a dreaded disease. In contrast, it is not unusual for individuals with panic disorder to describe experiencing anxiety and panic in situations where no clear trigger was present. Indeed, unlike most external cues, internal cues can be difficult to discern. The person who has an unexpected panic attack while sitting on the sofa at home, for example, may report the absence of any observable panic trigger. However, careful assessment may reveal the presence of internal cues such as a racing heart and a hot flash that occurred shortly before the attack started. As we describe in later chapters, with education and careful self-monitoring, patients can often learn to identify even subtle internal fear-evoking triggers.

Intrusive Thoughts, Ideas, Doubts, Images, and Memories

Fear and anxiety may also be triggered by mental events, that is, certain types of thoughts, ideas, images, impulses, doubts, and memories that the person experiences as unwanted, unacceptable, repugnant, embarrassing, upsetting, harmful, threatening, or disgusting. Contemporary conceptual models of anxiety regard these "intrusive thoughts" (which are often triggered by situational cues) as normal and harmless cognitive events (i.e., "mental driftwood"). Some anxious individuals conceal or try to suppress their fear-provoking thoughts, believing that thinking them would increase the probability of a corresponding negative event. As an example, one woman with sexual obsessions refused to describe to her therapist her unwanted impulses to kiss her female lab partner during class because she thought that saying this idea aloud would lead her to act on it. Other individuals conceal their thoughts because they are ashamed or embarrassed by their content. For example, a man with posttraumatic stress avoided discussing his memory of being attacked because he felt ashamed that he had been overpowered by his attacker.

Describing these noxious thoughts may be a great challenge for the patient. Therapists must remember to rely on active listening, showing empathy, and normalizing the patient's feelings to encourage him or her to share the necessary information. The therapist may find it helpful to offer educated guesses about the patient's particular fears so that the patient can confirm or deny their presence rather than having to explain the embarrassing or upsetting thoughts. Patients are often comforted when they learn that the content and frequency of their unwanted thoughts and memories is not shocking to the therapist. For example:

THERAPIST: It sounds like you're having trouble telling me about your upsetting intrusive thoughts. Based on what we've talked about, can I guess that you have sexual thoughts that you're very ashamed of and don't want to talk about?

PATIENT: Yes, that's right.

THERAPIST: Okay, thanks for saying so. I know it's hard to talk about those kinds of thoughts. One of the things I want to teach you is that most everyone has strange thoughts just like yours at times. You probably don't realize it because people don't just walk around talking about their own sexual thoughts, but it's true. Maybe as we work together and you start to feel more comfortable with me, you'll be able to tell me a little more about your unwanted thoughts. But I want you to know that as strange or dirty as you think your thoughts might be, they're just thoughts and they're completely normal.

Questions to help the clinician gain an understanding of the nature and intensity of mental fear cues are as follows:

- "What upsetting thoughts or memories do you have that trigger anxiety?"
- "What thoughts do you try to avoid, resist, or dismiss?"
- "What is it that triggers these thoughts (or memories)?"
- "Tell me about the form of these thoughts (memories). Are they images? Are they impulses to do something terrible?"
- "What about these thoughts (memories) is scary for you?"
- "What makes you feel that it is bad to think them?"
- "Do the thoughts appear in nightmares or only when you're awake?"
- "What else can you tell me about the thoughts?"

FEARED CONSEQUENCES
OF EXPOSURE TO ANXIETY CUES

The cues associated with anxiety are one of the main sources of information for developing an exposure therapy program. Another comes from assessing beliefs associated with these cues. As we have described in Chapter 3, the cognitive-behavioral model of anxiety distinguishes between feared stimuli and the meaning that patients give to these stimuli. The model further proposes that anxiety and fear arise from dysfunctional beliefs, interpretations, and assumptions about situations and stimuli that objectively pose little risk of harm (such as overestimates of the likelihood or severity of a disaster). Because modifying these mistaken perceptions is a key aim of exposure therapy, the clinician must be aware of these thinking patterns so that he or she can design strategies to address them. The chapters in Part II address the feared consequences that are characteristic of different types of fears.

At the most basic level, assessing cognitions begins with determining what the patient is afraid will happen if he or she confronts a fear cue or doesn't perform avoidance or safety behaviors. Most individuals with anxiety problems can describe fairly specific disastrous consequences that they believe might occur under such circumstances. For example, a man with claustrophobia may be afraid that if he were in a closet or other small room, he would have a panic attack and die of suffocation. A woman with PTSD symptoms might believe she is extremely vulnerable and that she'd be attacked again if she were to go out at night. A man with panic attacks and agoraphobia might be afraid that if he drives, he'll experience a panic attack, lose control of his car, and have an accident. A woman with obsessional thoughts about desecrating her synagogue may fear that she will act on this thought, while another with contamination obsessions may fear that she will become extremely sick.

Individuals with similar fear cues may differ with respect to their feared consequences. Therefore, it is important to identify the specific details of the feared consequences so that an exposure program can be developed to modify the patient's individual beliefs. For example, an exposure for a socially anxious patient who avoids casual interactions for fear of people noticing that he is very anxious will be different from an exposure for someone whose avoidance of casual interactions is based on the fear that she won't be able to think of anything to say. Similarly, someone with obsessional fears of contamination from urine because of the possibility of becoming ill will practice different exposures than someone with this type of obsession who is worried about spreading "urine germs" to the rest of his family.

Examples of questions that can help the clinician assess feared consequences include:

- *"What is so frightening for you* about using public bathrooms?"
- *"What do you tell yourself* if you experience those scary bodily sensations?"
- *"What makes it so bad* for you to go to someone's home where there is a dog?"
- *"What are you concerned might happen* if you volunteer an answer in class?"
- *"What is the worst-case scenario* that could happen in this situation?"

It is important to assess all of the patient's specific fears and to continue questioning until each feared consequence is well understood. We have observed novice therapists make the mistake of ending their questioning at a general level (e.g., "I am afraid of going to parties") before reaching the "ultimate" underlying feared consequence (e.g., "I will have nothing to say and people will think that I am strange"). The *downward-arrow technique* described by Burns (1980) can be used to determine the fundamental feared consequence, in other words, the absolute *worst* thing that could happen as a result of confrontation with a fear cue. This technique involves repeatedly asking (in a genuine way) questions such as "If that were to happen, what would that mean to you?" or "If that were true, what would be so bad for you about that?" The dialogue below demonstrates the use of the downward-arrow technique with a patient with social anxiety. Note the sequence of questions used by the therapist to get to the "bottom-line" feared consequence.

> THERAPIST: You mentioned that you were afraid of speaking to your department chair. Can you tell me what makes that frightening for you?
>
> PATIENT: I'm afraid that I'll babble and forget what I'm going to say.
>
> THERAPIST: Okay; and if that actually happened, what would be the worst thing about it?
>
> PATIENT: She'll think I'm not very smart.
>
> THERAPIST: I see. And let's say she really *did* think that. What would that be like for you?
>
> PATIENT: Well, then she wouldn't take me seriously.
>
> THERAPIST: Okay; and what would that mean for you?
>
> PATIENT: It means I'll never get a promotion and that she'll go around telling all of the other department chairs that I'm a stupid idiot. I'll probably get fired.
>
> THERAPIST: How much do you believe that's true?
>
> PATIENT: I see what you're getting at. It seems a little unreasonable, like I'm overreacting. But when I'm anxious that's what goes through my mind.

When preparing for exposure therapy the downward-arrow technique is used to understand the patient's fundamental feared consequences so that they can be tested through exposures. This is often straightforward, as in the example above. Sometimes, however, the feared consequences involve disasters that won't occur for a long time in the future. For example, one woman with religious obsessions and compulsions had the fear that she would go to hell when she died. How could this fear possibly be tested through exposure? As we discuss in detail in Chapter 10, when fears of long-term consequences are present, the clinician should consider that the patient's current anxiety is triggered by an intolerance of *uncertainty*—that is, the aspect of "not knowing for sure" whether the feared disaster will materialize. Another tricky situation arises when the patient cannot identify a specific feared consequence and reports that he or she will "just be very anxious." This is particularly common in children. The clinician should consider that the feared consequence is nothing more than being overwhelmed with unending anxiety, possibly leading to physical or mental breakdown. Some people with obsessional fears of contamination or with specific phobias (e.g., insect phobias) describe overwhelming feelings of *disgust* rather than fear. Fortunately, fears of unending anxiety or disgust, as well as intolerance of uncertainty, can be addressed in exposure therapy, as we will explore in Part II.

SAFETY-SEEKING BEHAVIORS

During the functional assessment, the therapist also must compile a comprehensive list of active and passive strategies the patient uses to try to control or reduce anxiety and bring about a feeling of safety, protection, or security (i.e., safety behaviors). Safety behaviors often represent long-standing habits. It is important to understand the role they play in the maintenance of inappropriate fear and anxiety, as discussed in Chapter 3. These behaviors will be targeted in the response prevention component of treatment. Table 4.2 lists five categories of safety-seeking behaviors.

When assessing safety behaviors it is important to understand not just the form or topography of the action (repeating a behavior 26 times, extensive avoidance, five emergency room visits in 1 week), but the *function* or *purpose* of the behavior—that is, *why* the individual performs such behavior and in what situations it occurs. In other words, what feared consequences does it prevent and how does the patient believe the safety behavior works? To illustrate, a woman with GAD was concerned that her husband, a trucker, would be fatally injured while driving. To prevent this from happening, she would call her husband repeatedly and warn him to be careful. The patient believed that this behavior reduced the probability of her husband getting into an accident by alerting him to potentially unsafe drivers. The therapist used this information to construct exposure exercises in which the patient refrained from calling her husband, which allowed her to learn that such actions were unnecessary to prevent harm.

Whereas some anxious individuals have no trouble reporting their full array of safety behaviors to an interviewer, others have more difficulty doing

**TABLE 4.2. Types of Safety Behaviors Observed in Individuals
with Pathological Fear and Anxiety**

Type of safety behavior	Description and examples
Passive avoidance	The deliberate failure to engage in a low-risk activity associated with a feared cue. Avoidance can be obvious or subtle. • Refusing to go on a hike through the woods for fear of snakes • Not eating in public for fear of embarrassment • Avoiding a cancer unit for fear of coming down with this disease • Holding one's breath while driving past a construction site • Avoiding driving close to pedestrians on the roadside
Checking and reassurance seeking	Subtle or overt behaviors aimed at confirming or verifying what is usually already known about a fear trigger or feared consequence. • Returning home several times to make sure the doors are locked and the lights have been turned off • Searching the Internet for information about signs of a feared medical condition • Repeatedly asking a religious authority whether an innocent behavior is actually a sin (e.g., swallowing "too much" saliva during a religious fast day) • Brief visual inspection of the electrical outlets • Mentally reviewing conversations to be sure one didn't use racial slurs by mistake • Asking parent, confessing
Compulsive rituals	Repetitive behaviors, often performed according to certain self-prescribed rules and aimed at reducing anxiety, "undoing" or removing a perceived danger, or preventing feared consequences. Rituals can be observable behaviors or mental acts. • Compulsive, rule-driven hand washing after using the bathroom • Rehearsing what one is going to say before asking a stranger for directions • Repeating simple behaviors (e.g., going through a doorway) • Repetitive praying until it is perfect • Needing to perfectly visualize a "good" outcome in response to thoughts of a bad outcome
Brief, covert (mini) rituals	Nonritualistic (e.g., brief) attempts to reduce feelings of anxiety, remove or escape from feared stimuli, and prevent feared disasters. These may be behaviors or mental rituals, and under some circumstances may be adaptive.

(*continued*)

TABLE 4.2. (*continued*)

Type of safety behavior	Description and examples
Brief, covert (mini) rituals	Applied in the context of pathological fear, however, these behaviors are unnecessary and they further contribute to the persistence of fear and anxiety. • Repeatedly mentally replacing a "bad" word or image with a "good" one • Trying to *suppress* upsetting thoughts, images, or memories • Attempting to *distract* oneself from the fear trigger • Using relaxation techniques to reduce feelings of anxiety. Sitting down to prevent fainting during a panic attack. Putting one's hands in one's pocket to prevent acting on an unwanted impulse
Safety signals	Stimuli associated with the absence (or reduced likelihood) of feared outcomes. Even if these items are not *used*, their mere *presence* can artificially reduce anxiety and make the individual feel as if he or she is safer than he or she would be if such items were not present. • Cell phone, hospital, "safe" person, medical equipment, benzodiazepine medication, water bottle

so. One reason is that some safety behavior is so subtle (e.g., mental compulsive rituals) or routine (e.g., taking antianxiety medication, asking for assurances) that it is not recognized as part of the problem. To clarify the impetus for such actions, patients should be asked what would happen if they did *not* engage in these behaviors. This aspect of the assessment can be facilitated by introducing the concepts of avoidance and safety seeking as protective responses, as in the dialogue below with a panic attack sufferer.

THERAPIST: People with anxiety, who fear that something bad is going to happen, tend to take action to protect themselves and to get rid of the anxious feelings. We call these kinds of actions "safety behaviors" because they make you feel safer. *Some* steps that we take to feel safe make good sense. Buckling your seat belt when you get into a car, for example, reduces the risk of severe injury if you have an accident. This is an example of a true safety aid. Do you see what I mean?

PATIENT: Sure.

THERAPIST: Good. When people have problems with panic attacks, they use safety behaviors because they feel like something awful—like a heart attack or embarrassment—will happen if they don't protect themselves. For example, if you're about to leave the house and you feel anxious and think to yourself, "What if I get so anxious that I have a breakdown and can't get to the phone to call for help?," a safety behavior might be to avoid going out at all or to only leave home with someone you trust. Can you tell me about the strategies you use to reduce your fear of a panic attack? What are your safety behaviors?

PATIENT: I always search the Internet for information about heart attacks. It makes me feel relieved somehow. I also use my water bottle to make me feel better when I'm driving. If I can take a sip of water, I know I'm still in control.

THERAPIST: Good going—those are perfect examples. I noticed a few others from our discussion, too. One is asking your wife for reassurance that "it's *just* a panic attack" and another is checking your pulse. Do you see how these are all done in response to your fear of having a panic attack?

PATIENT: Yes. I do.

A good question for assessing safety behaviors is, "What (*else*) do you do to try to make yourself feel more comfortable when you anticipate, or actually are confronted with, your fear triggers?" Next, we discuss each of the five categories of safety seeking.

Passive Avoidance

The situations and stimuli that patients avoid are often easy to predict based on their fear cues and feared consequences. For example, fears of death might lead to avoidance of funerals; fears of water might lead to avoidance of swimming pools; social fears might lead to avoiding speaking in front of groups; and so on. Some avoidance strategies are intricate and complicated, or not immediately obvious. They might also involve rules devised by the patient. Hence, rather than assuming what the person avoids, the clinician must carefully assess the specifics. The following questions can help to ascertain the nature of avoidance:

- "What do you avoid because of your fears of _____?"
- "How do you avoid _____?"
- "What situations do you stay away from because of your anxiety?"

Some patients use avoidance strategies only in certain circumstances. To illustrate, one man avoided speaking in work meetings *unless there was no one in the room that he believed was an "expert" on what he was speaking about.* Some patients ask others to engage in avoidance as well, such as in the case of a man with OCD who forbade his wife to shop in a certain "contaminated" food store. These examples underscore the importance of understanding the parameters of avoidance.

Checking and Reassurance Seeking

When a clinically anxious person is unsure whether a threat has been reduced or removed, he or she often engages in repeated checking to try to ensure that all is safe and thus prevent future negative consequences. In this way, checking is a preventative behavior, the intensity and duration of which is determined by the sense of responsibility, perceived probability of harm, and anticipated severity of the harm (Rachman, 2002). Specifically, checking is designed to remove uncertainty and attain a guarantee of safety regarding what usually amounts to obscure or unlikely disasters (e.g., a house fire resulting from a light being left on).

Checking behavior can be overt (e.g., measuring one's pulse, flipping light switches to make sure they're off) or covert (e.g., mentally reviewing a doctor's response to a health-related question). In addition, checking can be carried out by proxy in the form of unnecessary or repeated requests for reassurance (e.g., "Are you sure the pain in my stomach isn't stomach *cancer*?") or by asking others to perform the checking (e.g., requesting that one's partner check that the doors are locked before coming to bed). Reassurance seeking can also include repeatedly asking others to answer the same (or similar) questions over and over; repeated doctor visits for exams and consultations; reviewing information such as medical reports; and searching references such as textbooks or the Internet for the most definitive information (e.g., about a feared disease). Checking might also involve inspection of external or internal parts of one's own body (e.g., looking for signs of skin cancer, inspecting one's own feces). Since it is carried out in an attempt to prevent (often obscure or unlikely) dreaded future events, the checking behavior often has no natural terminus and thus can be prolonged, leading to severe slowness and lateness.

It is important to obtain information about the frequency, duration, and precise method of checking and reassurance seeking, as well as the relationship between checking and anxiety. The following questions are often helpful:

- "Do you check that [a feared consequence] won't happen [or hasn't happened]?
- "Do you ask other people for assurances that something bad won't happen?"

- "Can you tell me exactly what you do when you check _____?" [The patient can even be asked to demonstrate the checking if applicable.]
- "Are other people involved in your checking? If so, whom?"
- "What gives you the feeling that you need to check? How do you know when to stop?"
- "What might happen if you didn't check?"
- "How do you feel after you've checked? What makes you feel that way?"
- "How does checking prevent your feared consequences from occurring?"

Compulsive Rituals

Compulsive rituals are intentional, repetitive, and stereotyped actions that are performed in response to a sense of pressure to act, often according to certain rules (Rachman & Shafran, 1998). Rituals can be overt behaviors, such as hand washing in a certain way or finger tapping to a certain number. They might also be mental acts such as praying repeatedly until it is "perfect" or conjuring up a "good" image to replace an unacceptable or anxiety-provoking one. Patients may feel driven to repeat such rituals over and over with the purpose and expectation of gaining relief from anxiety or preventing feared outcomes. Essentially, rituals are "active avoidance strategies." They serve the same purpose as avoidance and checking.

It is important to distinguish the purposeful compulsive behavior displayed by patients with anxiety problems—such as OCD—from mechanical, robotic, repetitive behavior observed in other disorders, notably neurological problems such as Tourette syndrome and autism. Compulsive rituals are also distinct from the repetitive behaviors that typify impulse control disorders, such as repetitive hair pulling (i.e., trichotillomania), gambling, and stealing (kleptomania). Compulsive rituals that are driven by fear and anxiety are essentially maneuvers to reduce the perceived probability of feared consequences and thereby reduce subjective distress (i.e., they are *negatively* reinforced by the reduction in distress). In contrast, impulsive behaviors are performed because they bring about (at least in part) a pleasurable state (e.g., Grant & Potenza, 2004). In other words, impulsive behavior is *positively* reinforced.

The clinician should obtain information about the precise nature, frequency, and duration of compulsive rituals. When practical, it may be useful to have the patient demonstrate the ritual. Some rituals are embarrassing to describe, such as excessive wiping after using the toilet. In such cases, the therapist should inquire in an understanding yet straightforward way. For example, "Many people with fears of bodily waste take a lot of time using the bathroom because they have to make sure they are entirely clean. Is that a problem for you?"

In addition to the *form* or *topography* of rituals, it is important to know about the specific purpose of the ritual: What are its triggers and why does the person feel the need to perform it? Accordingly, the clinician should assess the relationship between rituals, fear triggers, and feared consequences. Inquiry might include questions such as the following:

- "What makes you want to do this ritual? Why do you feel it is necessary?"
- "What are you afraid will happen if you don't do this ritual?"
- "How do you feel after you have completed the ritual? How well does it work?"
- "When you finish doing the ritual, how do you feel about the risk of [specify the feared consequence]?"

Covert Rituals

Some rituals are very brief and subtle, or they are performed mentally (covertly), which makes them a challenge to accurately recognize. Nevertheless, a patient's continued use of such rituals can attenuate the effects of therapy and make the patient vulnerable to relapse. It therefore is worth spending time assessing and educating the patient about these types of rituals. The following script can be used to introduce the concept of covert rituals for someone with OCD.

"Sometimes people with OCD have very subtle and covert strategies to try to cope with their unwanted obsessional thoughts—for example, trying to kick the thought out of your mind, testing yourself to see if the thought is really true, analyzing the thought to try to figure out what it means, and distracting yourself by getting involved in something else. These strategies might help you deal with the thought in the short term, but usually the obsessional thoughts come back later on. Can you tell me about the subtle strategies you use that seem like the ones I just described?"

Follow-up questions that the clinician might ask to obtain information about subtle or covert rituals include the following:

- "Do you perform any types of brief or subtle mental or observable actions to keep you safe?"

- "Do you spend time trying to analyze unwanted thoughts, or thinking them through?"
- "Do you throw yourself into an activity to try to distract yourself when you become fearful?"
- "Do you do anything else that hasn't been covered? What do you do?"
- "What are you afraid would happen if you didn't do these types of things?"
- "How well do these strategies work for you?"

Safety Signals

Although up until this point we have focused on actions that patients perform, the clinician will also want to pay attention to cues or "signals" in the environment, the mere presence of which the patient associates with feeling safe. Common safety signals include certain places (e.g., being at home), people (e.g., spouse/partner or parent), and objects (e.g., cell phone or Medic Alert bracelet). One need not actively *use* a safety signal for it to play a role in the maintenance of anxiety. For example, some patients with recurrent unexpected panic attacks keep antianxiety (benzodiazepine) medication with them at all times, but don't necessarily use the pills. Such individuals, however, believe they need the medication nearby "just in case" a panic attack occurs (which they believe would result in a serious medical emergency). Because safety signals sometimes operate in such a passive way, patients do not always recognize these cues as part of their problem—especially when the safety cues become routine or can be justified in other ways.

For example, a man with health anxiety carried a bottle of water with him at all times because he believed he might need it if his throat began "closing in." When his therapist explained how the water bottle served as a safety cue, this patient justified his behavior by appealing to the health benefits of drinking water: "Having the water bottle isn't a bad thing. Water is good for you. Everyone should drink 48 ounces per day." Similarly, a woman with health anxiety carried a bright red card in her purse with the names and telephone numbers of 10 relatives to contact in case she suffered a stroke. She justified this by saying that it was a "good idea" since she was getting older (she was only 38 years old with a clean bill of medical health). While containing a kernel of truth, these rationalizations miss the point. These patients were using the safety signals to prevent feared consequences, the likelihood of which was grossly overestimated. Thus, the safety signal prevented the patients from recognizing the senselessness of their fears. Some questions to help identify safety signals are:

- "Are there other things you do to protect yourself from [specify the feared consequence]?"
- "Are there any objects or people that make you feel comfortable or that reduce your anxiety?"
- "Do you carry anything with you to help you feel safe?"
- "What precautions do you take so that you are prepared in case something terrible happens such as [specify the feared consequence]?"

SELF-MONITORING

To complement the functional assessment, we recommend also asking patients to keep a real-time log of their symptoms through self-monitoring. Such ongoing self-assessment often yields information not obtained in the functional assessment. It may also improve overall mood by encouraging a more objective sense of self-awareness to replace negative affect-laden self-statements such as "It happens *all the time*" and "This is the worst it has ever been." Self-monitoring can further be used as an outcome measure that assesses the frequency, intensity, and duration of current symptoms before and after treatment.

For the purposes of exposure therapy, self-monitoring involves recording instances of fear, anxiety, and avoidance or safety-seeking behavior as they occur in real time. It is an important tool since it furnishes the patient and the clinician with precise information about the situational cues, frequency, intensity, and duration of these symptoms. A model self-monitoring form appears in Figure 4.2. Clinicians should provide a rationale for self-monitoring that emphasizes the importance of accurate and timely recording of symptoms. This should include acknowledging that the task may require substantial effort by the patient (indeed, many individuals have difficulty with adherence to self-monitoring). The following is a sample rationale for self-monitoring in the case of a woman with OCD and compulsive checking rituals:

"I realize that using these self-monitoring forms might be demanding. After all, you've probably never tried to keep track of your problems this closely before. It's hard work. But let me give you three reasons why I am asking you to self-monitor your symptoms this week and why doing this hard work will pay off for you in the long run. First, keeping track of your symptoms will give us accurate information about the problems you are having with obsessions and rituals in your daily routine. Since I can't follow you around with a clipboard and take note of every time you do checking rituals, it's up to you to keep track of

FIGURE 4.2. Self-monitoring form.

Date	Time	What provoked the fear or anxiety? (brief description)	Fear level (0–100)	Safety/coping behavior	Time spent

the various triggers and thoughts that evoke these problems, and how much time they take up. Second, self-monitoring helps us assess your improvement. In other words, as we progress in treatment, we'll be able to look back and see changes in how often and how much of the time these rituals occur. Finally, self-monitoring can actually help you reduce your anxiety symptoms right away. I've seen many people who say that just knowing that they have to write it down actually helps them resist doing compulsive rituals. So, I encourage you strongly to do an honest job and I will be looking forward to seeing your completed forms at the beginning of the next session. In fact, the first thing we will do next time will be to review the forms together."

It's important to review the completed forms at the next session to reinforce to the patient the value of self-monitoring. If necessary, the clinician can ask for more in-depth information and clarification about a few representative episodes. It is most critical to obtain specific information about:

- How fear and anxiety is triggered (e.g., "You wrote that you became anxious when you were driving. What was it about driving that worried you?").
- What specific situations are avoided (e.g., "Do you avoid all forms of public transportation, or just trains?").
- Why the patient avoids these stimuli ("What do you think might happen if you tried petting the neighbor's dog?").
- How the patient responds to fear and anxiety ("What else, besides praying and washing your hands, do you do when you think you've had a wet dream?").

Self-monitoring provides an additional source of information that helps the clinician clarify the patient's fear, avoidance, and safety behaviors and the associations among them. These associations should be clear to the therapist; if not, further examples should be reviewed until they are elucidated.

CONCLUSIONS

The functional assessment is a critical aspect of exposure-based therapy for anxiety. Without complete and detailed knowledge of the patient's symptoms and the functional relations among them, it is very difficult to develop an effective exposure treatment plan. Importantly, the collecting of information about these symptoms need not be limited to the planning stage of treatment. The therapist should continue to collect information about the cues, feared consequences, safety behaviors, and the links between these symptoms throughout the course of treatment. This information can be used to update or revise the treatment plan as therapy proceeds. In the chapters in Part II, we discuss aspects of the functional assessment as they apply to specific sorts of fears.

5
Treatment Planning II

Hierarchy Development
and Treatment Engagement

After completing the functional assessment outlined in Chapter 4, you should have sufficient understanding of the patient's fears to formulate a treatment plan. The current chapter details how to devise the fear hierarchy, which serves as the therapeutic road map, using the information collected during the assessment. Before an effective hierarchy can be developed, however, the therapist must get the patient to buy into the conceptual model and treatment approach. Toward this end, engaging the patient in exposure first requires presenting him or her with a clear rationale for understanding his or her problem and for how therapeutic exposure can be beneficial. To illustrate the clinical strategies introduced in this chapter, we present Darnell, who suffered from a disabling fear of heights.

> Darnell was a 33-year-old married man with one infant daughter. While he met DSM criteria for specific phobia, natural environmental type, a detailed functional analysis revealed that he avoided the following situations: going above the ground floor in most buildings, looking out of windows that were high off the ground, climbing open staircases, standing on balconies, and driving to the higher floors of parking garages. Just anticipating having to confront these situations triggered an anxiety response that included a racing heart, feelings of dizziness, and shortness of breath. Darnell sometimes thought that if he got too anxious, he would lose control, faint, or have some sort of medical emergency which he couldn't specify. In addition to extreme avoidance

(e.g., parking garages), Darnell's safety behaviors included holding on to sturdy or fixed items if he was near a window or ledge, and keeping benzodiazepine medication with him at all times "just in case" he began to feel uncomfortable.

Darnell had always been a somewhat anxious person, but his fear of heights became a significant problem when he was 23 and experienced a panic attack while visiting the observation deck of the CN Tower in Toronto, Ontario, Canada. At that time, he described lightheadedness, butterflies in his stomach, and the frightening feeling that he might lose control and jump through the window. Darnell had to leave the building immediately and was rushed to the emergency room. The physicians determined that Darnell was medically healthy and referred him for CBT.

PRESENTING A CONCEPTUAL MODEL OF ANXIETY AND ITS MAINTENANCE

After completing the diagnostic interview and functional assessment, the therapist should begin socializing the patient to a cognitive-behavioral model for understanding the present problems with anxiety. This involves synthesizing the information collected during the assessment and, in a transparent and collaborative way, placing the patient's difficulties within the cognitive-behavioral conceptual framework described in Chapter 3. Doing so helps the patient understand how exposure therapy will ultimately be beneficial, even if it sounds like a challenging therapy in the short term. We find that when therapists report that their patients are having problems maintaining adherence to exposure therapy, it is often the case that they have spent too little time helping the patient understand his or her problem in terms of the conceptual framework.

The first point to convey is that it is well understood how the symptoms of anxiety work, how they become a vicious cycle, and how that cycle can be disrupted and weakened using certain therapeutic techniques. The therapist next describes how certain types of thinking patterns lead to feeling anxious in the context of feared stimuli (external or internal). Then, the therapist explains how these anxious feelings lead to urges to reduce anxiety by using avoidance and safety behaviors. But, whereas these *seem* like useful strategies in the short term, they are counterproductive in the long run.

Darnell's therapist began by asking Darnell about what *he* thought about the nature and origin of his anxiety. After listening to Darnell describe his own hypothesis about how his phobia developed (i.e., Darnell believed it was caused by his parents' divorce), the therapist acknowledged that it is difficult to tell for sure what exactly causes phobias and then presented the cognitive-behavioral conceptual model of the fear of heights as follows:

THERAPIST: As you know, your problems with anxiety fit into the category of a specific phobia of heights. Phobias are defined as excessive anxiety and fear that have become associated with a situation or object that is not actually very threatening or dangerous. For you, Darnell, heights, and even the anticipation of going up to a high place, triggers strong levels of anxiety even though being in such places is realistically pretty safe. As a result of your anxiety, you avoid high places and use certain strategies to reduce your distress or make yourself feel safer if you can't avoid being near a window or balcony. Let's take a few minutes to talk about how we understand phobias, because we know a great deal about them, and how they can be treated. Okay?

DARNELL: Sure.

THERAPIST: Even though we don't know the exact causes of problems like phobias—most likely they are caused by a combination of biological and environmental factors—we do understand how the *symptoms* of phobias work, and why they don't go away on their own.

Extensive research shows that phobias involve a vicious cycle that stems from two maladaptive patterns that are difficult to stop without help. The first pattern involves certain types of automatic thinking that intensifies anxiety. For example, you told me how you are convinced you would have a panic attack and feel dizzy if you went to the top of a tall building, and that when you feel dizzy you think this means you're going to lose control and jump from a high place. Certainly, *anyone* who thinks these things would feel anxious about heights. So it's not surprising that this occurs for you. Do you see how your thinking intensifies your anxiety?

DARNELL: Yes, I do.

THERAPIST: Okay. The second pattern has to do with how you react when you're feeling anxious or anticipating being in a frightening situation. Anxiety is inherently uncomfortable because it's the body's way of motivating you to get out of harm's way. So, when you become very anxious, it's only natural to want to do whatever you can to feel safer and reduce the anxiety right away. So, for you, avoiding high places is one sure way to keep anxiety at bay. However, the problem with avoidance is that you never have a chance to find out whether or not your fear is valid. What if heights aren't really that dangerous? What if the worst thing that happened was that you just got very anxious for a little while, and that you didn't have any medical emergency, loss of control, or nervous breakdown? What if your anxiety eventually calms down if you just give it some time, rather than causing you to lose control or jump? If you're always avoiding, you never have a chance to see for yourself, and so the vicious cycle of your phobia just goes on and on. You continue to be afraid. Do you see what I mean?

DARNELL: Yes. Avoiding only makes things worse. I know that.

THERAPIST: That's right; and there are other things you told me about that have a similar effect. You said that when you start to feel anxious about heights, you look for something sturdy to grab onto— even if it's another person. This might make you feel safer immediately, but it prevents you from finding out what would happen if you didn't grab hold of anything. What if you weren't going to lose control and jump? You'll never know if you always grab hold of something sturdy. The same is true, I'm sorry to say, with your antianxiety medication. If you take these pills whenever you have to go to a high floor in a building, you'll never have the opportunity to find out that maybe you could cope with the anxious feelings better than you thought. Maybe the anxiety goes away on its own. Does that make sense?

DARNELL: Yes. These reactions keep me from finding out that I don't need to be so afraid.

THERAPIST: That's exactly right. Now, the treatment techniques we're going to use are based on this understanding of your phobia— they're called exposure and response prevention. These techniques are designed to weaken the thinking and reacting patterns that contribute to the vicious cycle of your phobia. *Exposure* means gradually, and with my help, practicing confronting situations you've been avoiding. When you confront these situations repeatedly, you'll weaken the maladaptive thinking patterns that provoke so much anxiety for you. In other words, you'll change your mind about how dangerous high places are because you'll see for yourself that they're not as bad as you thought. *Response prevention* means that, again with my help, you'll practice not using maladaptive safety behaviors to reduce your anxiety. This will help you learn that you don't need to go to any great lengths to reduce anxiety or to prevent anything awful from happening. In other words, you'll change the way you react to high places.

Although it is critical to present this kind of explanation at the very beginning of treatment, the clinician will find him- or herself reiterating this information throughout therapy to keep the patient working within the conceptual framework. Note also that the therapist illustrated the points above using specific examples from Darnell's functional assessment. This helps the patient to understand how it applies to his or her specific problems.

PRESENTING THE RATIONALE FOR EXPOSURE

When it is clear that your patient understands the conceptual model of anxiety and its maintenance, you should present the rationale for using exposure-based treatment. Specifically, by gradually facing feared situations and discontinuing safety behaviors, the patient learns that not only do phobic fear and anxiety diminish naturally, but that feared consequences are unlikely to occur. A coherent rationale for exposure therapy is crucial because it helps the patient understand why he or she should seemingly take a large risk by repeatedly facing frightening situations without a safety net. The rationale must therefore spell out the logical links between the patient's problems with anxiety, the treatment procedures, and the anticipated outcome. It should also be individualized according to the patient's idiosyncratic symptoms. To illustrate a prototypical rationale for exposure, we continue with the example of Darnell and his phobia of heights. Within the various chapters of Part II, we provide outlines and examples of analogous rationales for conducting exposure to the various other types of anxiety-provoking stimuli.

It is important to note that the purpose of exposure therapy is *not* to persuade or reassure the patient that he or she is *absolutely* safe or that feared consequences are *out of the question* whatsoever. This approach fails because it is akin to helping the patient seek reassurance, which (as discussed in Chapter 3) maintains inappropriate anxiety. It is also *impossible* to completely reassure most patients about their fear—they are usually adept at identifying even the most minute source of risk or uncertainty, which they amplify and use to rationalize avoidance behaviors. Thus, it is better to explain to the patient that the purpose of exposure is to help him or her learn that any risks associated with feared situations and stimuli are *acceptably low*, and that safety behaviors are therefore unnecessary or redundant. We suggest reiterating throughout therapy that a goal of exposure is for the patient to learn to tolerate acceptable levels of risk and uncertainty. Darnell's therapist introduced these concepts in the following way:

> THERAPIST: To reduce your fear we will help you confront it in a structured and organized way. When you face the situations that provoke your fear of heights, and you remain there instead of avoiding or running away, you'll see that your anxiety gradually subsides on its own. I know this may sound strange, so let's think of another fear that you might be familiar with—like the fear of dogs. Let's

say I'm terrified of dogs and I avoid them because I'm afraid they'll bite. How would you suggest that I get over this fear?

DARNELL: Well, I guess I'd bring you around lots of dogs so you could see that they're not going to bite you.

THERAPIST: Right. That's *exactly* what we'd do. Maybe I'd start by first looking at a dog in a cage, then I might approach and play with a small dog and work my way up to a big one.

DARNELL: I see. I need to go to high places to see that I'll be okay, that I can handle it.

THERAPIST: Exactly. So just like we would gradually expose me to dogs to get over my fear, I'm going to gradually help you practice entering high places that you've been avoiding so that you weaken your fear of heights.

DARNELL: Okay, that makes sense.

Next, the therapist provided a concrete explanation for how exposure works to reduce the fear of heights:

"As I mentioned, the technique of helping people get over their fears by gradually facing them is called exposure therapy. When you gradually confront situations that trigger your fear of heights, with my help, you will see that in time these situations provoke less and less anxiety. Eventually, with lots of practice, you won't need to avoid them. So, for example, I will help you to practice confronting things you told me you've been avoiding, like staircases, parking garages, and tall buildings.

"The basic ideas behind exposure therapy are simple. First, you will learn that your anxiety does not stay at high levels forever or spiral "out of control." In fact, your feelings of anxiety will actually decrease as you repeatedly enter these situations and remain there for an extended period of time. This process is called *habituation*. You can think of habituation as similar to what happens when you get into a swimming pool when the water feels cold. If you stay in the water, it seems to warm up after a few minutes. But the water isn't actually changing temperature—your body is getting used to being in the water. The same thing happens when you confront a situation like a high place. At first, you'll feel anxious, but if you give it some time, you'll start to calm down just by remaining there. In other words, you'll get used to it. You probably have never discovered this habituation on your own since you usually avoid high places. So, you've never given yourself the chance to see that your fear will naturally subside. When we do exposure therapy, you'll have the chance to see this.

"The second thing you'll learn from exposure is that the things you're afraid of are much less likely to happen than you have been thinking. So, you will see that things like losing control, jumping from high places, and getting sick or fainting are not likely to happen despite your thoughts that they *could*. This learning is what reduces the phobia.

At this point it is useful to draw a graph for the patient (or present him or her with a handout) depicting the expected pattern of habituation over the course of several sessions of exposure. On a whiteboard in the office, Darnell's therapist drew and briefly explained the graph in Figure 5.1.

"When it is done correctly, exposure therapy is very helpful for reducing phobias like the fear of heights. But exposure is hard work and you should expect to feel anxious at times, especially when you start going into the feared situations. Fortunately, this anxiety will be temporary. Let me show you on this graph what you can expect when you practice exposure. The first time you enter a feared situation you will probably feel very uncomfortable, and it's at this point that you typically leave the situation and reduce your anxiety immediately. But if you

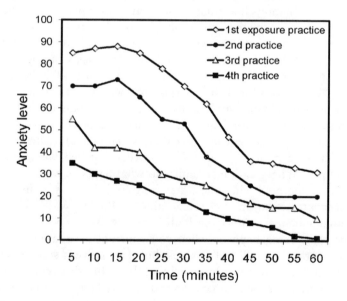

FIGURE 5.1. Pattern of anxiety reduction (habituation) during repeated and prolonged exposure practice.

make yourself stay for more than just a few minutes, you'll see that your anxiety level begins to decline—this is *habituation*. Then, the next time you try exposure, you will initially feel uncomfortable, but your anxiety will subside more quickly because you've learned that habituation occurs. The more you practice staying in the feared situation until anxiety goes down, the less your beginning anxiety level will be, and the quicker it will subside. In other words, you'll be weakening the connection between the situation and fear.

"Of course, all of this only happens if you remain exposed and do not try to reduce your anxiety level artificially by using any avoidance or safety strategies like stepping back or holding on to something to make you feel more secure. You have to force yourself to go *toward* the anxiety and remain long enough for habituation to occur. As I like to tell people, you must invest anxiety now in order to have a calmer future.

"Of course, I will do what I can to make the exposure exercises as easy for you as possible without compromising the effectiveness of the therapy. My job is to help you to succeed, and you'll have a large say in when we conduct each exposure. We'll plan these exercises together ahead of time so that there are no surprises. I will also be there to support and coach you through each exposure practice. Nevertheless, you will still have to tolerate some anxiety, at least initially, as you learn to weaken your fear of heights. Do you have any questions?

The therapist then described the nature of the therapeutic relationship so that Darnell knew exactly what to expect:

THERAPIST: A good way to think of me is as your coach and cheerleader. As your coach, my job is similar to that of a trainer or teacher. Did you ever take lessons to learn how to play a sport or a musical instrument?

DARNELL: Yes, I took drum lessons for a while when I was a kid.

THERAPIST: Great. So, when you were learning how to play the drums, your teacher probably watched your technique and looked for things you were doing well and things that needed to be corrected. He probably gave you pointers for how to improve and had you practice certain exercises over and over to help you learn to read music, keep the beat, and so on. Now, if you didn't listen to these pointers or practice these exercises the way the teacher taught you, you wouldn't have improved your drum playing. Also, your teacher probably never *forced* you to practice the drums. You made up your mind to practice on your own since you wanted to be a good drummer.

The treatment of your fear of heights works in much the same way. As your coach or teacher, I know how to help you get the best possible results. Together, we'll build a list of situations for exposure—a treatment plan. If you follow this program the way that I show you, chances are you will see improvement. But, if you decide not to practice the exercises in the correct way, the chances are you will not improve as much as you would like. I'll never force you to do the exercises—this is your therapy and the decision has to come from you. However, I might try to help you see that your feared situations are not as dangerous as you think, and that it is in your best interests to approach rather than to avoid your feared situations.

I said that you could think of me as both a coach and a cheerleader. In my role as cheerleader I will be behind you every step of the way as you complete this challenging therapy. We are a team and I will give you my support and do whatever I can to help you complete the exercises in a therapeutic way. If you feel very scared, or if you feel like you're having trouble with the exercises, I want you to let me know so I can help you. Also, if I see that you're having a difficult time, I'll step in and help you out. What questions do you have for me?

DEVELOPING EXPOSURE (FEAR) HIERARCHIES

In planning for exposure practices, it is up to the clinician to arrange opportunities in which the patient encounters the cues that provoke the fear of disastrous consequences, but where such consequences do not materialize. Through these experiences the patient gradually learns that the stimuli are not as dangerous as he or she had thought and that anxiety subsides naturally. The exposure treatment plan, or *fear hierarchy*, is a list of rather specific feared stimuli (e.g., situations, objects, thoughts, bodily sensations) that the patient will confront during therapy. Prolonged exposure to each hierarchy item, one at a time, is conducted repeatedly (without safety behaviors) until distress levels reduce to the point that the patient can manage adaptively with the situation. In this section, we discuss the fundamentals of developing fear hierarchies using Darnell's phobia as an illustrative example. The chapters in Part II, however, cover specific issues related to hierarchies when working with particular types of feared stimuli.

As a general rule, fear hierarchy items must match the specific *situational*, *cognitive*, and *physiological* elements of the patient's fear as closely as possible. Darnell, for example, must confront situations in which he (1) is in a high place; (2) experiences physiological arousal—especially feelings of dizziness and shortness of breath; and (3) believes he might lose control, lean over the edge, jump, and fall. If balconies of *tall* buildings trigger these experiences, he must practice exposure to *tall* buildings; low buildings will not be sufficient. If walking up to the edge (railing) and looking down provoke discomfort, this is what he must do—standing back from the edge and keeping his eyes closed, for example, will not be effective. This is because when his feared consequences don't occur (e.g., loss of control, jumping, ever-increasing anxiety), Darnell could attribute this to his avoidance, rather than learning that such events are simply unlikely. The importance of closely matching hierarchy items to the patient's fear can not be overemphasized: a person afraid of dogs must confront the types of dog he or she is frightened of. Someone afraid of germs from hospitals must confront items *in a hospital*. Someone afraid of starting a fire because she has left a light on in her house must turn many lights on and leave the house, and so on. Individual chapters in Part II discuss issues relevant to matching exposure items with the various types of fear cues.

Once chosen, the exposure hierarchy items are ranked according to the level of distress the patient expects to encounter when confronting each item. For Darnell, exposure to relatively low balconies was less anxiety-provoking than exposure to higher ones. Darnell's therapist introduced the concept of the fear hierarchy in the following way:

"Our goal for today is to begin planning for exposure. To start with, we need to make a list of the specific situations and body sensations that trigger anxiety and that you avoid. I'll need your help in making this list because you know best what triggers your fear of heights. Once we have our list I'll ask you to rank each situation according to how uncomfortable you think it will make you. Then I'll help you arrange the situations in order from the least to the most anxiety-provoking. In other words, you'll choose when you confront each situation, although I might make certain recommendations to ensure that we get the best possible results. This list of situations is called a *fear hierarchy* and you can think of working through the hierarchy as climbing up a ladder. During each session you'll take another step up the ladder until you reach the top. I will also ask you to continue practicing exposures between sessions. Treatment will be most effective if we plan to go gradually, yet steadily, up the ladder. Remember that I will help you at each step."

After the general concept of a fear hierarchy has been described, the therapist and the patient together generate items to be confronted. Considerations for developing hierarchies for situational, imaginal, and interocep-

TABLE 5.1. General Considerations for Preparing Exposure Hierarchies

Situational exposure

- Consider exposure "field trips" for confrontation with stimuli outside of the office
- Specificity of hierarchy items should be at the therapist's discretion
- Each hierarchy item should have an identified rationale and target a feared consequence
- Choose items that represent an acceptable level of risk
- Consider using a *graded* approach that begins with moderately distressing items
- Include the *worst* fear in the hierarchy
- Use SUDS ratings to monitor the patient's anxiety

Imaginal exposure

- Use the same guidelines as with situational exposure
- Primary imaginal exposure—exposure to the actual fear-evoking thoughts aided by written or recorded verbal material
- Secondary imaginal exposure—visualizing feared consequences of not performing rituals
- Preliminary exposure—imagining the confrontation with feared stimuli before engaging in actual exposure

Interoceptive exposure

- Less disturbing body sensations should be confronted before highly frightening ones
- Primary interoceptive exposure—feared body sensations are deliberately provoked and maintained repeatedly in the therapy session and for homework until habituation
- Secondary interoceptive exposure—provoking feared sensations by confronting other triggers that are avoided because they trigger feared sensations

tive exposure appear in Table 5.1 and are discussed in the remainder of the chapter.

SITUATIONAL (*IN VIVO*) EXPOSURE HIERARCHIES

Choosing Hierarchy Items

Thoughtful and creative planning are the cornerstones of an effective exposure therapy program. Therefore, developing the situational exposure hierarchy requires careful inquiry. Informed by the information collected during the functional assessment and information-gathering phases (see Chapter 4), the therapist and patient collaboratively generate a list of situations that evoke the anxiety and fear that will be confronted during exposure sessions. Many of these items may not exist within the office, so the therapist should be prepared to make "field trips" into the community (e.g., to a parking garage or high-rise building). The number of items on the hierarchy will necessarily vary based on the range of different stimuli that the patient fears. Situations that are avoided, that evoke safety behaviors, and that cannot be confronted without the use of safety behaviors should be considered for inclusion on the hierarchy. The Exposure Hierarchy Form, which appears in Figure 5.2, provides space for recording hierarchy items. Specific recommendations for generating hierarchies for different types of fears appear in the chapters of Part II.

Specificity

The therapist must make decisions regarding how specific the hierarchy items should be. Although including items that match core elements of the patient's fears is the overall goal, the hierarchy does not necessarily need to contain every possible fear cue or every possible exposure variation. As an example, consider an OCD patient with obsessional fears that while driving he might have injured a pedestrian without realizing it. In this case, "driving" might be a single hierarchy item. Alternatively, this might be broken down into multiple items of varied difficulty: "driving on a deserted street," "driving where pedestrians are walking (e.g., a crowded parking lot)," and "driving where pedestrians are walking *at night*." We suggest building an initial hierarchy with enough detail to advise the patient (and the therapist) of the nature and difficulty of the exposure exercises, but which is general enough to leave open the option to modify the specific task(s) in accord with the patient's particular concerns. This allows greater flexibility in developing exposure tasks of varying degrees of difficulty if needed, some of which might not be conceived until the particular exposure is begun.

To further illustrate, consider a college-age social anxiety patient with fears of speaking to strangers. Whereas some types of strangers pose only moderate difficulty for this individual (e.g., older people, members of the same sex), others are extremely frightening (e.g., people around the same age, members of the opposite sex, authority figures such as police officers). Thus, "strangers" was included as a hierarchy item, which allowed the therapist to help the patient begin with "easier" strangers (e.g., in a nursing home or hospital waiting area) and gradually work up to more difficult ones (e.g., campus fitness center, campus police station) within a few sessions.

FIGURE 5.2. Exposure hierarchy form.

	Description of the exposure task	SUDS	Session
1.			
2.			
3.			
4.			
5.			
6.			
7.			
8.			
9.			
10.			
11.			
12.			
13.			
14.			
15.			
16.			
17.			
18.			
19.			
20.			

Rationale

The patient and therapist must both understand how each exposure task is designed to modify expectancies of danger. This ensures that each exposure is a mutually agreed-upon undertaking rather than something the therapist simply *makes the patient do*. During the treatment planning process, the reasons for selecting each hierarchy item should be made clear to the patient, as in the following example:

THERAPIST: What is it specifically about being up high that is so distressing for you?

DARNELL: Heights just make me feel weird. I start to get all dizzy, short of breath, and my heart pounds. It's like I'm going to lose control and fall or jump from the high place. And I can't look down because that just makes it feel worse.

THERAPIST: So, you either avoid high places or you hold on to something sturdy and try not to look down if you can't avoid them, right?

DARNELL: That's right.

THERAPIST: Okay, then it sounds like a helpful exposure practice for you would be to stand near the edge of a high place—maybe a balcony or the top of a stairwell—and look down.

DARNELL: Oh man ... I don't know if I can do that. I'll get so anxious. I'm afraid I'll lose it up there.

THERAPIST: I understand it's difficult for you to think about doing that right now because you see it as very scary. But remember that one of the goals of exposure is to help you learn that the probability of these bad things happening is much lower than you think. You're also going to learn that your anxiety won't stay forever. But the only way to learn this is by trying it out to see what happens. I guess it means taking a leap of faith to some extent. Do you see what I mean?

DARNELL: Well, that will be a tough one, but I need to get over this problem.

Targeting Feared Consequences

As the previous dialogue illustrates, hierarchy items should be chosen with one or more particular feared consequences or catastrophic misinterpretations in mind. In this case the belief was Darnell's prediction that his anxiety would cause him to lose control and jump or fall. Essentially, he was afraid of heights because he didn't like the way he felt when in such situations.

A good way to think about exposure practices is as experiments in which patients put their faulty beliefs and assumptions to the test.

Pushing the Envelope: Where to Draw the Line?

Although patients clearly overestimate the probability and severity of potential danger associated with their fear cues, this does not preclude the presence of at least *some* element of actual risk. This raises the issue of where to draw the line in exposing patients to "risky" situations. As a general rule of thumb, the clinician should choose exposure tasks that represent no more than "acceptable" or "everyday" levels of risk—in other words, situations that people might find themselves in either purposefully or by accident without any severe consequences. We will provide numerous examples in the chapters of Part II, but to illustrate here, consider an individual whose OCD symptoms involve obsessional fears of "urine germs." The actual risks associated with incidental contact with urine are sufficiently low; most people, in fact, come into contact with urine on a daily basis and it is generally sterile. Thus, the therapeutic benefits of putting a few drops of urine on the skin are justified by the benefit likely to be obtained by learning that urine is not a generally dangerous substance. Conversely, immersing one's hand in a dirty public toilet would be unnecessarily excessive.

If the reader is struggling with the concern that a particular hierarchy item may be too dangerous for exposure therapy, we suggest asking the rhetorical question: "Do regular people ever *inadvertently* confront this item (perhaps without even realizing it)?" As a general rule, if the answer is "yes," then the exposure is probably safe. Consider, for example, that people routinely embarrass themselves, answer a question incorrectly, become highly anxious, ride elevators, think of distressing, obscene, or traumatic subjects, leave appliances running while sleeping or away from home, handle money without washing their hands, encounter the number 13, make contact with garbage cans, step in dog feces, and so on. The difference is that with exposure, these experiences are systematically planned and carefully executed, rather than occurring randomly or by accident. Thus, purposeful confrontation with such situations is very instructive for patients who feel they must go to great lengths to reduce the potential risks associated with such things.

Gradual versus Rapid Exposure

Research has not clearly established whether it is more effective to gradually increase the difficulty of exposures (i.e., progress through the hierarchy from easier to more difficult items) or to move quickly through the hierarchy (or even begin with the most anxiety-provoking item). From a clinical perspective, however, a gradual approach is usually (but not always) more palatable to patients and is most likely to engender his or her engagement in exposure exercises. On the other hand, if progress up the hierarchy is too slow, it may compromise the momentum of therapy and attenuate fear reduction.

We generally recommend a gradual approach that begins with moderately distressing stimuli and progresses to more and more difficult exposures as soon as the patient is ready (as indicated by a demonstrable reduction in reported fear of the previous hierarchy items). There are, however, instances when a more rapid approach is appropriate, and even recommended. Many specific phobias (e.g., fears of balloons), for example, can be treated effectively and efficiently in a single prolonged session of rapid exposure (e.g., Ollendick et al., 2009). A more rapid approach is also called for when the patient's fear is circumscribed enough that all relevant exposures can be accomplished in a single session; when the patient wishes to undergo a more rapid approach; and when gradual exposure is impractical due to geographic or time constraints.

Incorporating the Worst Fear

Although research suggests that the order in which exposure hierarchy items are confronted has little bearing on the efficacy of treatment (Hodgson, Rachman, & Marks, 1972), from a purely practical standpoint most patients are happy to begin with less threatening items and gradually move to more disturbing ones (i.e., graded exposure). However, situations or stimuli that evoke the patient's fundamental (worst) fears *must* be included on the hierarchy and confronted during therapy. Failure to do so can leave the patient believing that some aspects of his or her fear really *are* valid and should be avoided. To explain to patients the importance of confronting highly distressing situations, we often use the metaphor that in therapy "we must bulldoze the anxiety over, or else, like weeds in a garden, the symptoms will grow back." Most individuals understand this and, although they may initially resist, can usually be encouraged to keep an open mind. It may also be useful to point out that success with less frightening exposures often makes the more anxiety-evoking situations less difficult.

Using the Subjective Units of Discomfort Scale

Once an initial list of exposure situations and stimuli has been generated, the patient gives each item a rating using the *Subjective Units of Discomfort Scale* (or "SUDS" for short). This is a scale that ranges from 0 (no anxiety) to 100 (extreme anxiety) and enables the therapist and the patient to communicate about how much distress an exposure item might provoke. The therapist can introduce the concept of SUDS as follows:

"Now that we have a list of potential exposure situations, the next step is to rank them according to how much anxiety they provoke. To do this, we will use SUDS—SUDS stands for Subjective Units of Discomfort Scale. It's an imaginary scale that goes from 0 to 100 and it helps you tell me your level of anxiety or fear. If your SUDS level is 0, then you are not anxious at all—like you're watching a funny movie or relaxing at home. If your SUDS is about 20 or 30, it means you have a mild degree of anxiety or distress. If your SUDS is 50, you are moderately distressed. A rating of 70 to 80 SUDS means a high degree of distress. And 100 SUDS is like experiencing the worst possible anxiety you could think of—like you're tied to the railroad tracks and the train is coming around the bend. Usually when people have a high SUDS rating they're also experiencing physical reactions like a pounding heart, shortness of breath, sweating, or an upset stomach."

Next, the therapist should help the patient calibrate his or her SUDS ratings by giving and asking for examples:

"It can take some practice to get the hang of SUDS ratings since it might seem difficult to quantify your feelings at first. But there's no 'right' or 'wrong.' It's your own personal rating system. So, a 65 for you is different than a 65 for someone else.

"Right now, *my* SUDS is about 15. Overall I feel relaxed, yet I know some of the things we are discussing are probably making *you* feel anxious. Tomorrow, however, I have a dentist appointment. When I think about that, my SUDS goes up to about 30 because I'm a little uneasy about visiting the dentist. How about you? What's your SUDS level right now? What kinds of situations might make it higher (or lower)?"

If necessary, the therapist should help the patient make adjustments in SUDS by pointing out when numerical ratings do not seem to correlate with other variables (e.g., "You don't look as anxious as I would expect you to look with a SUDS of 80. I wonder if you are overestimating your SUDS"). Once the patient is able to provide reliable and valid SUDS ratings, the situations and stimuli on the exposure hierarchy can be ranked. (Figure 5.2 has a column for indicating SUDS ratings for each exposure hierarchy item.) Darnell's therapist initiated this process as follows:

THERAPIST: I'd like you to give each item on the hierarchy a SUDS rating so we can see which ones are more and less distressing for you. Let's start with standing at an open window on the second floor of a building. What would your SUDS be if you were in this situation?

DARNELL: That wouldn't be so bad. I guess my SUDS would be about 25.

THERAPIST: Good. How about going onto a balcony or deck that's only two floors up?

DARNELL: That would be a little worse. Maybe 40.

THERAPIST: How about if you went to a higher balcony, like at a high-rise hotel?

DARNELL: That would be much scarier—like about 75.

IMAGINAL EXPOSURE

As we have described, for many individuals with anxiety problems fear is associated with mental stimuli such as unacceptable intrusive thoughts, doubts, and images (e.g., images that go against one's religion or sexual preference), memories of traumatic experiences (e.g., a violent or sexual assault), and unwanted impulses to act improperly (e.g., to hurt a child or yell curse words). The aim of imaginal exposure is to help patients confront fear-evoking mental stimuli and weaken the associated anxiety through habituation and the correction of catastrophic (mis)interpretations of the presence and significance of such thoughts.

To illustrate, consider the case of Martha, a 45-year-old heterosexual female with OCD who, despite being married for almost 20 years, experienced unwanted and upsetting obsessional doubts that she was a lesbian (she had no history of homosexual behavior). If Martha caught herself admiring another woman (e.g., nice clothes, hairstyle, figure), she began to wonder whether this was actually "sexual attraction." This was highly disturbing to Martha. As a safety behavior, she mentally checked herself to be sure she wasn't experiencing sexual arousal while thinking of other women (and to be sure she still felt aroused when thinking of men). Martha also asked her husband for frequent reassurance that she was heterosexual.

Although situational exposure sometimes implicitly evokes fear-provoking thoughts (e.g., exposure to a certain area evokes thoughts of the traumatic event that occurred there), imaginal exposure gives the therapist a systematic method for exposing the patient to the key fear-evoking elements of his or her feared mental stimuli. In Chapter 10, we discuss the specific methods for conducting this type of exposure, but it usually involves the patient either recounting his or her upsetting thoughts and images, writing and reading scripts containing the distressing material, or making a recording of the anxiety-provoking material that is replayed until habituation occurs. The last two strategies in particular allow for continuous confrontation with an otherwise covert event and, if necessary, manipulation of the content of the stimulus. Moreover, the repetition of fear-evoking material (i.e., via a recording) is incompatible with engaging in safety behaviors (e.g., mental rituals, thought suppression). The use of recorded stimuli also ensures that self-supervised (homework) exposure will incorporate confrontation with the correct stimuli.

Types of Imaginal Exposure

We have previously described three ways of using imaginal exposure (e.g., Abramowitz, 2006), the choice of which depends on the specifics of the patient's symptoms.

Primary Imaginal Exposure

In primary imaginal exposure the individual directly confronts the repugnant, distressing, frightening thoughts, memories, images, or impulses that are associated with fear, avoidance and safety behaviors. Examples include confronting memories of a traumatic event (e.g., a violent assault), distressing images of harming a loved one, and unwanted thoughts contrary to one's sexual preference (as in the case of Martha described above).

Secondary Imaginal Exposure

This type of imaginal exposure is used to augment situational exposure when confrontation with actual situations evokes fears of disastrous consequences that cannot be confronted in real life. In these instances, imaginal exposure is begun during or after situational exposure, and should involve visualizing the feared outcomes or focusing on uncertainty associated with the risk of feared outcomes. For example, following situational exposure to using the stove for a person with OCD-related accident obsessions, imaginal exposure might involve imagining a house fire that destroys everything the person owns. Martha practiced imaginal exposure to "turning into a lesbian" after situational exposure to watching attractive women working out at the health club.

Preliminary Imaginal Exposure

This third form of imaginal exposure entails visualizing confronting a feared stimulus as a preliminary step in preparing for situational exposure. For example, someone with a phobia of birds might vividly *imagine* confronting a bird before actually entering this situation. Someone with a fear of trash cans might initially picture touching such objects before actually touching them.

Therapists can adapt the following introduction to imaginal exposure (for posttraumatic intrusions following a brutal attack) for use with their patients:

> THERAPIST: In addition to practicing situational exposure to things that remind you of the attack, we will also conduct exposure in imagination. The goal of using imaginal exposure is to help you reduce the intense anxiety and distress associated with thoughts and memories of the attack by having you confront them. When you stay with these memories, instead of pushing them away, you will find that the anxiety and fear decreases. It's natural to want to avoid painful experiences such as memories, feelings, and situations that remind you of the attack. However, trying to avoid or push the thoughts away hasn't worked for you since you keep experiencing these thoughts. Actually, it doesn't work for most people. Let me show you what I mean. For the next 10 seconds, I want you to think about anything in the world that you want to, except whatever you do, don't think about a white bear. ... Did it work?
>
> PATIENT: No. I started thinking about white bears as soon as you told me not to.
>
> THERAPIST: Right. That's what people say when I ask them to try what you just did. Can you tell me how that experiment might be relevant to your thoughts about the attack?
>
> PATIENT: It's like you said. I'm trying to push those memories away, and it's just impossible. That's why they keep coming back.
>
> THERAPIST: Exactly. So, we want to try this new strategy of confronting the thoughts and going toward the anxiety and distress, rather then trying to avoid them. Do you have any questions about this?

Imaginal Exposure Hierarchies

Scenes and scenarios for imaginal exposure are chosen from the list of unwanted, intrusive thoughts, ideas, images, and memories, as well as the feared consequences of confronting exposure stimuli, that were obtained during the functional assessment (see Chapter 4). As with planning situational exposure exercises, imaginal exposure must involve confrontation with the precise stimuli that trigger excessive fear and anxiety—the difference, of course, being that the stimuli will be cognitive. For example, someone with anxiety-provoking images of his own funeral must visualize this event in therapy with the same detail that he experiences when the image intrudes in his daily life. A woman with doubts that she might have pushed an innocent bystander into traffic without realizing it must confront such doubts as vividly as possible. The victim of a violent crime who experiences posttraumatic stress symptoms must relive this event in his or her imagination and incorporate each detail.

Primary Imaginal Exposure

Primary imaginal exposure hierarchy items might include articulations of the distressing thought, such as an explicit narrative of an unacceptable sexual encounter, description of a horrible accident, or repetition of an upsetting phrase. The thoughts can be articulated in written form, or verbally using a recording device. The therapist and patient should outline the content of each imaginal item before beginning each exposure so that both are aware of the desired content and expected distress level.

Sometimes, patients' apprehension about confronting their seemingly horrific, immoral, or obscene intrusive thoughts and images can interfere with discussing and planning imaginal exposure hierarchies. If such a problem arises, the therapist can assess how the patient is *interpreting* the frightening thought in such a way that it leads to a desire to conceal the cognition. Next, cognitive therapy techniques (e.g., Wilhelm & Steketee, 2006) can be used to normalize the experience of distressing thoughts, modify mistaken beliefs about their importance or dangerousness, and help the patient overcome the need to conceal them. The therapist should also compassionately reiterate that the purpose of treatment is to work on *confronting*, rather than *avoiding*, feared thoughts, which will necessarily provoke anxiety.

On a related note, patients' upsetting intrusive thoughts can be extremely offensive, unsettling, and graphic. For example, we have worked with obsessional patients with extremely vulgar sexual images (e.g., graphic thoughts of having sex with animals), highly blasphemous and sacrilegious thoughts (e.g., of Jesus masturbating while hanging on the cross), and descriptions of very violent and horrific acts (e.g., sexual assaults involving death threats). It will behoove the clinician to prepare for such extreme thoughts and to regulate his or her response to hearing a patient describe his or her intrusive thoughts. Some patients may be concerned that their intrusive thoughts will "freak out" the therapist. Thus, even a hint of alarm, horror, or disgust on the part of the therapist could reinforce such maladaptive beliefs. An appropriate response to admittedly distressing intrusive thoughts and memories is to acknowledge in a nonjudgmental way that it is easy to see how the patient could be disturbed by the idea, but that nevertheless even highly distressing thoughts are "just thoughts." As a final point, there is no evidence that repeated exposure to patients' descriptions of their horrific thoughts and memories causes either the patient or the therapist to become traumatized, as some authors have espoused (e.g., Stamm, 1999).

Secondary Imaginal Exposure

Secondary imaginal exposures are conducted in combination with situational exposures that trigger the target thought, doubt, image, or idea. The most practical way of presenting the fear-evoking material is by using a scripted narrative of the feared consequences associated with the corresponding situational exposure. This script can be spoken by the patient or the therapist. As an example, consider a patient with obsessional fears of the number 666 who also performs prayer rituals to reduce the associated anxiety and her perceived risk of being possessed by the devil. After exposure to the number 666 (e.g., writing it on a piece of paper and putting it in her pocket), this patient might confront the following thought for imaginal exposure by repeatedly listening to it as recorded using a digital voice recorder:

> "I wrote the number "666" over and over on pieces of paper and put them in my pocket and under my pillow. Now I'm afraid I will be possessed by the devil. I feel like I need to pray to God to save my soul. But this time, I'm not going to do it. I'm going to let the devil come and take my soul. I'm taking a huge risk. I won't know whether my soul really belongs to the devil until after I die. Maybe I'm possessed. Maybe I will burn in hell because I am confronting 666.

Preliminary Imaginal Exposure

We don't recommend including preliminary imaginal exposures on the fear hierarchy since they are best used only if a patient is having difficulty confronting an actual feared stimulus. For example, if a patient with the fear of vomiting is planning to eat a certain feared food, but is having difficulty getting up the courage to do so, he or she might agree to *imagine* doing this exposure as a precursor to the actual exercise. Studies indicate that all things being equal, situational exposure is more potent than imaginal exposure for reducing fears of tangible situations and other external triggers (e.g., Rabavilas, Boulougouris, & Stefanis, 1976). Thus, preliminary imaginal exposure should be undertaken with the patient's understanding that it is a stepping-stone toward the corresponding actual exposure.

INTEROCEPTIVE EXPOSURE

Because the experience of anxiety and fear includes the physical sensations associated with the fight–flight response, it is possible for these sensations themselves (e.g., racing heart, dizziness) to become fear triggers (Barlow, 2002). Moreover, some people catastrophically misinterpret the presence and meaning of unexpected body sensations (e.g., headache = brain tumor). Other patients fear bodily sensations for other reasons, such as those with social anxiety who worry that their physiological symptoms of fear will be noticeable to others. These individuals begin to anticipate feeling frightened and this triggers uncomfortable (yet harmless) bodily sensations, which trigger high levels of anxiety, and so on.

Systematic exposure to body sensations that provoke anxiety, known as "interoceptive exposure," was initially developed by Barlow and colleagues (1989) to help panic patients confront sensations that occur as part of panic attacks. Interoceptive exposure involves intentionally re-creating feared body sensations (e.g., running in place to increase heart rate, hyperventilating to create feelings of dizziness) and allowing the patient's fear to habituate. Through this process the patient learns that (1) the sensations are not dangerous and (2) the sensations (and anxious feelings) do not persist indefinitely or spiral "out of control."

Providing a Rationale

Many anxious patients become focused on *external* fear triggers and are not aware that fear triggers can also be *internal*. We therefore find it useful to spend time discussing this phenomenon before introducing the concept of interoceptive exposure. We, for example, provide a "crash course" on the nature and purpose of the fight–flight response (e.g., Abramowitz & Braddock, 2008; Deacon & Abramowitz, 2006b) to help the patient recognize that the sensations he or she experiences when he or she becomes anxious may be *uncomfortable*, but are not *dangerous*. Then, we discuss the importance of confronting these sensations to foster this learning. As with exposure to situations and thoughts, patients may initially find it counterintuitive to purposely induce the very sensations that trigger their anxiety. This highlights the importance of a clear and convincing rationale for therapy, such as the one Darnell's therapist provided:

> THERAPIST: As you told me before, when you even think about being in a high place, you begin to notice certain feelings and sensations inside your body. You said that your heart speeds up, you feel lightheaded or dizzy, and you feel as if it's hard to catch your

breath. You also said that it you're afraid you will lose control or that something awful is going to happen to you. It's very common for people with a fear of heights to be afraid of how they feel when they're in a high place. Does that make sense?

DARNELL: Yes. I've never thought about it that way.

THERAPIST: Good. So along with helping you get used to being in high places, we also need to help you get used to the uncomfortable body sensations that accompany fear. To weaken this kind of anxiety we will help you confront the body sensations in a planned and careful way. When you repeatedly confront these feelings, you'll learn that you're able to manage them better than you had thought. You will also learn that they are not harmful. You probably won't lose control or have any medical emergencies. In other words, confronting these feelings will help you see that there is no basis for the fear associated with the bodily sensations.

Planning

As with situational and imaginal exposure, a hierarchy-driven approach to interoceptive exposure is recommended in which less-disturbing body sensations are confronted before the most upsetting ones. Planning for interoceptive exposure also requires determining how the feared sensations will be evoked. Procedures for producing many of the commonly feared bodily signs and sensations associated with anxiety are presented in the relevant chapters within Part II.

Interoceptive Exposure Techniques

Primary Interoceptive Exposure

In primary interoceptive exposure the therapist helps the patient deliberately provoke feared bodily sensations in the office using a variety of techniques and maneuvers—for example, rapidly breathing through a straw to produce feelings of breathlessness (further examples are described in Chapter 11). The sensation(s) is maintained or repeated during the session until habituation occurs. During the exposure, the patient is instructed not to engage in any safety behaviors or other activities that would reduce the intensity of the sensation or prevent a feared outcome (e.g., holding on to prevent fainting). Instead the patient is encouraged to make the sensations as intense as possible.

As with situational and imaginal exposures, interoceptive exposures should first be performed in the session with the therapist present. In fact, we encourage clinicians to perform the exposure alongside the patient so that both individuals can compare their physical experiences and so the clinician can model a calm response to the sensations. Subsequently, the patient is instructed to practice the exercise repeatedly either inside or outside the session. Cognitive therapy techniques (e.g., Taylor, 2000) can also be used to identify and modify catastrophic beliefs about the dangerousness of the feared bodily sensations.

Secondary Interoceptive Exposure

Secondary interoceptive exposure involves confronting feared bodily sensations by engaging in activities that have been avoided *because they produce the feared sensations*. The possible situations and stimuli for this type of exposure are therefore highly patient-specific and must be identified via a thorough assessment. Some patients, for example, avoid drinking soda or champagne *because of the fear of feeling bloated*. Others avoid vigorous exercise *because they fear heart palpitations, sweating, feeling flushed, or weak*. Darnell avoided high places because of the feelings he experienced inside his body: lightheadedness, trouble catching his breath, and so on. Further examples include avoidance of eating spicy or high-fiber foods for someone afraid of stomach and lower GI sensations, and jogging outside on a cold morning for a patient afraid of throat pain (i.e., from the cold, dry air).

As others have pointed out (Abramowitz & Braddock, 2008; Taylor & Asmundson, 2004), the distinction between this form of interoceptive exposure and situational exposure is clinically and conceptually important—even if it may not be evident from a practical standpoint. We assert that the difference lies in the *intent* and *emphasis* of the exposure task. Whereas the focus in *interoceptive* exposure is on the intense bodily sensations that are produced, *situational* exposure focuses on confronting feared situations regardless of whether or not strong bodily sensations are produced.

RESPONSE PREVENTION:
ENDING SAFETY BEHAVIORS

Although response prevention is often considered as a treatment technique for OCD (i.e., "exposure and response prevention") in which the patient resists performing compulsive rituals, as we have discussed, rituals are part of a broader class of safety behaviors that are present in one form or another across clinical anxiety problems. As a result, response prevention is an important component of exposure treatment for most types of anxiety and fear. Whether they occur in the form of compulsive rituals, subtle mental maneuvers, reassurance seeking, or safety signals, safety behaviors reinforce pathological anxiety and must be targeted for stoppage during exposure therapy. If patients do not terminate their safety behaviors, then, rather than demonstrating that anxiety subsides on its own and that feared consequences are unlikely, the outcome of exposure tasks will be interpreted as meaning that safety behaviors are necessary to prevent disasters. Recall from our earlier discussion (Chapter 3) that safety behaviors are reinforced (and therefore develop into strong habits) because they sometimes lead to an immediate reduction in distress. Thus, they can be difficult for the patient to stop on his or her own.

Response prevention is a technique in which patients are helped to voluntarily refrain from maladaptive safety-seeking behaviors. The specific strategies used (e.g., rules and guidelines) are highly variable depending on the patient's particular fears and safety behaviors. Guidelines for response prevention should therefore be determined collaboratively and only after a thorough functional assessment has been conducted. Whereas some patients are able to immediately cease all safety behaviors at the start of treatment, others require a gradual approach.

The individual chapters in Part II provide details regarding response prevention for patients displaying specific types of fears. Here, we discuss some general considerations for arranging a response prevention plan. As with exposure, it is important for the clinician to provide a clear rationale for response prevention. The reader can revisit our rationale presented earlier in this chapter that describes the negative effects of safety behaviors and the reasons for stopping them as part of treatment. It is also helpful to emphasize that not performing safety behaviors is a difficult choice—it represents choosing to be anxious in the short run, rather than trying to feel safe immediately. If relatives or friends are involved in the patient's safety behaviors, encourage their help with refraining from such activities. Finally, it can be useful to ask the patient to keep a record of all safety behaviors performed as a measure of success. Figure 5.3 includes a self-monitoring form that patients can use to document safety behaviors and their triggers.

Darnell's therapist enacted a response prevention plan during each exposure practice wherein Darnell was not to hold on to anything sturdy that prevented him from feeling like he might lose control. The therapist also consulted with Darnell's prescribing physician, who agreed that response prevention would also involve refraining from the use of benzodiazepine medication during the treatment period.

CONCLUSIONS

We have seen our fair share of beginning therapists describe anxious patients who stall when it comes time to do exposure, simply refuse to confront their

FIGURE 5.3. Safety behavior monitoring form.

Date	Time	Situation that provoked the safety behavior (brief description)	Description of safety behavior

fears, or worse, drop out of therapy when it comes time to begin exposure. Yet upon close assessment of the therapeutic process, it is often the case that such patients have not been given a clear enough explanation and rationale for the use of exposure therapy. This underscores the importance of carefully planning and obtaining the patient's "buy-in" before proceeding with treatment. Of course, not all patients readily agree to confront their fears; balking and arguing are not uncommon occurrences (see Chapter 6). Yet, by providing a convincing case for the use of exposure, many such problems can be circumvented. When the patient understands why exposure is necessary to reduce pathological or phobic fear, he or she will likely be ready to help plan for exposure and engage in this treatment.

6

Implementing Exposure Therapy

An Overview

In this final chapter of Part I we provide a general overview and guiding principles for the practice of exposure therapy for anxiety. We also describe a number of common obstacles to successful exposure and make recommendations for how to navigate such hurdles. As in Chapter 5, we use Darnell's case to illustrate how exposure procedures are commonly implemented. Readers are reminded that while this chapter represents a general overview, specific information regarding how to plan and implement exposure to particular types of fears are presented in Part II.

OVERVIEW: THE STRUCTURE
OF EXPOSURE SESSIONS

While many adequate exposure sessions can be conducted within the typical 60-minute therapy session, in many instances it is best to allot 90 minutes. This is usually enough time to allow sufficient habituation to occur.[1]

---

[1]Whereas some authors use the terms "habituation" and "extinction" interchangeably, many learning theorists define *habituation* as a reduced response to repeated presentations of an unconditioned stimulus and *extinction* as a reduced response to a conditioned stimulus. In this book, we use the term "habituation" to refer to the process of anxiety reduction *during* exposure sessions and "extinction" as the desired *outcome* of exposure therapy (i.e., a reduction in fear of the conditioned stimulus).

Each therapy visit should begin with a 5- to 10-minute check-in and review of the past session's homework assignment, which includes examination of any self-monitoring forms and exposure practice forms (discussed later in this chapter). Next, the agreed-upon exposure task is introduced. The actual duration of an exposure session is determined by the patient's anxiety level—the exposure is terminated when the patient's anxiety level (i.e., SUDS) has decreased to at least 50–60% of its initial (or peak) level. Ideally, the patient should remain in the feared situation until he or she experiences only a mild sense of subjective distress. About 15 minutes at the end of each session should be allocated for debriefing, assigning homework practice, and discussing the next session's exposure task.

EARLY EXPOSURE SESSIONS

Getting the Patient Ready and Managing Cold Feet

During the first few exposure sessions the therapist should begin with a brief review of the rationale for exposure. We find it helpful to "quiz" the patient (e.g., "How will facing the situations you are afraid of help you with your phobia?"). The handout How to Make Exposure Therapy Work (Figure 6.1) helps to clarify expectations for how exposure sessions should proceed and can be reviewed with patients before getting started.

Therapists should be prepared to offer comfort and encouragement if the patient reports apprehension when beginning the first exposure. Darnell's initial exposure involved going to the second floor of a shopping mall, standing at the railing, and looking down at the first floor. When he expressed trepidation about beginning this task, his therapist explained how the session would proceed.

THERAPIST: You look apprehensive, Darnell. What's going through your mind?

DARNELL: I'm a little scared. I don't know what to expect and I don't like feeling anxious.

THERAPIST: Sure, I understand. Would it help if I told you how I think we should proceed?

DARNELL: Sure.

THERAPIST: First, you will be in the driver's seat. My job is only to help you get the most benefit from the exercise. So, I'd like us to go up to the second floor and walk over to the railing where you can look down at the first floor. Then, we'll just stay there for a while. I'll help you monitor your anxiety level by asking you where you are on the SUDS scale. I'll also be helping you resist any urges to

FIGURE 6.1. Patient handout: How to make exposure therapy work.

1. **Prepare to feel anxious.** It is normal to feel uncomfortable when doing exposure therapy. In fact, if you become anxious it's a sign that you are doing exposure correctly. Your job is to remain in the situation until your anxiety subsides on its own.

2. **Don't fight the anxiety or fear.** If you try to resist or fight the anxiety, you'll only make things worse. Instead, let the anxious feelings just be there. Remember that they're temporary. The worst thing that will happen is *temporary* distress.

3. **Do not use safety behaviors before, during, or after exposure.** In order to work properly, exposure practices must be completed without safety behaviors, reassurance seeking, distraction, medications, alcohol, or other strategies that make you feel safer or that prevent you from becoming anxious. Even very small or brief safety behaviors will spoil exposure.

4. **Test out negative beliefs about the consequences of facing your fear.** Before starting an exposure practice, ask yourself what you're afraid might happen when you confront this situation. Then, like a scientist, test out whether your fearful prediction is true by doing the exposure. Afterward, consider what the experience taught you. What evidence did you gain? Have your thoughts about the situation changed?

5. **Keep track of your SUDS.** During exposure practices monitor how distressed you become using the SUDS scale from 0 (calm) to 100 (extremely anxious). Pay attention to whether your level of fearfulness changes as time goes by.

6. **Stay in the exposure situation until you feel a significant reduction in anxiety.** Remain exposed to the feared situation until your anxiety subsides, no matter how long this takes. If you leave the situation when you are still very anxious, you will only make your fear and anxiety stronger.

7. **Repeat exposures until they no longer make you very anxious.** The more you practice an exposure, the more your anxious feelings will decrease and the easier it will be to feel comfortable with the feared situation.

8. **Practice exposure in different settings.** Confronting your fears in new and different settings helps to solidify your improvement. Practice with your therapist, with family members (if applicable), on your own, and in different places that trigger your fear.

step back away from the edge. At first, I expect that you will feel uncomfortable. But you will see that your distress subsides over time. We'll stop when your anxiety has decreased considerably from the starting level. Then we'll talk about what you learned from doing the exercise and come up with some situations for you to practice on your own before our next session. How does that sound?

DARNELL: It sounds difficult, but I know it's what I have to do if I want to get over this.

Introducing the Exercise

The therapist begins by describing how the feared stimulus will be confronted, for how long, and what kinds of safety behaviors the patient should work on resisting. A brief description of the exercise can be entered on the Exposure Practice Form (Figure 6.2), which is used to keep a record of SUDS levels during the exposure session. Darnell's therapist introduced Darnell's first exposure as follows:

"Let's start gradually so you can ease yourself into it, but my goal is for you to get right up to the railing and look down. We can start back a few paces and gradually approach the railing. Your job will be to practice not holding on or moving backward. I will be asking you to rate your SUDS level every 5 minutes, so have a number between 1 and 100 in mind."

Discussing Feared Consequences and Mistaken Beliefs

Based on the functional analysis, the therapist should be able to anticipate the patient's concerns regarding the feared consequences of exposure to the selected hierarchy item(s). These specific fears should be clarified as much as possible since they will be "put to the test" during the exposure task. Vague consequences are more difficult to disconfirm than more specific ones. Darnell's therapist had the following discussion about Darnell's feared consequences:

THERAPIST: During exposure, we'll be putting your fear to the test. So, before we start, what are you afraid might happen if you approach the railing and look out over the first floor?

DARNELL: What if I get very anxious and lose control? What if I feel like my head is swimming and I faint? What if I go crazy and just jump off the second floor?

FIGURE 6.2. Exposure practice form.

Date: _____

Time: _____

1. Description of the exposure practice:

2. Feared outcome of exposure:

3. Safety behaviors to prevent:

4. Every _____ minutes during the exposure, rate SUDS from 0 to 100:

5. SUDS when beginning exposure (0–100) _____

SUDS	SUDS	SUDS	SUDS	SUDS
1. _____	7. _____	13. _____	19. _____	25. _____
2. _____	8. _____	14. _____	20. _____	26. _____
3. _____	9. _____	15. _____	21. _____	27. _____
4. _____	10. _____	16. _____	22. _____	28. _____
5. _____	11. _____	17. _____	23. _____	29. _____
6. _____	12. _____	18. _____	24. _____	30. _____

6. What was the outcome of the exposure? What was learned?

THERAPIST: Okay. We're going to test out those possibilities when we do the exposure practice, just like a scientist tests a theory or *hypothesis*. It will require you to be brave and take a little bit of a leap of faith, but you can do it. My guess is that things won't be as bad as you think. But I guess you'll have to see for yourself. So, are you ready?

DARNELL: Well, I know it's a silly thing for me to be afraid of. My rational mind tells me I'll be okay. And you said we can go slowly. Yes, I think I'm ready.

Introducing the Feared Stimulus

The therapist obtains a baseline SUDS rating (Darnell's was 65). Then the therapist introduces the patient to the feared situation or trigger. It is a good idea to begin exposures gradually and observe how the patient responds. If he or she eagerly "jumps in," praise his or her initiative and follow his or her lead. If things progress more slowly, some words of encouragement might be needed. If necessary, the therapist can model exposure to the feared stimulus. In doing so, be sure to demonstrate calmness in order to help the patient feel less fearful or self-conscious about engaging in a seemingly fearful or potentially unusual or embarrassing task (e.g., touching the floor, stuttering while conversing with others, thinking about or looking at distressing or vulgar material). Patients' early successes with exposure can set the tone and increase confidence in the treatment, thereby motivating the patient to persist when confronting more distressing stimuli.

Darnell and his therapist took the elevator to the second floor and walked toward an area that overlooks the first floor. It is important for patients to *fully* confront the feared situation without any avoidance or safety behaviors. Patients are also encouraged to focus on the exposure stimulus; thus regularly asking questions such as "How are you feeling now?", "What are you telling yourself?", and "What's your SUDS?" is a good way to maintain this focus and continually assess thoughts and feelings during the exercise.

THERAPIST: I'd like you to walk as close to the edge and railing as you can.

DARNELL: (*Hesitates*) ... Okay. (*Takes a few steps toward the edge.*) There, I'm doing it.

THERAPIST: Great job. ... How are you feeling?

DARNELL: My head is spinning a little. I'm nervous. I don't want to look down or fall.

THERAPIST: Sure. You're doing great. We'll just have to assume the spinning feelings are part of anxiety, right? That would make sense to me, huh? Remember you're feeling anxious because you've avoided situations like this for so long. Now, you're fighting your fear. What's your SUDS level?

DARNELL: About 65.

THERAPIST: Okay; this is great. Do you feel like you need to grab something?

DARNELL: I feel a little unsteady, but I think I can manage to stay up without holding on to the railing.

THERAPIST: You're doing a fantastic job. Keep it up.

Note how the therapist responded to Darnell's report of his head spinning by amplifying his uncertainty about the meaning of these sensations, while modeling a noncatastrophic response with a more realistic interpretation. This maneuver helps patients consolidate new, helpful ways of thinking about feared stimuli and risk taking (i.e., uncertainty). Note also the use of praise for following through with exposure tasks. This is an important rhetorical strategy for encouraging adherence.

Careful Observation and Ongoing Assessment

The clinician should continually be on the lookout for subtle (and not-so-subtle) safety behaviors or other curious maneuvers that most individuals under similar circumstances probably wouldn't do. Patients who appear to "space out" during exposure should be asked whether they are engaging in mental strategies such as praying, distracting, or analyzing. These safety behaviors limit the effectiveness of therapy because they protect the patient from direct exposure to his or her feared stimuli and thereby prevent the natural habituation of anxiety. These behaviors might also have become so habitual that they occur without the patient's awareness. Accordingly, they should be brought to the patient's attention whenever they are observed and strongly discouraged.

The therapist should also continually be attentive to the possibility that additional situations may need to be incorporated into the exposure plan or targeted in homework practices. Patients often make impromptu remarks about characteristics of feared stimuli that they find especially frightening or distressing. These comments usually reflect catastrophic beliefs and need to be addressed. Darnell, for example, mentioned during an exposure session that he would feel especially anxious if he had a full bladder while practicing in this situation. He believed that he was likely to soil himself if he became very anxious. The therapist must be attentive to such comments (and encourage the patient to be open in reporting them) so that exposures can be designed to target the patient's fears as specifically as possible. Accordingly, later in the session, Darnell and the therapist stopped for a large cup of water and then resumed the exposure with Darnell feeling somewhat like he had to use the bathroom.

Using Cognitive Interventions during Exposure

The therapist takes an active role in facilitating cognitive change during exposure. In other words, one does not simply sit and wait passively for habituation to occur. Instead, cognitive therapy interventions (e.g., Beck, Emery, & Greenberg, 1985) should be used to help the patient challenge problematic beliefs about the feared consequences and other risks associated with the current exposure task. This can lead into a discussion about risk taking and embracing acceptable, everyday levels of uncertainty. Therapists should emphasize that the practicalities of taking such low-level risks outweigh the consequences of avoiding or trying to eliminate all risk in order to procure an absolute guarantee of safety (which is not feasible). Informal Socratic questioning and discussions of the evidence for and against mistaken beliefs is one of the most useful cognitive interventions to be deployed in the context of exposure. Toward the end of Darnell's first exposure session, the therapist engaged him in a Socratic discussion about changes in his anxiety level.

THERAPIST: So, let's review what you've done in the last hour. You went up on the second floor of the mall—which you'd been avoiding for a long time—and even went up to the edge and looked over the railing. And you did all of this without holding on to anything, without taking any medication, and even with a full bladder! Nothing catastrophic has happened to you, and as a matter of fact, your SUDS level even dropped to 20! What's going on? How did that happen?

DARNELL: I guess I got used to it. This isn't as bad as I thought.

THERAPIST: Yeah, that's right. But how would you have ever learned that if you never did exposure?

DARNELL: I probably wouldn't have learned it. I would just go on avoiding and being scared of heights.

THERAPIST: That's exactly right. When you face your phobia head on, and you resist safety behaviors, your SUDS level eventually goes down and you learn that your fears are unrealistic.

As a rule, therapists should avoid trying to reassure the patient that exposure situations are "not dangerous." This is for the patient to discover for him- or herself through experience. Instead, we recommend describing risk levels as "acceptably low" rather than "zero." Some patients will seem to need a *guarantee* of safety and engage in subtle reassurance seeking or checking strategies (e.g., watching the therapist's facial expression closely). We recommend that questions about risk in a given situation be answered only once. After that, the patient should be asked to recall (to him- or herself) what the therapist previously said about the situation.

ASSIGNING HOMEWORK EXPOSURE PRACTICE

At least 1–2 hours of daily homework exposure practices are assigned following each in-session exposure. Early in treatment, homework assignments can include repetition of the in-session exposure exercises. As therapy progresses, however, homework can involve exposure to situations and stimuli not confronted during the session. As the patient becomes more and more accustomed to the procedures for doing exposure, he or she can be encouraged to take a more active role in designing homework exposures. Homework exposure practice should be conducted in the same manner as in-session exposure (i.e., using the handout in Figure 6.1). Instructions for each exercise should be clearly described, including how the specific task is to be performed, where, when, and for how long. Recording this information on a copy of the Exposure Practice Form that is given to the patient also promotes adherence (multiple copies will be necessary if multiple assignments are given).

It is also important for the therapist to review the patient's homework practice forms at the start of each subsequent session. This reinforces the importance of such assignments and sends the message that practicing exposure between sessions is a significant part of treatment that the therapist takes seriously. Particular attention should be paid to making sure that adequate habituation has occurred and that the patient was able to consolidate new information about the feared stimulus. Verbal reinforcement (i.e., praise) for successfully completed homework should be given liberally. Instances where homework was attempted but habituation did not occur can be labeled as common (but temporary) outcomes when trying to change long-standing habits. Normalizing the failure to habituate places the blame on technical factors rather than on the patient or the therapy itself. A detailed analysis of failed exposures should be undertaken to determine whether or not the exercise was performed correctly. If the patient did not attempt the assigned practice at all, the therapist should problem-solve and help the patient complete the task before moving on to more difficult hierarchy items.

CONDUCTING CHALLENGING EXPOSURES

For many patients, success with early exposure exercises prepares them to complete higher level exposures without undue difficulty. For others, however, the process is more challenging. Patients may require hefty doses of encouragement and praise for their efforts when confronting their worst fears. The therapist should, on the one hand, take a firm stand that such exposures are a necessary part of therapy as agreed upon during treatment planning; yet, on the other hand, the therapist should convey sensitivity and understanding that these tasks are likely to evoke high SUDS levels. Patients can be reminded that distress during exposure is a temporary side effect. It might be useful for the therapist to model difficult exposures before they are attempted by the patient. Informal discussions of evidence collected from previous exposure exercises can also be helpful when patients are hesitant to begin more difficult tasks, as can discussions regarding the importance of learning to take acceptable risks and tolerate uncertainty. Under no circumstances, however, should the therapist attempt to reassure the patient that "everything will be okay."

Research indicates that fear reduction is most complete and long-lasting when exposure is practiced in varied settings (e.g., Bouton, 2002). For some patients, it will therefore be important to conduct exposure to the most feared situations in many different contexts. For example, suppose a patient with OCD who has blasphemous obsessional thoughts has become relatively comfortable confronting such thoughts in the therapist's office using imaginal exposure. He might next practice evoking these obsessions in situations that he has been avoiding, such as in a place of worship or a cemetery. A patient with social anxiety who fears being rejected by members of the opposite sex might practice talking with such individuals in different settings such as school, the mall, on the telephone, and at the doctor's office waiting room. The assessment of each patient's idiosyncratic fear triggers and avoidance patterns will be especially important for determining the specific contexts in which exposure needs to occur.

IMPLEMENTING RESPONSE PREVENTION: ELIMINATING SAFETY BEHAVIORS

It might be easy to overlook the importance of eliminating escape and active avoidance strategies (e.g., safety behaviors) that serve to maintain clinical anxiety problems. Yet patients are not "recovered" if they continue to use such strategies to deal with excessive anxiety and fear. Therefore, in addition to helping patients confront their fear triggers, therapists must also help patients to refrain from using their maladaptive safety behaviors so that they can learn that these strategies are not required for coping with fear. *Response prevention* is the name commonly used to describe instructions to abstain from compulsive rituals and other safety maneuvers.

The optimal response prevention strategy is to instruct the patient to drop all safety strategies at once, "cold turkey." Although such strategies are under the patient's control (i.e., they are performed *deliberately* in response to exposure [or anticipated exposure] to fear cues), this expectation is sometimes overwhelming to the patient. It might also be difficult to reconcile with a graduated exposure approach. That is, a patient may have unplanned encounters with feared stimuli which evoke very strong urges to perform safety behaviors, but which have not yet been practiced in exposure sessions. Thus, as an alternative to implementing "complete" response prevention from the first session, therapists might consider a gradual approach in which instructions to refrain from safety behaviors parallel progress up the exposure hierarchy (with the eventual goal being complete abstinence). Indeed, some authors (e.g., Rachman, Radomsky, & Shafran, 2008) have argued that the practice of gradually fading safety-seeking behaviors, rather than abruptly prohibiting them, might make exposure therapy more acceptable and tolerable to patients without reducing its effectiveness.

STYLISTIC CONSIDERATIONS

As we have suggested, conducting exposure-based therapy is at once a science and an art. Scientifically, the treatment procedures are firmly based on well-understood principles of human learning. Moreover, as we reviewed in Chapter 2, substantial research evidence indicates that therapeutic exposure causes significant reductions in pathological fear. Less well studied, but probably equally important, is the "art" of implementing this technique. In this section, we describe a number of tactics clinicians can use to help patients get the most out of exposure therapy.

Building on Early Successes

As mentioned above, many patients experience higher levels of anticipatory anxiety as the difficulty level of exposures increases. To encourage patients to confront more challenging situations, therapists should heed, rather than disregard, the patient's distress while affirming the importance of *choosing* to persist with these exercises. For example, when preparing for difficult exposures, Darnell's therapist reminded him of the outcomes of previous successful tasks. Specifically, they had a discussion about how conducting a higher level exposure task would likely have the same consequences as previous easier exposures.

Refining the Fear Hierarchy

Adhering to the collaboratively developed exposure plan reinforces the systematic nature of the therapy and places clear expectations on the patient. This consistency probably helps patients to cultivate trust and confidence in the therapist and favors continued patient commitment to the therapy. Nevertheless, important details of the patient's fears are sometimes not revealed until well into treatment. Therefore, in addition to progression up the fear hierarchy as planned, exposure sessions should involve continued assessment and adjustments to the exposure hierarchy depending on the specifics of the patient's fear that may be unearthed as treatment progresses.

Conducting Exposures Outside of the Office

The idiosyncratic fears and avoidance patterns of anxious patients often require that exposure be conducted outside the therapist's office. Examples include visiting public bathrooms or the pesticide aisle of a home improvement store for individuals with contamination obsessions, going to restaurants and interacting with servers for someone with social anxiety, going to the site of a traumatic event for someone with PTSD and going to crowded places or grocery stores for someone with agoraphobia—to name just a few possibilities. Some patients' symptoms even require that exposure be conducted in their own home or on public transportation. It is therefore advantageous to have the flexibility of being able to leave the office to accompany patients on such "field trips."

Although exposures in public places typically can be conducted surreptitiously and with anonymity, the patient's permission must be obtained. Plans for how the exercise will proceed should also be discussed beforehand so that potentially embarrassing and attention-drawing incidents can be minimized or avoided and the patient can feel comfortable about confidentiality. In situations where there might be less anonymity, we recommend seeking permission and providing advance warning to anyone else who might be inadvertently involved in the exposure. On occasion, the other party will want an explanation of the therapeutic activity, and as a rule (as long as the patient consents), honesty is always the best policy. For example, one patient with OCD treated in our clinic had obsessional thoughts of death and required exposure to a funeral home. When planning this exercise, the therapist telephoned a local funeral home to inquire about a visit. The director, perhaps thinking he was getting a new client, asked about the purpose of the appointment. Fortunately, the patient had given the therapist consent to disclose the actual nature of the proposed visit. After a brief description of the purpose and procedures of exposure therapy, the director was happy to give the therapist and patient a "tour" of the funeral home.

We find that many patients are willing to go out in public with their therapist once they understand the importance of doing so. However, it is advisable to take the time to discuss and plan for potential contingencies, including a cover story and strategy for expeditiously handling awkward encounters with friends, relatives, or others while out in public places. Liability issues are also a reality in today's world, adding another dimension of precaution for the therapist. For example, in our clinics, therapists are generally not permitted to drive patients to exposure destinations. Thus, plans for meeting at specific destinations are arranged ahead of time.

Using Distraction during Exposure

The informed reader might recognize that using distraction techniques during exposure therapy (i.e., to make exposure practices more "bearable") effectively amounts to avoidance behavior and therefore is counterproductive. In studies directly comparing exposure sessions in which patients distract themselves (e.g., by playing a video game while confronting the feared stimulus) to exposure with attention focused on the feared stimulus (e.g., by discussing with the therapist their thoughts and feelings about confronting the feared situation), attention-focusing conditions appear more effective, especially when it comes to maintaining improvement from one session to another (e.g., Grayson, Foa, & Steketee, 1982; Sartori, Tachman, & Grey, 1982). On the other hand, experimental evidence indicates that engaging the patient in stimulus-irrelevant conversation (often considered a distraction) that does not prevent him or her from attending to and processing what is being learned during the exposure does not appear harmful and may even enhance the effectiveness of exposure therapy (e.g., Johnstone & Page, 2004).

The potential benefit of stimulus-irrelevant conversation raises the possibility that it is at times appropriate to use this form of distraction during exposure. Practically speaking, temporary distraction techniques can be helpful in order to demonstrate to the patient that he or she can carry on a conversation or complete some other task (i.e., he or she can function normally) while anxious, or when in the presence of the feared stimulus. It is important, however, to always "bring the patient back" to the exposure task by pointing out that he or she is still confronting a feared situation and yet is able to get other things done. On the other hand, distraction is maladaptive when it is used to completely take the patient's focus off of the exposure task. For example, if Darnell were to distract himself by imagining being on a relaxing beach instead of overlooking the first floor of a mall, it would be counterproductive.

Training the Patient to Become His or Her Own Therapist

Research suggests that patients who complete all exposure tasks under the therapist's supervision are more vulnerable to symptom relapse relative to those whose therapist-guided exposures are followed by self-guided exposure practices (e.g., Emmelkamp & Kraanen, 1977). Self-guided exposure probably promotes autonomy and helps the patient gain confidence in his or her ability to combat fear whether or not the therapist is present. Thus, after formal treatment ends, patients who have practiced implementing these skills on their own are likely to be better off than those who have not. These results highlight the importance of homework exposure. They also suggest it is therapeutic to use a *fading* procedure across treatment sessions. That is, while close management of the initial exposure exercises is imperative, the therapist should consider stepping back and encouraging patients to become "their own therapist" when it is clear they have learned to effectively implement the treatment techniques. This entails allowing the patient to select (from equally fear-evoking stimuli), design, and implement exposure tasks. The therapist, of course, maintains the role of coach and lends his or her expert guidance during each exercise.

Promoting "Programmed" and "Lifestyle" Exposure

From the first exposure session, the patient should be taught to think of exposure as a new lifestyle that is conducive to gaining control over, rather than being controlled by, anxiety and fear. To promote this new set of habits, we find it useful to differentiate between *programmed* and *lifestyle* exposure. Programmed exposure includes carefully developed hierarchy-driven exercises that the patient agrees to conduct under specified circumstances, at predetermined times, and in particular locations in and between sessions. Lifestyle exposure, on the other hand, refers to making choices to take advantage of additional opportunities to practice confronting, rather than avoiding, fear cues (i.e., focus on *choosing to be anxious*). The patient is encouraged to be opportunistic and to view situations in which fear is triggered unexpectedly as occasions to practice exposure techniques and work on his or her problem, rather than as situations to be avoided or endured with great distress. Patients can often be reminded that every choice they make regarding whether to confront or avoid a fear cue carries weight. Each time they choose to confront such a situation without using avoidance or safety behaviors, they are helping themselves become less fearful in the long run. Alternatively, each time a decision is made to avoid, they are strengthening their fear.

Using Humor

The use of humorous comments or modest laughter to lighten the mood during awkward exposures, or to help the patient's anxiety to habituate, is often appropriate and can even be beneficial. Nevertheless, it is not advised if the patient appears highly distressed. In such instances, the therapist should convey understanding of how difficult exposure can be, and that with time and persistence the exercises will ultimately become more manageable. The therapist must be a keen judge of when the use of humor is befitting. A good rule of thumb is to follow the patient's lead and ensure that he or she understands the therapist is laughing *with*, and not *at* him or her. Remarks should remain relevant to the exposure situation and should not serve to distract the patient from the task.

Determining Session Frequency

The number of exposure sessions will depend on the length of the fear hierarchy and how rapidly the patient's anxiety habituates, allowing progress from item to item. Exposure for a specific fear of, say, balloons, might require from one to three exposure sessions. On the other hand, for someone with OCD with numerous types of fear triggers, 12–16 (or more) exposure sessions might be required.

The optimal rate of exposure practice sessions is unclear. Studies with individuals suffering with agoraphobia and specific phobias (e.g., Chambless, 1990), as well as with OCD (Abramowitz, Foa, & Franklin, 2003), indicate that spacing the treatment sessions out over time does not necessarily detract substantially from the short-term effectiveness of massed sessions or "intensive" therapy. At follow-up, no differences in relapse rates were observed among phobic patients, and no differences in severity were present among patients with OCD. It is possible, however, that patients receiving less intensive therapy were conducting more home-based exposure practice which might account for their similar rates of improvement relative to intensively treated individuals.

An interesting line of experimental research has looked at the short- and long-term effects of massed versus spaced learning trials. This work suggests that while longer and more varied intervals between practice trials may impede learning in the short run (i.e., during the *acquisition* phase), it actually *enhances* long-term retention of the learned material since it provides more opportunities to rehearse what has been learned in varied contexts (Schmidt & Bjork, 1992). Conversely, massed practice (i.e., sessions held very close together in time), which maximizes immediate performance, may result in the loss of some learned information once the massed practices are stopped. This would argue for the use of an "expanding spaced" schedule of exposure therapy sessions in which initial sessions are massed together to promote learning, followed by gradually increasing the time interval between sessions to prevent the return of fear. Initial research looking at this type of treatment schedule with individuals with specific phobias has been encouraging (e.g., Rowe & Craske, 1998).

COMMON OBSTACLES TO USING EXPOSURE

In this section, we describe several common barriers to the successful implementation of exposure therapy. Solutions are presented to help the clinician effectively overcome these obstacles. Additional obstacles relevant to working with complex symptom presentations are discussed in Chapter 16.

Nonadherence

The most common obstacle to successful exposure is the patient's refusal to confront his or her feared stimuli or resist safety behaviors whether in the session or for homework. Because exposure and response prevention represent the active ingredients in therapy, such difficulties must be addressed immediately. Luckily, many problems with adherence can be circumvented by being proactive. First, it is crucial that patients grasp the conceptual model of anxiety and understand how their own symptoms are maintained according to the conceptualization outlined in Chapter 3. Second, the rationale for exposure must be very clear so that patients understand how engaging in difficult and frightening therapy exercises will reduce their fear and anxiety in the long term. These two points underscore the importance of the psychoeducational component of exposure therapy. As we have mentioned, many therapists gloss over this material and do not adequately prepare their patients to get the most out of exposure practice. A third strategy for avoiding adherence problems is to ensure that the patient feels involved in the selection and planning of exposure exercises.

When the patient fails to follow through with exposure tasks, the therapist should first inquire as to why. Sometimes nonadherence can be addressed with problem solving, such as making more time available for home exposure. The clinician should also make sure that the patient perceives that the exposure task as relevant—that is, it addresses the patient's fears and dysfunctional beliefs. When the patient understands the purpose of the exercise and expects that his or her anxiety will temporarily increase before habituation occurs, the therapist is in a strong position to successfully encourage patients to "invest anxiety now for a calmer future."

If the patient is skeptical about exposure on the basis of previous failed attempts to confront feared stimuli, the therapist can draw a distinction between *typical exposure* and *therapeutic exposure.* That is, whether deliberately or by accident, most patients at some point find themselves in the situations they fear. In most cases, however, they manage to use safety behaviors and subtle avoidance strategies to escape from anxiety and "protect" themselves against feared consequences. We would refer to this as "typical" exposure because it is characteristic of how the patient has usually used maladaptive strategies to handle confrontation with fear triggers. In contrast, *therapeutic exposure* is well planned, is performed without avoidance or safety behaviors, involves rational thinking, and lasts until anxiety subsides on its own. *If the patient experiences a sense of relief only after terminating exposure, then it is not therapeutic.* Exposure that is terminated before anxiety habituates only reinforces avoidance habits as well as the belief that feared consequences are likely. Conversely, therapeutic exposures must be repeated until they no longer evoke distress.

We sometimes observe that therapists become tempted to suspend or postpone scheduled exposures when the patient becomes highly anxious. Rather than suspending or postponing exposure, we recommend refining the exposure hierarchy and adding intermediate items (e.g., trying to find a stimulus that the patient is willing to confront). We discourage postponing exposures altogether since this can reinforce avoidance patterns and send a message that the task is too dangerous or difficult. We suggest instead that therapists emphasize the patient's control over exposures—it is ultimately his or her choice to perform the tasks. However, this choice has important consequences: choosing not to complete the exercise as directed is essentially the decision to remain fearful. The therapist can use motivational interviewing techniques (e.g., Miller & Rollnick, 2002) to create and amplify, from the patient's point of view, the discrepancy between nonadherence and his or her broader values and goals. When nonadherence is perceived as conflicting with important personal goals (such as self-image, happiness, or success), change becomes more likely (Miller & Rollnick, 2002).

Arguments over the Risks of Exposure

As a result of feeling very anxious, patients sometimes become contentious and argue that the suggested exposure exercise is too risky. If such discussions take a combative turn, the therapist should summarize the discussion and reach a conclusion that the patient *could* be correct in his or her assertion about such risks, but that rather than taking anything for granted, it is important to closely examine the facts or test them out. For example, if a socially anxious patient strongly states that she "couldn't handle" feeling embarrassed, this should be honestly considered. However, the ensuing dialogue should include Socratic questions about past experiences. For example, has the patient ever felt embarrassed before, and if so, what was the outcome? Was it temporarily very uncomfortable, or so horrific that the patient's entire present and future livelihood were affected? Do you know other people who have been embarrassed? What was it like for them? Is there any way (besides avoiding all social situations) to make sure that one will never again have to face being embarrassed? Would it be more helpful to learn how to manage such uncomfortable situations rather than trying to avoid them at such high costs? This approach highlights the importance of maintaining a collaborative relationship.

Our advice is to refrain from debates with patients over the potential risks involved with doing exposure exercises and stopping safety behaviors. Not only are such arguments fruitless, but they reinforce the anxious patient's patterns of spending too much time analyzing and worrying about risk and uncertainty. Moreover, when patients perceive that the therapist is frustrated, angry, or trying to coerce him or her into compliance , they tend to lose motivation (e.g., "You can't *make* me do this"). When a reluctant patient attempts to engage in rational argument about risk and danger, the best course of action for the therapist is to step back and recognize that the decision to engage in treatment is a difficult one. Motivational statements such as the following are often persuasive: "Remember that we both agreed on a plan for the exposures that you would practice. I hope you will hold up your end of the agreement" and "You're in treatment for yourself—not for me. So I won't argue or debate with you. This is entirely your choice. I will, however, point out that you could gain relief from your symptoms by trying these exercises and enduring the short-term anxiety. On the other hand, you are the one who has to live with the anxiety problems if you choose not to do the therapy."

Suspending or Terminating Exposure

If, despite much effort to resolve arguments or disagreements over exposure tasks, the patient persists in refusing to cooperate, it may be suitable to suspend therapy. For some clinicians, this might mean shifting the focus of treatment to some other problem or working on increasing motivation for working on anxiety and fear. For others, this might mean ending therapy altogether. If this becomes inevitable, it should be done in a sensitive (as opposed to a punitive) way, and the door should be left open for the patient to return at some point in the future. Discussing nonadherence as indicative of "bad timing" often works well, as in the following monologue:

> "For whatever reasons we're not getting very far with exposure therapy. I know this treatment can be very difficult, and you're clearly having a hard time working on the exercises that will help you with your anxiety problems. When this is the case, treatment can't be as effective for you as it should be. My guess is that now is just not the right time for you to be doing this kind of therapy. So it is best that we stop at this point. Maybe at some point in the future it will be a better time for you, and you will be able to do the exercises you need to do to benefit. I would be happy to work with you at that point."

Therapist Discomfort with Using Exposure

Lastly, it is normal for therapists who use exposure techniques—especially newly minted exposure therapists—to feel some trepidation when asking fearful patients to purposely confront stimuli that evoke more fear. Perhaps the exercises seem unnecessarily painful. If the reader falls into this category, here are some points to keep in mind. First, a solid foundation of research demonstrates that exposure therapy is the treatment of choice for fear- and anxiety-based problems and that without this technique patients have little hope of improving. Ultimately, reducing pathological anxiety requires temporarily evoking the patient's anxiety and urges to perform the unwanted behaviors. Second, there is no evidence that it is dangerous or harmful to provoke the kind of temporary anxiety that is experienced during exposure. The distress evoked during therapeutic exposure is short-lived. When this anxiety decreases patients are left with important knowledge about situations they once believed were dangerous and about their own ability to manage their own subjective distress. Third, and contrary to some popular myths, reducing fears by exposure will not cause "symptom substitution" of additional symptoms. Fourth, and finally, although exposure requires that the therapist purposely help the patient to become anxious, we find that when the rationale for this technique is made clear, and the treatment plan has been established collaboratively, the intervention engenders a warm and supportive working relationship that further authenticates the patient's courage and progress.

CONCLUSIONS

Hopefully by this point we have built a strong foundation for (1) why exposure therapy is the treatment of choice for problematic anxiety and (2) the general framework for implementing this treatment. This chapter provides a generic step-by-step overview of the use of exposure therapy. In the next part, we outline how to apply exposure treatment to a wide variety of anxiety symptoms.

Part II

Implementing Exposure Therapy for Specific Types of Fears

Part I of this book provides a general overview of the theory and practice of exposure therapy. The chapters in Part II focus on the practical aspects of using exposure techniques for a wide range of particular feared stimuli that treatment providers who work with anxious clients are likely to encounter. Thus, readers will find examples, case illustrations, and lessons learned from clinical practice to help them design and implement effective exposure-based therapy for a variety of fears. These chapters are all organized in the following manner: First, we present an overview of the symptom presentation or clinical picture in which the particular type of fear is likely to occur. Second, we discuss the basis for using exposure techniques, including theoretical considerations and their implications for exposure. Third, we provide step-by-step guidance for how to conduct a functional assessment of the common cues, feared consequences, and safety behaviors associated with the particular type of fear. The next sections contain suggestions for how to present the rationale for exposure to the patient, tailor the fear hierarchy, and conduct and implement exposure and response prevention for the corresponding fears and safety behaviors. These discussions feature numerous examples from our own clinical experiences to illustrate the application of exposure for particular feared stimuli. Each section concludes with a discussion of important hints and pitfalls that are sometimes encountered and an in-depth case description illustrating an exposure-based treatment program for a representative problem with the particular fear covered in that chapter. Each chapter also contains a list of suggested resources that provide more in-depth information on how to incorporate exposure strategies into a broader empirically supported cognitive-behavioral treatment framework for the particular problem.

7

Animal-Related Fears

CLINICAL PRESENTATION

This chapter focuses on how to use exposure therapy for fears of animals (such as dogs and insects) that are typically classified as specific phobias. Because these fears are relatively tangible they can be one of the most straightforward problems to treat with exposure. Some individuals may present with relatively circumscribed concerns, such as wanting to decrease their fear of snakes so that they can more comfortably enjoy camping. Others, however, may be experiencing more severe impairment, such as children who won't play outside for fear of being stung by a bee. Although animal-related fears are common in both children and adults, those seeking treatment are primarily children. Table 7.1 presents some basics facts regarding the types of specific fears covered in this chapter.

Even within this relatively straightforward group of anxiety-provoking stimuli, there exists significant heterogeneity. Some patients experience discreet periods of intense fear when they are confronted by an animal, such as if they unexpectedly disturb a spider while cleaning. Others describe more continuous worry about encountering the feared object, such as heightened vigilance for bugs while spending time outdoors. Still others may focus on the frustration or embarrassment associated with avoiding certain routine tasks, for example, the inability to go to a friend's home without requesting that the dogs be locked in the basement. Patients may also report a variety of emotional reactions to feared stimuli. Anxiety regarding predatory animals such as sharks or bears appears to be related to fears of being attacked. Fears of other animals, such as spiders or bugs, appear to be related primarily to disgust, the fear of contamination (Matchett & Davey, 1991), or the fear of feeling afraid (i.e., anxiety sensitivity). Some animals, such as snakes,

TABLE 7.1. Quick Reference Overview: Animal-Related Fears

Fear-evoking stimuli
- Animals with potential for aggression
- Disgust-provoking animals

Prototypical examples
- Dogs
- Snakes
- Spiders
- Bees
- Rats

Safety behaviors
- Avoidance of animals or situations in which they might be encountered
- Presence of parents or companions
- Reassurance seeking

DSM-IV-TR diagnostic category
- Specific phobia

Treatment overview
- Typical length: four to six sessions; may be conducted in a single 3-hour session
- Begin with assessment and psychoeducation
- Begin exposure by second treatment session
- Use cognitive strategies to address overestimation of danger

Obstacles
- Generalization
- Locating targets for exposures
- Managing inherent danger
- Working with children and families

may be associated with both fear and disgust. Examples of specific fears are listed in Table 7.2.

BASIS FOR EXPOSURE THERAPY

Theoretical Considerations

Many commonly feared animals, such as dogs and snakes, do pose some inherent danger: people are sometimes attacked by dogs and bitten by snakes. Of course, this is not uniformly true of the items covered in this chapter as it is difficult to imagine how a ladybug is likely to inflict serious

TABLE 7.2. **Examples of Animal-Related Fears**

Category	Examples
Fear animals	• Dogs • Sharks • Bears • Horses • Birds
Disgust animals	• Spiders • Insects and other bugs • Snakes • Dead animals • Rats and mice • Bats

harm. However, regardless of the presence or absence of intrinsic danger, the problem lies not in the *likelihood* of danger itself, but from the *misappraisal* of the likelihood of danger. In reality there is no guarantee that the neighbor's dog won't bite you or that the snake you encounter in the woods is not poisonous. However, the fear and avoidance displayed by people with phobias vastly outstrips the object's actual danger. Alternatively, some people with phobias can acknowledge that danger is unlikely but nonetheless can still think that the idea of contact with the object, such as a spider crawling through their hair, is overwhelming. For these individuals, *disgust* may be more of an issue than *fear*, and they may be overestimating the intensity and duration of their emotional reaction, rather than the threat of bodily harm from the animal itself. In either case mistaken beliefs regarding the consequences of confrontation with the feared object are important factors in the maintenance of the problem.

In response to their intense feelings, individuals typically avoid contact with the feared animal, as well as situations in which they perceive an increased chance of encountering the animal. As with other types of excessive fears, this avoidance prevents the natural extinction of the physiological and cognitive aspects of the fear reaction. For instance, if a child never remains in the same room as his friend's dog he won't have the opportunity to learn that the dog is much more likely to sniff him than to bite him. When complete avoidance is not feasible, the individual may rely on others, such as parents, to provide "protection." Since these safety behaviors successfully (and immediately) reduce anxiety, the next time the individual is confronted with the feared object he or she is likely to respond in the same manner, thus perpetuating the cycle.

Implications for Exposure Therapy

Consistent with this conceptual model, reducing animal phobias requires learning that the phobic stimulus and related emotional responses are not as dangerous, persistent, or catastrophic as anticipated. The most powerful method for learning such lessons is through repeated and prolonged direct experience confronting or interacting with the feared animal. Through gradually spending increasing amounts of time with the animal in the absence of a feared consequence (e.g., being bitten or stung), a patient begins to learn that the animal isn't as dangerous as he or she once believed. For individuals with phobias associated with *disgust* (e.g., phobias of rats or cockroaches), the patient learns that these unpleasant emotions dissipate (or are bearable) without needing to resort to avoidance. As with other types of feared stimuli, exposures must last long enough for the patient's fear or distress to decline while in the presence of the phobic stimulus; otherwise the phobia will persist.

FUNCTIONAL ASSESSMENT

This section presents a functional analysis of animal fears. Table 7.3 summarizes the highlights of this discussion.

Fear Cues

External Situations and Stimuli

Fear associated with specific animals or objects is predominantly cued by one of three stimuli: the animal itself, reminders of the animal, or situations in which the animal might be found. For example, a child with a fear of dogs may become anxious and decide to cross the street (avoidance) if a neighbor with a dog approaches. Alternatively, an adult with a fear of sharks—an animal that is rarely, if ever encountered—may become very nervous while at the beach. Another individual may be so terrified of horses that he becomes nervous even around equine toys or decorative figurines. In addition to visual cues, verbal stimuli may also elicit anxiety. For some patients, the mere mention of bees, rats, or roaches may be sufficient to induce a fearful whimper or an outspoken demand for the conversation to cease immediately.

Internal Cues

Research suggests that for some individuals, animal fears are associated with how the person *feels* when confronted with the animal (i.e., the fight–

TABLE 7.3. Functional Assessment of Animal-Related Fears at a Glance

Parameter	Common examples
Fear cues	
External situations and stimuli	The feared animal, pictures or videos, talking about the object, situations in which the object might be found
Internal cues	Physiological responses (i.e., anxious arousal) in the presence of the animal
Feared consequences	Fear that the animal will bite, sting, or otherwise hurt the person; fear that the animal will contaminate the person; fear that the person will be overwhelmed by fear and do something embarrassing
Safety behaviors	
Avoidance patterns	Staying away from the specific animal or situations in which it might be present (e.g., outdoors, lakes, friends' homes)
In-situation safety behaviors	Asking other people to remove the animal, asking questions for reassurance, checking
Beliefs about safety behaviors	Avoidance and in-situation safety behaviors protect one from being harmed by feared animals and prevent intolerable levels of fear and/or disgust, which may be seen as leading to psychological or physical harm.

flight response) as much as with the fear of being attacked (e.g., McNally & Steketee, 1985). Thus, functional assessment should include questions to assess internal fear triggers such as arousal-related body sensations.

Feared Consequences

As mentioned previously, there are two categories of feared consequences associated with these types of phobic stimuli: physical harm and emotional discomfort. The former includes pain or physical injury from incidents such as being bitten by a dog, stung by a jellyfish, or kicked by a horse. For some objects, anxiety stems from secondary consequences of the encounter, such as choking to death from an allergic reaction to a bee sting. The latter type of feared consequence includes intense anxiety or disgust.

Sometimes patients, especially children, have difficulty articulating specific feared consequences associated with their feared stimuli. For phobias involving disgust, a patient may report that the feared stimulus (e.g., rats, snakes) is "gross" or "slimy." In such instances, the implicit feared consequences include the possibility of contamination, as well as the concern that their emotional and physical reaction (e.g., disgust, nausea) will persist indefinitely or spiral to unbearable levels. Similarly, the fear of anxious arousal and its consequences (as discussed in Chapter 11) can play a role in animal phobias. For instance, a man may fear that the anxiety experienced in the presence of a cockroach will spiral into a loss of consciousness, thereby placing him at risk of harm and negative evaluation from others.

Safety Behaviors

Avoidance Patterns

In order to prevent feared consequences (including those feared to occur as a result of emotional reactions) of exposure to the feared animals or objects, individuals avoid these phobic stimuli. A child with a fear of dogs may be brought to therapy by parents concerned that she won't play outside or go to her friends' houses. Adults may avoid camping, swimming, hiking, or other outdoor activities because of animal phobias.

In-Situation Safety Behaviors

When avoidance of feared stimuli is not possible, safety behaviors may take the form of relying on others, such as parents, for assistance. For example, someone afraid of grasshoppers might have her sister walk ahead of her to root out the little green bugs. Another common safety behavior is reassurance seeking, which may involve repeated questioning, as with the child who repeatedly asks if there are any bears in the woods, or the woman who asks her husband to check the basement for spiders before she can go downstairs.

Beliefs about Safety Behaviors

Individuals who fear animals and other objects often believe their safety behaviors have the power to directly prevent feared catastrophes from occurring. For example, the child afraid of dogs may attribute the nonoccurrence of a dog bite to his or her vigilant avoidance of dogs. Unfortunately, such avoidance prevents the individual from learning that exposure to the feared stimulus is most likely harmless and tolerable. Similarly, safety behaviors may be performed with the intention of escaping from one's own negative emotions, typically fear or disgust. In such cases, individuals may believe that safety behaviors have the power to prevent intolerably high negative affect which they fear may lead to adverse psychological ("nervous breakdown") or physical (heart attack) consequences.

PRESENTING THE RATIONALE
FOR EXPOSURE THERAPY

The main points to cover when adapting the rationale for exposure therapy to individuals with animal phobias are as follows:

- Reduce the stigma of having a specific fear by explaining that approximately 50% of people have some fear over their lifetime that clearly exceeds the actual level of danger (Curtis, Magee, Eaton, Wittchen, & Kessler, 1998).

- Further normalize the experience by emphasizing that fears are an understandable result of avoidance patterns, which prevent the person from learning two things: (1) that the feared animal is actually safer than the person thinks, and (2) that anxiety, fear, and disgust are tolerable and will subside on their own if the person gives them time.

- Explain the importance of the anxiety response as a necessary and effective system for detecting danger and motivating protective action.

- Emphasize the necessity of learning *from personal experience* that the patient is overestimating the likelihood or severity of harmful or catastrophic outcomes.

- Clarify that the patient and therapist will collaboratively decide at what pace the patient proceeds up the exposure hierarchy and thus moves closer to making contact with the feared object.

- Remind the patient that although the exposures involve low risk (i.e., a level similar to situations that people encounter on a daily basis), there is no *guarantee* that feared consequences won't occur. Thus, an important lesson to be learned from exposure is how to become comfortable with everyday levels of uncertainty and unpredictability where animals are concerned.

DEVELOPING THE EXPOSURE HIERARCHY

When designing exposure hierarchies for fears of animals, there are typically two dimensions to manipulate: proximity and salience (representativeness). Hierarchies based on proximity can be developed by initially determining how closely the patient can approach the feared animal before treatment.

Building the hierarchy then involves breaking down the distance between the patient and the feared stimulus into manageable steps (i.e., hierarchy items), for instance, walking closer to a dog or sliding one's hand nearer to a bug. Some fears are more amenable to exposure hierarchies that increase the fear value of the target rather than the proximity. For instance, exposure for a fear of sharks may begin with confronting drawings of sharks, before progressing to photographs and then videos. Of course, both proximity and salience can be manipulated within a single hierarchy as well, such as gradually approaching a garter snake and then repeating the process with a larger "scarier" snake (perhaps at a zoo or pet store). Both variables can even be altered within a single stimulus, such as having a child pet a dog's back while it looks the other way before petting it on the head while looking at its face.

If a patient is not able to approach the actual feared stimulus, no matter its proximity, exposures can begin with pictures, stories, mental images, or even words. The final steps of the hierarchy should always include confrontation with the most frightening aspect of the feared stimulus in the most vulnerable manner possible, keeping in mind objective safety. For example, one might have a spider crawl on one's hand (e.g., while visiting the zoo) or watch the movie *Arachnaphobia* alone in the basement. Table 7.4 includes additional ideas for exposure items.

CONDUCTING EXPOSURE THERAPY SESSIONS

A strong therapeutic relationship is invaluable when conducting exposures for specific fears. Facing your greatest fear is hard work. Patients may gain a great deal of strength and motivation from their therapist. The therapist should validate the patient's anxiety while simultaneously encouraging him or her to face his or her fears. Modeling is an effective technique for accomplishing both aims, as in this example involving a 34-year-old nurse with a snake phobia.

> THERAPIST: So, Rachel, today we had planned to have you put your hands inside the cage and touch the snake. Does that still sound good?
>
> PATIENT: I don't know. That seems really hard; maybe I could just put my hand against the cage today.
>
> THERAPIST: Touching the snake is a big step. Remember how successful you were last week at approaching the cage and touching the glass by the snake's head? That wasn't easy. Tell me what you are afraid would happen if you touched the snake today.

TABLE 7.4. Examples of Exposure Exercises for Different Types of Animal-Related Fears

Type of animal	Exposure stimuli
Bugs (and bees)	Look at pictures of bugs; touch plastic bugs; look at dead bugs in a plastic bag; touch dead bugs; let bugs that don't fly walk around on hand and work up to face; let bug fly around office; also may include exposures to being outside
Sharks	View pictures of sharks swimming, pictures showing teeth; leaf through a new book on sharks to practice being startled by new pictures; watch video of shark jumping out of water and attacking a cage; observe sharks at aquarium; go swimming in pools, lakes, and ocean
Spiders	Look at pictures, look at household spider in a jar, put hand in jar and let spider walk on hand; go to a zoo or science center and approach larger exotic spiders in glass cage, put hand in cage, let spider walk on hand and in hair

PATIENT: Well, for starters it might bite me, but, I don't know … it just looks so gross and slimy.

THERAPIST: What if we broke it down into smaller steps. First, we could stand by the cage with the top open, then you can put your hand in the empty end of the cage, and then finally, when you are ready, you can touch the snake starting with the tail.

PATIENT: I can try that, but I still don't think I can touch it. Are you sure it is safe?

THERAPIST: Remember what we learned about this kind of snake?

PATIENT: Yeah, yeah, I know, they're not poisonous.

THERAPIST: Right. What if we agree that I will complete each step first and you will follow? That way we can both have disgusting "snakiness" on our hands and try to survive it together.

PATIENT: Okay, that sounds fair.

Note how the therapist reacted to Rachel's doubts about completing the exposure by validating her feelings. The therapist also reminded Rachel of her previous success and then broke the task into smaller, more manageable steps. Finally, note the use of modeling to encourage Rachel to agree to a plan. Although modeling is a valuable tool, it is one that should be faded out as therapy progresses so that (as we have previously mentioned) the patient does not use the therapist for seeking reassurance of safety.

When patients express fear and hesitation about exposure, the therapist should fall back on the collaborative relationship to help the patient *choose* to move forward. In addition to modeling actual confrontation with the exposure stimulus, the therapist can model how to manage negative emotions such as fear and disgust. While acknowledging that exposures may be difficult, scary, disgusting, unpleasant, and so on, therapists can also convey that these exercises are low risk, tolerable, and ultimately invaluable in overcoming fears of animals.

IMPLEMENTING RESPONSE PREVENTION

Since avoidance is the primary safety behavior in animal fears, elaborate response prevention plans are typically unnecessary. However, as discussed above, some patients rely on the presence of others to keep them "safe." In order to fully be exposed to their fear, these individuals need to conduct exposures alone following therapist-supervised exposure. Therapists should also refrain from giving verbal reassurance, and instead prompt the patient to answer any of his or her own questions about risk. Finally, some patients may temporarily tolerate an exposure to an object that elicits disgust by focusing on their ability to wash or clean themselves afterward. This pattern is similar to fears of contamination and is dealt with in detail in Chapter 12.

HINTS, TIPS, AND POTENTIAL PITFALLS

Managing Safety

Since many specific fears have some basis in reality (e.g., people are occasionally bitten by snakes, dogs, and spiders), the objective danger involved in exposures needs to be considered. For example, it is not advisable to conduct exposures to dogs bred to fight, poisonous snakes, or venomous spiders. For the most part, the limits of safe exposures are fairly intuitive. Sometimes, however, it can be difficult to determine where appropriate precautions end and problematic anxiety begins. For instance, a fear of bees in a young woman with an allergy to bee stings presents some unique challenges. Although responding to bee stings is medically necessary, avoiding the front yard in the summer is excessive. In this and similar situations, it is advisable to consult with an expert (e.g., an allergist) when designing the exposure hierarchy to avoid unnecessary risk. With children it is often best to address any uncertainties with parents outside of the child's presence in order to avoid having the parent inadvertently model overanxious behavior.

Generalization

It is important for patients to confront their feared stimuli repeatedly and in different contexts to ensure generalization of treatment effects. For example, to truly conquer a fear of spiders, a patient needs to be able to able to confront spiders at home, on vacation, at work, and elsewhere. The clinician should explain this concept early on in treatment and strongly emphasize the importance of self-guided exposure practice. Initially, patients can restrict home practice to repeating the exposures completed in session. However, as therapy progresses, they should try new steps at home before, or without, doing them under the therapist's supervision. This teaches the patient that he or she can manage fear independently.

Locating Animals in the Community

Public libraries are excellent sources of books and movies featuring commonly feared animals. The Internet is also an abundant and readily available source of helpful pictures and videos. To maximize the effectiveness of exposure therapy, however, it is often necessary to access live animals. Many feared animals, such as dogs, cats, or birds, are commonly kept as pets and are relatively easy to procure for exposures. For therapists working in hospitals or other settings that prohibit the presence of pets, therapy dogs and their trainers make excellent exposure partners. Field trips to pet stores, animal shelters, and nature centers are also useful. To facilitate at-home practice, encourage individuals to work with friends, family members, or neighbors who have the desired pets. Individuals with a fear of dogs might go to a local dog park. More exotic animals such as lizards, snakes, sharks, and spiders may be found in pet stores, zoos, aquariums, and nature centers. For these animals it will likely be necessary to conduct therapy sessions out of the office. It may even be possible to work with the staff at some zoos and nature centers to handle these animals. Insects, grasshoppers, other bugs, and worms can be gathered from basements, porches, and garages and are also sold at bait shops and at pet stores as food for other animals.

Addressing Unavailable Targets

Sometimes it is not possible to conduct exposures to an actual exemplar of the feared object. This may occur if the potential danger associated with an animal is very real and not suitable for exposures, such as bears, sharks, or rattlesnakes. In other circumstances, it may not be possible to do exposures because the object is unavailable or doesn't exist, such as Dracula, werewolves, or mummies. To address these fears it is important to conduct a thorough functional analysis. For fears of very dangerous animals such as sharks or bears, *excessive* avoidance of situations in which confrontation with the feared animal is *possible* but not necessarily *probable* (e.g., the beach, the woods) should be targeted in exposure. For stimuli that do not exist, such as zombies or monsters, the clinically relevant concern is the fear evoked by distressing images. Thus, exposure can involve confronting pictures, movies, or stories about the feared object.

CASE ILLUSTRATION

John was a 7-year-old first grader who had been afraid of dogs since witnessing a frightening episode when a neighbor's large dog attacked a terrier that was walking with its owner. John had been playing in the yard and ran inside terrified. After that incident he had become increasingly avoidant of dogs. During the initial assessment, the therapist determined that John's biggest fear was that a dog would "jump on him and bite his face." Thus, John avoided dogs, even though that meant declining invitations to friends' homes. He had even stopped playing in his front yard because some of the neighbors had dogs. John also relied on his parents to decrease his fear by hiding behind them in situations where dogs might be present. After completing a functional analysis, the therapist made a simple diagram of the conceptual model of anxiety (Figure 3.1) to explain John's symptoms in cognitive-behavioral terms to John and his father.

At the beginning of treatment John's therapist worked with John and his father to design a fear hierarchy that included rewards for meeting treatment goals. Initially, John didn't think he would be able to come to the therapist's office if there was a dog present, but agreed to try if the dog was held tightly by its owner. This served as the first step of John's hierarchy. John agreed that lying on the ground and having a dog eat a treat off his forehead was about the scariest thing he could imagine (this was so frightening that John initially refused to put it on the hierarchy, although he allowed his therapist to include it just in case John felt up to trying it later in treatment).

John's exposure hierarchy was as follows:

Description of the exposure task	SUDS
Enter office with dog firmly held by owner	45
Stand next to dog held by owner	50
Pet the dog's back and head	60
Have dog walk around on leash	75
Let the dog off leash	85

Feed dog a treat	90
Have dog jump up and put paws on chest	95
Lay on ground and let dog eat treat off forehead	100

At the next session, John's therapist arranged for a golden retriever named Leo to be present for the exposures. John and his therapist set the goal for John to pet the dog on its head. If John was successful he could have a friend over for dinner that evening. John began by slowly entering the room while Leo was held by his owner. This took about 5 minutes because John repeatedly dashed out of the room when Leo shifted positions. When he first entered the room John stood on the couch behind his father; over time he was able to stand on the floor on his own and cautiously approached the dog. After another 5 minutes and several aborted attempts, he was able to pet Leo's back. Throughout the process the therapist asked John for the level of his anxiety (SUDs) to help him notice that his distress did indeed decline as he spent more time with the dog. John gradually worked his hand up the dog's back until he pet Leo briefly on his head. The therapist and John's father congratulated him on his success and made plans for inviting a friend for dinner. Between sessions John and his father were asked to continue to practice doing what he had accomplished in the session. They identified a neighbor's beagle as a good dog with which to practice.

The therapist began the next session by reviewing the home practice with John and his father. John was eager to begin and thought he would be able to let the dog walk around by the end of the session. However, when Leo was brought into the room, John's anxiety increased and he needed to repeat the steps that he had accomplished the week before. The therapist pointed out, however, that John was able to pet Leo in much less time than in the previous session. When they began working on having Leo walk around the room, John would periodically scream and jump on the couch. The therapist generally ignored this reaction and complemented John for staying in the room. By the end of the session John was able to tolerate Leo walking around the office without a leash. The therapist ended the session by reviewing with John that he had learned spending time with dogs gets easier with practice.

At the beginning of the third session, the therapist prompted John to begin working on feeding Leo. Since John, like many people with dog phobias, was most afraid of the dog's mouth, the therapist broke this goal into separate steps: touching the dog's nose, touching the dog's mouth, letting the dog lick his hand, and feeding the dog. John required multiple attempts at each step before he was successful. During this time, the therapist remained patient and firmly encouraged John to keep trying. In addition, he praised John each time he got closer to his goal. When John stated that he was afraid, the therapist replied "That's okay, it will get easier with practice." Although he wasn't able to complete his goal of feeding Leo during the third appointment, John fed and walked Leo during the fourth session.

By the fifth session John was feeling fairly comfortable with Leo and wanted to complete his hierarchy so he could earn his ultimate reward: a sleepover with two friends. The last two items on his hierarchy were designed to address his worst fears. Through having Leo jump up on his chest he was able to face the aspect of his main fear that could readily happen when meeting a friend's dog. By lying on the floor and having Leo eat kibble off his forehead, John gave up all his safety behaviors and left himself be completely vulnerable to the dog. The therapist helped him realize that if he could do the top items on his hierarchy he could easily do other activities with dogs under normal circumstances.

ADDITIONAL RESOURCES

Antony, M. M., Craske, M. G., & Barlow, D. H. (2006). *Mastering your fears and phobias: Workbook* (2nd ed.). New York: Oxford University Press.

Craske, M. G., Antony, M. M., & Barlow, D. H. (2006). *Mastering your fears and phobias: Therapist guide* (2nd ed.). New York: Oxford University Press.

8

Natural Environments

CLINICAL PRESENTATION

The fears included in this chapter largely fall under a diagnosis of specific phobia, natural environmental type (American Psychiatric Association, 2000). Common presenting complaints include anxiety in situations in which one could be harmed, such as in a tightly enclosed or crowded place, standing on a balcony, driving in a car, being in or on water, or in a thunderstorm. In addition to fearing external harm in such environments, some individuals are concerned with internal threats associated with the experience of anxiety. For instance, they may fear having a panic attack and being unable to escape or get help in enclosed malls, open spaces, crowds, or stadiums. Many individuals fear danger from both the environment itself and from their internal reaction. For instance, Darnell, whose case was discussed in Chapters 5 and 6, was not only afraid that he might fall from high places, but also that he might be overcome with anxiety and lose control. Others fear enclosed spaces because of the feeling of being trapped in addition to fearing that they will "run out of air" and suffocate. Table 8.1 provides an overview of environmental fears.

When presenting for help, patients may focus their complaints on the degree to which their activities have been restricted, rather than on their specific fears. For instance, some are unable to attend movies or go to crowded restaurants, and others become trapped in their homes because of the fear of having panic attacks. Still others cannot use elevators or undergo important medical procedures such as having an MRI (magnetic resonance imaging).

TABLE 8.1. Quick Reference Overview: Environmental Fears

Fear-evoking stimuli

- Places
- Natural phenomena
- Situations

Prototypical examples

- Storms
- Airplanes
- Driving
- Large crowds
- Enclosed spaces, such as elevators
- Heights

Safety behaviors

- Avoidance of situations
- Companions

DSM-IV-TR diagnostic categories

- Specific phobia
- Panic disorder with agoraphobia
- PTSD

Treatment overview

- Typical length of treatment varies widely (1–12 sessions)
- Begin with assessment and psychoeducation
- Incorporate exposure by sessions 2 or 3

Obstacles

- Traveling for exposures
- Identifying safety behaviors

BASIS FOR EXPOSURE THERAPY

Theoretical Considerations

Fears of harm in specific locations typically reflect unrealistic beliefs regarding the likelihood and severity of negative events. Overestimates of likelihood usually relate to the probability of rare (although *possible*) occurrences, such as a plane crash, elevator accident, drowning, or lightning strike. Overestimates of severity typically pertain to beliefs about the consequences of experiencing anxiety symptoms in the feared situation. For instance, a man who avoided riding escalators believed that if he became too anxious, he would lose control and wildly push people out of his way in his attempt to escape. Fearful individuals attempt to mitigate their concerns through a variety of methods including avoidance, carrying antianxiety medication, or enduring the experience only because they know escape will occur shortly. Unfortunately, although these responses decrease anxiety in the short run, they prevent learning that the feared outcome is unlikely to occur and that anxiety is temporary and harmless. Thus, the safety behaviors become habitual responses that maintain the person's phobia.

Implications for Exposure Therapy

Based on this understanding of environmental fears, treatment must provide the patient with corrective learning experiences. Only through remaining in the feared situation until anxiety decreases can a patient learn that he or she is overestimating the likelihood and severity of danger. Through spending time in the feared situations, the patient can learn that the chances of being on a bridge when it collapses, in an elevator when it malfunctions, or in a plane when it crashes are extremely (and acceptably) low. Moreover, although the experience of anxiety can be very unpleasant, it is highly unlikely that it will cause the patient to lose control, become dangerous, or embarrass him- or herself. Rather, he or she is more likely to be able to endure this discomfort until it passes. Thus, exposure also helps the individual learn that anxiety is not dangerous. Once the patient's anxiety repeatedly decreases while he or she remains in the feared situation, that environment's salience as a cue for anxiety diminishes. As this connection is weakened, the acute fear response to the situation, as well as the anticipatory anxiety regarding potential future confrontations, decreases.

FUNCTIONAL ASSESSMENT

Table 8.2 provides an overview of the cognitive-behavioral parameters of fears of natural environments. The next sections describe these parameters in detail.

Fear Cues

External Situations and Stimuli

Anxiety reactions are typically cued by being in the feared situation or by the realization that one will have to encounter the situation in the near future (i.e., anticipatory anxiety). For example, people may fear being in MRI machines, cellars, or elevators; ascending tall buildings, ladders, or

TABLE 8.2. Functional Assessment of Environmental Fears at a Glance

Parameter	Common examples
Fear cues	
External situations and stimuli	Certain situations, locations, or places
Internal cues	Physiological sensations associated with anxiety (changes in breathing, increased heart rate, muscle tension, and tremors)
Feared consequences	Being injured in the situation, losing control or having a medical emergency due to too much anxiety, embarrassment and negative evaluation resulting from observable anxiety symptoms
Safety behaviors	
Avoidance patterns	Remaining inside, using public transportation rather than driving, avoiding roads with bridges, driving rather than flying, taking the stairs in tall buildings, wearing loose-fitting clothing
In-situation safety behaviors	Planning escape route, staying in close proximity to loved one, distraction, reassurance seeking
Beliefs about safety behaviors	Essential to maintain control and avoid harm

stairwells; driving on highways, across bridges, or through tunnels; riding in buses, planes, or trains; or being in water, fields, or shopping malls. Some fears are not of specific *places* but rather of *situations* that can occur anywhere. For instance, an impending storm may provoke anxiety in someone with a fear of thunder, lightning, or tornados regardless of location. In addition, this fear may be triggered by a variety of external stimuli including tornado sirens, dark clouds, or ominous weather reports. Similarly, an individual may not fear shopping malls unless they are crowded or being in small rooms unless they are locked.

Internal Cues

Physiological symptoms of arousal can also trigger increased anxiety, especially if these body sensations are interpreted as a sign that one is in physical danger or is losing his or her composure. For instance, one woman maintained that there was nothing frightening about balconies except the "funny feeling" in her stomach as she looked over the edge. Others may interpret shakiness in their arms (due to muscle tension) or other arousal-related sensations (e.g., lightheadedness, loss of concentration) as signs that they are about to lose control of their car and have an accident (e.g., drive off of a tall bridge). Similarly, an increase in heart rate, difficulty breathing, or an upset stomach can be interpreted as signs that one is actually in danger or will have a panic attack and lose control.

Feared Consequences

The fear of being out of control, either of the situation itself or of one's reaction to it, lies at the heart of many environmental fears. Individuals may be concerned that they will be harmed by events they are incapable of stopping, such as bridges collapsing, suffocating in a small room, having an accident while driving, or having one's home destroyed by fire from a lightning strike. Similarly, some fears focus on the safety of other people, such as hitting a pedestrian while driving. Internal cues can also be interpreted as signs of danger, such as difficulty breathing or chest tightness being interpreted as indicating that one is suffocating from lack of oxygen while in a small room or an MRI scanner. Other times, individuals do not fear death or harm but rather the physical reactions themselves. For example, one might be concerned about the embarrassment of having a panic attack at a mall or losing one's composure if trapped in an elevator. The same situations can be related to diverse consequences for different patients, which highlights the need for a thorough functional analysis of the fear symptoms.

Safety Behaviors

Avoidance Patterns

Although avoidance is often limited to specific feared locations or types of situations, in the most severe cases it can trap patients in their homes. It is important for therapists to understand the full range of situations and stimuli that are avoided, as well as the *reasons* for avoidance. As noted above, some individuals avoid situations because of the fear of harm from external circumstances, such as a plane crash, elevator accident, or lightning strike. But avoidance might also be based on the fear of internal consequences associated with anxious arousal, such as the common claustrophobic concern of running out of air and suffocating in enclosed spaces. Many individuals avoid certain environments because they are afraid of how they might *feel* in those environments or because they fear not having access to help or easy escape routes.

In-Situation Safety Behaviors

Many responses to environmental fears are intended to increase a person's sense of control. For instance, some individuals may ensure that they have an escape plan (e.g., knowing where the exits or bathrooms are, having an excuse to leave early) before they will enter feared situations such as malls, movie theaters, or restaurants. In situations where escape may not be easy or possible, safety behaviors may be used to manage anxiety symptoms, such as always keeping a full water bottle on hand to prevent dying of suffocation. Checking for signs of danger can also function as a safety behavior. For instance, an individual with a fear of tornados may continuously check the Weather Channel for reassurance that there are no storms on the horizon. Finally, some people may only venture into feared situations with a trusted companion or with a cell phone, making the companion or phone a safety signal.

Beliefs about Safety Behaviors

Patients with environmental fears typically believe their safety behaviors serve to keep them out of harm's way by either removing a perceived threat or by reducing the concern that anxiety will escalate to harmful levels. A patient who believed that remaining in her car during a thunderstorm was the only way to avoid being killed by lightning provides an example of the former. A man who carried antianxiety medication when traveling on airplanes because of his fear of having a panic attack and dying at 30,000 feet exemplifies the latter.

PRESENTING THE RATIONALE FOR EXPOSURE THERAPY

It is important for patients to understand that during exposure they will need to (1) enter situations that make them uncomfortable and (2) act in a manner that is precisely the opposite of what makes them feel at ease (drop their safety behaviors; i.e., response prevention). The purpose of exposure is often to demonstrate not only that feared situations pose low risk, but that anxiety does not spiral "out of control" or lead to disastrous consequences. Repeated and prolonged exposure to both internal and external cues is therefore essential. A dialogue with a patient to present this rationale might progress as follows:

> THERAPIST: You've said before that movie theaters cause you a great deal of anxiety.

PATIENT: That's right, I would love to go see movies again, but I just need to get rid of this anxiety first.

THERAPIST: I am confident that we can help you feel comfortable at the movies again. However, you will have to enter theaters so that you can see that your anxiety will decrease. Do you remember our conversation about exposure treatment?

PATIENT: Yes, it made a lot of sense for a specific fear, like of dogs, but I am not sure how it would work for me. I don't even know what I am afraid of, really; I just get nervous and have to get away.

THERAPIST: Although your fears are less concrete than a fear of dogs, our exposure treatment will work the same way. Based on our conversations it sounds to me that you are afraid that you will feel trapped in the theater and that it would be impossible, or very embarrassing, to get out if you needed to escape because of too much anxiety. Does that sound right?

PATIENT: Yes, that's a good way to describe it.

THERAPIST: Okay, good. Now we know the target of our exposures. Not only do we have to go to movie theaters, we need to make sure that you experience that trapped feeling. If we sit in the theater long enough, your fear will improve as you learn from your own experience that in fact your anxiety and trapped feelings ease up if given time.

In this exchange, the therapist clarifies that one of the challenges of exposure therapy involves entering situations despite feeling anxious. This also places the patient's own symptoms (fear cues, beliefs, and avoidance) into the conceptual model of anxiety presented in Chapter 3. Through this process the stage is set for designing exposure exercises that are tied to the patient's presenting problem.

DEVELOPING THE EXPOSURE HIERARCHY

Given the idiosyncrasies of environmental fears, exposures need to be based on a clear understanding of the patient's fear cues and the anticipated negative consequences. Some fears lend themselves nicely to gradations of intensity. For example, a fear of heights can be easily manipulated by going to progressively higher floors in a building. A fear of enclosed spaces can be gradually addressed through entering smaller and smaller rooms. A fear of bridges can be graduated by confronting longer or higher bridges (depending on the patient's particular fears). For someone afraid of being struck by lightning, exposure could progress from experiencing a storm in the basement, then from an interior room in the house, then from a room with windows, then from the porch, and so on. Because exposures can be designed relatively easily for some fear stimuli (e.g., heights and enclosed spaces), therapists can often treat these symptoms effectively in a single session (Ollendick et al., 2009).

Other exposure stimuli may be less controllable, such as the size of crowds in public places, weather-related stimuli (storm severity), or access to an airplane. In some cases it may be necessary to use imaginal exposure. When using imaginal exposure, the patient should be encouraged to repeatedly picture the feared outcome occurring—for example, having a panic attack while on a plane that leads to losing control—until that thought no longer provokes anxiety. The therapist can also manipulate the degree of safety behavior use. For example, a patient with a fear of crowded places could initially enter a mall with a "safe person." Gradually, this safety cue can then be reduced, such as by having the safe person walk behind the patient, stay by the door, and then not be present at all. Finally, some exposure hierarchies will need to include interoceptive exposures (which are discussed in Chapter 11). For instance, before standing on a balcony in a public place, a patient with a fear of heights might induce arousal using hyperventilation to learn that anxiety is unlikely to lead to fainting or losing control. Table 8.3 presents some examples of possible hierarchy items for exposure to common environmental fears.

CONDUCTING EXPOSURE THERAPY SESSIONS

During exposure, it is important for the therapist to continually communicate with the patient to ensure that the situation provokes anxiety and challenges the patient's beliefs about the consequences of becoming anxious. Therapists should also keep a close watch for the use of subtle safety behaviors that might reduce distress or lead to feeling secure. Consider how the therapist works with a patient who is afraid of driving on bridges and who believes that his intense anxiety will cause him to lose control and cause an accident.

THERAPIST: Okay, this bridge is pretty long. How are you feeling?

PATIENT: Not too bad. I am pretty nervous, but I am handling it.

THERAPIST: I see that you are gripping the steering wheel pretty tightly. Did you notice that?

PATIENT: I'm doing that so I don't swerve the car. It keeps me in control so I don't panic and drive over the edge.

TABLE 8.3. Examples of Exposure Exercises for Common Environmental Fears

Type of environmental situation	Exposure stimuli
Storms	Look at books, watch videos; during storm: stand by window, drive around, stand outside
Flying	Read about planes, watch planes take off and land, imaginal exposures to worst-case scenario flights (see Chapter 10 for more information on imaginal exposure), sit in plane, spend time in airport, take short commuter flight, take long flight
Driving	Drive slowly on empty side streets or in parking lots, in familiar neighborhoods, on city streets, during rush hour, on the highway; drive at night and in bad weather
Enclosed spaces	Remain in a small bathroom, closet, elevator, back seat of car, sleeping bag; wear turtleneck, scarf, or respirator; wear handcuffs or cover body with heavy blanket; breathe through straw, swallow quickly and repeatedly, hold breath, hyperventilate
Heights	Stand on balcony, hold railing, look over edge without holding railing, run toward railing with hands behind back, run backward

THERAPIST: How likely do you think it is that you would lose control and drive off this bridge?

PATIENT: Probably pretty unlikely.

THERAPIST: So griping the steering wheel makes you feel better, but doesn't really make you any safer. What does that sound like?

PATIENT: Yeah, a safety behavior. Do you think I should loosen my grip?

THERAPIST: Give it a try. If that goes well, next you could try with only using one hand on the wheel to prove that anxiety isn't dangerous.

IMPLEMENTING RESPONSE PREVENTION

When avoidance is the primary safety behavior, an elaborate response prevention plan may not be required. However, as discussed above, some patients rely on more or less subtle in-situation safety signals and behaviors to help them to feel safer in the context of their feared environments. In such instances, exposures must be conducted without the use of such maneuvers and safety cues. Therapists should also refrain from providing verbal reassurance and instead prompt the patient to answer any of his or her own questions about risk.

HINTS, TIPS, AND POTENTIAL PITFALLS

Leaving the Office

Exposures for environmental fears will often require the therapist to leave his or her office. To assist patients with exposures, therapists may need to travel to bridges, escalators, high-rise office buildings, open fields, tunnels, or movie theaters. In very severe instances patients may be confined to their home and unable to attend therapy sessions. In these cases treatment might need to begin at the patient's home. However, we recommend that therapists require the patient to come to the office (even if the visit requires the use of safety cues and behaviors) to demonstrate a minimum level of motivation for treatment. Working outside the office can bring up legal, billing, and safety issues, particularly when riding in a car with a patient, such as for driving exposures. Therapists are encouraged to familiarize themselves with state regulations, billing laws, institutional rules, and their own insurance policy. For instance, we encourage therapists to meet their patients at the site of out-of-office exposures rather then taking responsibility for driving the patient themselves.

When Situational Exposure Is Impractical

Sometimes situational exposures for environmental fears present logistical challenges that limit the therapist's involvement. For example, if an exposure involves a patient spending the night away from home, it would be impractical for the therapist to supervise the entire experience. Instead, he or she might assist at the beginning (e.g., helping the patient get settled in a hotel), or be available by phone. Other exposures, such as those for a patient afraid of flying, can be particularly challenging to implement. Available options for *in vivo* exposures include making arrangements with private pilots and flight schools, purchasing inexpensive plane tickets, and taking advantage of planned holidays. However, we find that discussion of mistaken cognitions about flying, the use of self-help books for individuals with this fear (e.g., Brown, 1996), and interoceptive exposure to internal fear cues (for those with the fear of panicking on the plane) go a long way toward reducing the need for repeated exposure to actual flights.

In other circumstances exposures may be impossible to control, such as when working with patients with fears of thunderstorms. Such fears may necessitate impromptu sessions or clear instructions to the patient and a family member for how to take advantage of the next storm. In general, if the therapist is not going to attend an exposure, he or she should thoroughly prepare the patient to conduct the exercise. Specifically, the therapist could provide written instructions for how to do the exposure, complete preliminary imaginal or related exposures with the patient, or role-play the planned exposure in the office. Being available by phone or e-mail is also likely to help with compliance.

CASE ILLUSTRATION

Bill was a 25-year-old accountant who sought treatment for a fear of elevators. He did not know when this fear began, but stated that it became problematic when he moved to a larger city with many multistory buildings. Although he was able to locate a second-floor apartment, he often found himself either taking the stairs at work or riding the elevator with great distress. When the therapist conducted a functional analysis, it turned out that there were a number of enclosed situations that triggered Bill's anxiety, including small meeting rooms and bathrooms. In general, Bill was afraid that he would run out of oxygen and not be able to escape before he panicked or passed out. His fears of elevators also included being trapped and falling. Given the specificity of his fears, Bill and his therapist planned to complete exposure treatment during a single 4-hour therapy session. During the initial appointment, Bill and his therapist developed the following treatment hierarchy:

Description of the exposure task	SUDS
Sit in back corner of small room	25
Stay in small dark closet	40
Ride elevator to third floor	65
Ride elevator to top floor	70
Ride older elevator	85
"Try" to make elevator get stuck	90

Because the therapist's office did not include the settings needed to complete his exposures, Bill met his therapist at the library downtown for the treatment session. They began the exposures by sitting in the back corner of a reading room in the library. During the exposure they unobtrusively recorded his SUDS levels in a small notebook. Although this exposure was not very challenging for him, Bill experienced mild anxiety that gradually decreased without leaving the room. For the second item on his hierarchy, Bill locked himself in small single-person bathroom and turned out the light. The therapist stood outside and periodically knocked on the door to get a SUDS rating. Once again Bill's anxiety decreased fairly rapidly. After approximately an hour practicing with small rooms Bill felt ready to work directly with elevators.

The first exposures were conducted at the library since the elevators only went up three floors and were not busy. Bill and his therapist began by riding from the ground floor to the third floor. Bill thought that this was manageable because he knew that it was a short trip. Thus, for the next step Bill and the therapist rode the elevator up and down continuously, without exiting, until Bill's anxiety decreased. After six or seven trips between the three floors, Bill began to relax and his anxiety about being "confined" in the elevator habituated. Toward the end of the exposure, Bill was confident enough to test his fear of the elevator falling by first walking around and then jumping up and down in the elevator. After conquering this fear, Bill and his therapist repeated similar steps in a 20-story office building that Bill had been avoiding, and finally in a building with an older elevator that Bill thought might be less safe. In addition, the elevators in these buildings received regular use and could be counted on to be fairly crowded, which exposed Bill to feeling trapped. Although Bill was initially concerned that they would receive odd looks for never exiting the elevator during the exposure practices, it quickly became apparent that people were minding their own business and hardly noticed. They did, however, limit jumping to when they were alone in the elevator.

By the end of this 4-hour session, Bill felt much more confident about riding in elevators and realized that his fears of running out of oxygen were unfounded. His therapist encouraged him to practice daily and challenge himself by riding elevators to higher floors then necessary. Approximately 3 months after his treatment session, Bill returned for a follow-up appointment to assess his progress. At that time he was regularly riding elevators and had even begun dating a woman with a 10th-floor apartment.

ADDITIONAL RESOURCE

Craske, M. G., Antony, M. M., & Barlow, D. H. (2006). *Mastering your fears and phobias: Therapist guide* (2nd ed.). New York: Oxford University Press.

9

Social Concerns

CLINICAL PRESENTATION

Shyness and social anxiety are common and do not by themselves necessarily indicate a psychological disorder. However, individuals whose social anxiety is extreme, distressing, or debilitating (i.e., they meet criteria for a diagnosis of social phobia; American Psychiatric Association, 2000) may benefit from treatment. People with social phobia may fear circumscribed social situations, such as public speaking or urinating in public restrooms, but more commonly present with fears of a variety of situations in which they might be observed by others, appear foolish, or be scrutinized. The range of distress and impairment caused by this problem extends from individuals who function highly despite a specific fear of public speaking to others who are unable to work, develop friendships, date, or even leave home due to pervasive social anxiety. Table 9.1 includes a brief overview of social concerns.

BASIS FOR EXPOSURE THERAPY

Theoretical Considerations

Cognitive-behavioral theories of social phobia (Clark & Wells, 1995; Rapee & Heimberg, 1997) highlight the role of maladaptive beliefs and safety behaviors in the maintenance of this disorder. Socially anxious individuals tend to view *themselves* as socially unskilled and *others* as critical and judgmental. They tend to believe that others pay close attention to them and are likely to notice even minor instances of imperfect speech or behavior, anxiety symptoms, or flaws in their appearance. Accordingly, individuals

155

TABLE 9.1. Quick Reference Overview: Social Concerns

Fear-evoking stimuli

• Interpersonal interactions
• Certain types of people
• Public places
• Performance situations
• Experiencing publicly observable anxiety-related symptoms

Prototypical examples

• Interacting with others at meetings, in classes, on the phone
• Dealing with authority figures (boss, police officer, teacher) or attractive people
• Social gathering including restaurants, bars
• Giving a speech, making a toast, playing sports

Safety behaviors

• Avoiding feared interpersonal and performance situations
• Minimizing interactions, including not making eye contact
• Hiding anxiety symptoms by keeping hands in pockets; wearing clothes to hide "defects" in appearance; growing a beard, wearing a hat, glasses, etc.
• Drinking alcohol or using drugs (e.g., marijuana)

DSM-IV-TR diagnostic categories

• Social phobia
• Avoidant personality disorder

Treatment overview

• Typical length: 12 individual therapy sessions
• Begin with assessment and psychoeducation
• Use cognitive therapy techniques to challenge beliefs about the dangerousness of social situations
• Begin situational exposures by session 3 or 4
• Use social mishap exposures in later sessions
• Consider combining interoceptive and situational exposure
• Decrease safety behaviors along with exposure

Obstacles

• Comorbid depression
• Patient lacks social skills
• Therapist social anxiety

---

with social phobia worry that others will detect their mistakes and imperfections and evaluate them negatively as a result. Although interpersonal criticism and rejection is rarely life-threatening, socially anxious individuals may perceive negative evaluation as catastrophic—perhaps on a par with serious injury or death.

The extreme focus on one's appearance and behavior in social situations prompts fearful individuals to adopt an "observer perspective" (Wells, Clark, & Ahmad, 1998). In other words, they imagine watching themselves from the point of view of a critical outside individual. Socially anxious patients closely attend to their own behavior, body sensations, and appearance, scanning for characteristics that might invite criticism from others. An unfortunate side effect of this heightened self-focused attention is that patients often fail to notice that others are *not* reacting negatively and in many cases are *indifferent* to them or have failed to notice them at all.

When socially anxious individuals believe that negative evaluation is likely, they experience cognitive, behavioral, and physiological symptoms of anxiety. These symptoms may directly exacerbate the very characteristics for which the patient fears negative evaluation, such as blushing, trembling, stuttering, or difficulty urinating. Avoidance and in-situation safety behaviors are used to reduce the possibility of being noticed, appearing foolish, and being negatively evaluated. These actions maintain excessive social anxiety by preventing patients from learning that others are generally unconcerned with their perceived mistakes and imperfections, and that the anxiety associated with social mishaps and the resulting negative evaluation is transient and manageable.

Implications for Exposure Therapy

This framework for understanding social anxiety has clear treatment implications. Specifically, treatment must assist the patient in approaching feared social situations, eliminating the use of safety behaviors, and acquiring corrective information that is incompatible with the maladaptive beliefs that maintain fears of social situations. Through the use of situational (*in vivo*) exposures, patients learn that others are generally unlikely to pay close attention to them in social situations and rarely display overt criticism or ridicule. By conducting exposure exercises that involve deliberately engaging in social mishaps (such as purposely mispronouncing a word), patients also learn that behaving imperfectly—or even *foolishly*—and actually being negatively evaluated by others is tolerable (albeit temporarily uncomfortable). Lastly, frequent opportunities to engage in social exposures allow patients to build and gain confidence in their social skills (e.g., how to make proper eye contact and start or end conversations), and realize that they are less likely to behave foolishly than they originally believed. This does not, however, rule out the possibility that some patients will require specific training in social skills as part of their treatment.

Response prevention demonstrates that safety behaviors are often unnecessary to prevent feared outcomes. It also assists patients in developing more adaptive coping strategies in social situations. Following a successful series of exposures to social mishaps, patients often realize that they can manage all right in social situations, which is of great value in helping them eliminate safety behaviors.

FUNCTIONAL ASSESSMENT

Table 9.2 includes typical examples for each parameter of a functional assessment of social anxiety. The next sections describe these parameters in detail.

Fear Cues

External Situations and Stimuli

Patients with social phobia tend to fear situations in which interactions with others are likely, or in which their performance may be evaluated by others. "Performance" should be interpreted broadly to include any action performed with an audience, including running on a treadmill, signing for a delivered package, eating a burger, or even walking in public. Particularly anxiety-provoking situations include giving speeches, interviewing for a job, asking a potential romantic partner out on a date, and conversing with others at a party. Other examples include eating in public, working out at a gym, and using public restrooms. Social anxiety may also be triggered by situations in which the individual is the center of attention, such as volunteering in class or speaking up at a meeting. Situations in which the patient might inconvenience others or experience conflict with them, such as returning an item at a store, may elicit social anxiety. Even being at home alone may not insulate a person from experiencing social anxiety. To illustrate, a 25-year-old woman was afraid to answer her phone because she feared sounding awkward and being negatively evaluated by the caller.

Internal Cues

Patients with social anxiety are often concerned that others will notice their anxiety-related body sensations and reactions. For some, reactions such as blushing are the primary source of social anxiety. Common internal fear triggers include heart palpitations, shortness of breath, and sweating. Outward manifestations of anxiety include shaky hands, blushing, difficulty urinating, and speech problems such as quivering voice, stuttering, and pausing (often referred to by patients as "freezing up"). It is therefore important to assess this aspect of social anxiety.

TABLE 9.2. Functional Assessment of Social Concerns at a Glance

Parameter	Common examples
Fear cues	
External situations and stimuli	Interpersonal interactions, performance situations, any place where others are present
	Certain types of people (e.g., potential romantic partners)
Internal cues	Anxiety-related body sensations and reactions that may be observed by others
Feared consequences	Being negatively evaluated, criticized, or rejected; appearing anxious, foolish, weak, or unintelligent to others
Safety behaviors	
Avoidance patterns	Situations and places in which the individual may be observed by others, or may have to interact with or perform in front of others
In-situation safety behaviors	Attempts to prevent interpersonal interactions or minimize their duration; hiding one's observable anxiety reactions; entering feared situations when few others are present; using alcohol or other drugs; excessively rehearsing what to say
Beliefs about safety behaviors	Prevent one from being noticed and negatively evaluated by others

Feared Consequences

For most people with social anxiety, the fundamental fear is that others will negatively evaluate, ridicule, or reject them. This may occur for different reasons and take a variety of forms. Some worry about being judged for appearing anxious, mentally ill, unintelligent, rude, strange, unattractive, or deviant. The person might fear that the negative evaluation will manifest simply in the disapproving thoughts and feelings of others or perhaps in overt ridicule or discriminatory behavior. One patient worried that dating partners would reject her once they learned of her anxiety problem. Another feared being fired from his job because his boss might conclude on the basis of his visible anxiety symptoms that he was "weird" and ineffectual. Male clients who have strongly internalized the masculine gender role often report concerns that they will be perceived as "weak" and not in control of their emotions if they tremble, sweat, blush, or otherwise appear anxious.

Safety Behaviors

Avoidance Patterns

Pervasive avoidance of social situations is often the most obvious symptom of social phobia. Patients may avoid speaking to all but their most trusted family members and friends. They may avoid public places such as grocery stores and shopping malls, or travel to them at times when few others are present (e.g., in the middle of the night). In extreme cases, individuals may scarcely be able to leave their homes due to fear of negative evaluation from others (as opposed to fear of having a panic attack as is characteristic of agoraphobia). In other instances, the avoidance may be more circumscribed. For example, a socially anxious student may put off taking a required speech class, even if it means delays in graduating. One 42-year-old patient with the fear of urinating in public would only use locked, single-occupancy restrooms when he was outside of his home, such as those found in gas stations. He avoided attending concerts and sporting events in which he would have no choice but to either hold his urine for long periods of time or urinate in the presence of others.

In-Situation Safety Behaviors

If avoidance is not possible, socially anxious individuals may use a variety of strategies to reduce the possibility of being negatively evaluated by others in social situations. Most commonly, they attempt to be as invisible as possible to avoid detection by those around them. They may sit in the back row, remain silent, escape at the first available opportunity, avoid making eye contact, say as few words as possible when spoken to, speak quietly, and deflect conversation topics away from themselves. At the same time, they may be unusually polite and excessively accommodating in their interactions in order to avoid criticism. Efforts may also be taken to reduce visible symptoms of anxiety. Patients may keep trembling hands in their pockets or wear baggy clothing to hide sweating. Some male patients grow thick beards and wear baseball caps to conceal blushing. To reduce the probability of saying something unintelligent, individuals may excessively rehearse speeches or conversations. Alcohol or other drugs (e.g., marijuana) may be used to reduce anxiety symptoms and facilitate more relaxed conversation. In some cases, the habitual use of these substances becomes a clinical problem in its own right.

Beliefs about Safety Behaviors

Avoidance and in-situation safety behaviors are believed to reduce the probability of being noticed by others and being negatively evaluated. There is some truth to this notion, as socially anxious individuals are often able to escape notice from others. Paradoxically, some safety behaviors aimed at preventing feared outcomes may actually *increase* the probability of being negatively evaluated by others. For example, patients who avoid eye contact, speak softly, and say as little as possible during conversations may actually invite others to view them as odd, unlikeable, or unintelligent.

PRESENTING THE RATIONALE
FOR EXPOSURE THERAPY

The rationale for exposure therapy for social fears begins with a discussion of the individualized conceptualization of the patient's social anxiety using information gathered during the functional assessment. The therapist describes how the patient's social anxiety is caused by maladaptive beliefs about his or her social incompetence and others' propensity to scrutinize and criticize his or her imperfections. The therapist adopts an open-minded, neutral stance regarding the validity of these beliefs and emphasizes that exposure may help the patient to accurately determine just how threatening social situations really are. Safety behaviors are described as preventing the patient from learning (1) whether or not others are likely to notice him or her and judge him or her for minor social mistakes, and (2) whether the discomfort caused by engaging in the occasional social mishap is really as terrible as the patient imagines.

By facing feared social situations without the use of safety behaviors, patients may test the validity of their beliefs about others, see that anxiety habituates in fear-provoking social situations, and gain experience and confidence in navigating social encounters. Thus, the typical results of well-conducted exposure and response prevention are the realizations that (1) one can generally perform adequately in social situations; (2) others are generally unconcerned with the subtle behaviors of those around them and are more inclined toward sympathy than criticism when others experience social mishaps; (3) committing the occasional social mishap and being negatively evaluated may be temporarily uncomfortable, but is tolerable; and (4) anxiety that occurs in social situations is temporary and will subside over time if safety behaviors are not used.

It should be emphasized that committing an occasional embarrassing faux pas, such as spilling a drink or forgetting an acquaintance's name, is unavoidable. Social anxiety is thus relatively unique among clinical anxiety problems in that the outcomes patients fear do occasionally come to pass. Because of this, it is not enough for patients to learn through exposure that social situations are not threatening *provided that* they behave in a competent manner and escape negative evaluation; this will not prepare them for the inevitable occurrence of an actual social mishap. Rather, the patient must also come to understand that behaving in an unskilled or foolish manner in a social situation, and perhaps even experiencing embarrassment and negative evaluation as a result, is also manageable. Thus, exposure therapy can be used to assist the patient in learning that he or she is able to cope with the temporary discomfort caused by appearing foolish to others. Patients who have learned not to fear social situations *without regard* to the quality of their behavior or the reactions of others will have the best outcomes in exposure therapy.

DEVELOPING THE EXPOSURE HIERARCHY

Hierarchy items typically consist of *in vivo* exposures involving social interactions, performance situations, and visits to social settings that have been previously avoided. Initial exposure tasks will consist of engaging in moderately distressing social situations. Depending on the functional analysis, such tasks may include asking strangers for the time, standing in a line, writing in front of others, or simply walking in a public place while making eye contact with others. Subsequent tasks will be of increasing difficulty and typically involve being the center of attention, interacting with particularly anxiety-provoking persons (e.g., asking strangers for directions, talking with potential romantic partners), returning items to a store, or high-pressure performance situations such as giving a speech. Often the most feared social situation includes genuine social evaluation, such as interviewing for a job or asking someone out on a date. It is important that the exposure hierarchy include the most feared situations.

Recall that patients with social anxiety overestimate both the *probability* and the *costs* of embarrassment and negative evaluation. Exposures therefore need to provide patients with corrective learning for both of these concerns. Social tasks in which the patient attempts to behave competently are useful in demonstrating that the patient is unlikely to act in a foolish manner. However, it is also important for socially anxious individuals to learn that the social cost of actually making a mistake or appearing anxious is less than expected and manageable. Indeed, exposures in which patients deliberately commit social mishaps may be the single most effective strategy in the treatment of social phobia (Hofmann & Otto, 2008). Thus, we recommend that early exposures consist of situations in which the patient attempts to behave normally or competently. As these initial hierarchy items are mastered, more anxiety-provoking exposures to making mistakes and appearing anxious can be conducted. In our experience, patients rarely volunteer ideas for such exposures, thus providing creative therapists an opportunity to design appropriate exposure tasks. Table 9.3 lists suggested expo-

TABLE 9.3. Examples of Exposure Exercises for Social Concerns

Type of concern	Exposure stimuli
Being in public	Shop in a crowded store, attend a concert or sporting event, read in a public place, work out at a gym, walk in a public place and make eye contact with others
Being the center of attention	Answer a question in class, drop change in public, speak loudly, wear unusual or out-of-place clothing (e.g., sombrero, mismatched outfit), join an aerobics class
Interacting with others	Speak to strangers, ask others for the time, strike up conversations with store employees, attend a social event, have friends over for a get-together, speak to friends on the phone, join a club or organization
Performing in front of others	Exercise in a crowded gym, give a speech, make a toast, eat alone in a crowded restaurant, sign a check or fill out an application with others watching, speak up at a meeting, interview for a job
Displaying anxiety reactions in front of others	Interact with others or go to a public place (1) while stuttering, pausing, or mumbling; (2) immediately following vigorous exercise; (3) with water splashed on armpit area of shirt to simulate sweating; (4) with hands noticeably trembling or shaking
Conflict	Return an item at a store, send food back at a restaurant, drive slowly in the left lane, pretend to forget money when purchasing an item, slowly use an ATM machine with others waiting
Appearing foolish in front of others	Ask for directions to an obvious location, order an item at a restaurant that is obviously not on the menu, incorrectly answer a question in class, purposely mispronounce a word during a conversation, slip or fall down while walking in a crowded area, drop a handful of coins on the floor in a shopping mall, attempt to purchase an item without sufficient money, engage a stranger in a conversation while trying to be as boring as possible or while making foolish statements, stand at a urinal in a public restroom and feign the inability to urinate (for male clients), call out the floors while riding in a crowded elevator

sure exercises for different kinds of social fears, including actually appearing foolish in front of others.

Interoceptive exposure exercises may also be beneficial for patients who fear the social consequences of appearing anxious in the presence of others. Tasks such as hyperventilation, running, breath holding, or caffeine ingestion may be conducted prior to entering social situations or in social situations themselves. For example, the patient might run on a treadmill in a crowded gym or hyperventilate immediately prior to initiating a conversation with a stranger. Other feared anxiety-related reactions, such as hand tremors or stuttering, may be simulated by the patient during situational exposures. See Chapter 11 for more information regarding interoceptive exposures.

CONDUCTING EXPOSURE THERAPY SESSIONS

Exposures to some social situations may be conducted in a prolonged manner until the patient's anxiety has habituated. For example, tasks such as eating alone at a restaurant, walking in a crowded area, and feigning the inability to urinate in a public restroom may be performed until the patient's anxiety has sufficiently decreased. However, many situational exposures involve relatively brief interactions with others. Exposures such as asking strangers for the time, filling out an application, and dropping change in a crowded lobby are quite brief and may last only a few seconds. In such cases, the patient's SUDS should be assessed following each trial, and the task should be repeated (perhaps in different situations) until the patient's anxiety has habituated. Each different exposure can be used as a test of the patient's beliefs and expectations, and changes in these cognitive phenomena should be tracked and discussed.

Practically speaking, it may not be possible to conduct therapist-assisted exposures to social situations that cannot be replicated in the therapeutic setting. Exposure to speaking at work meetings, answering questions in class, and speaking with coworkers at a holiday party must be conducted by patients on their own. Creative therapists may generate in-session tasks to approximate social situations that otherwise could only be conducted as homework assignments. Toward this end, we find it useful to enlist the help of colleagues to serve as conversational partners or audience members. In this manner, patients may practice exposures such as asking an attractive person out on a date or interviewing for a job in a relatively safe setting prior to conducting them in the real world. An additional benefit of using confederates is that they may, if desired, provide the patient with objective (and encouraging) feedback about his or her performance during the task.

Exposure therapy for social phobia is often conducted in groups. Compared to individual therapy, group treatment offers several advantages. These include the ability to implement a host of *in vivo* exposures in the therapy setting using group members as confederates, opportunities for patients to receive support and feedback from other group members, and the fact that attendance at therapy sessions by itself constitutes a potentially valuable form of exposure. Conversely, group treatment necessarily involves less individualized therapist attention for each patient, as well as fewer opportunities for in-session exposures owing to the need to allow patients to take turns conducting exposures during the treatment. Research indicates that both group and individual treatment for social phobia are effective. The choice of whether to implement group or individual treatment may be based on practical factors such as the ease of simultaneously recruiting sufficiently large numbers of patients to implement group therapy.

The tendency of socially anxious patients to focus on themselves rather than their surroundings in social settings has the potential to interfere with learning during exposure tasks. Patients whose attention is concentrated on their speech or anxious arousal may fail to observe that others did not pay attention to them while walking through a crowded lobby, or that others appeared more sympathetic than critical after they spilled a drink. The following dialogue illustrates the process of preparing a 34-year-old patient with social phobia for an exposure task:

THERAPIST: The exposure task we planned for today involves approaching strangers and asking them for the time. Are you ready to do this?

PATIENT: I think so, yes.

THERAPIST: Great. Before we start, let's talk about what you'll be doing and what you'll be able to learn from this. As we discussed, you'll be conducting this exposure in the walkway that connects our clinic with the hospital. There will be a lot of busy people walking quickly on their way to meetings and appointments. Your job will be to approach several people, walk up to them, and ask, "Excuse me, do you know what time it is?" You'll be wearing your watch, and remember that there is a big clock right near where you'll be standing. How does that sound?

PATIENT: A little scary. They'll probably be mad at me for wasting their time with such a dumb question.

THERAPIST: Perhaps, perhaps not—who knows? That's why you're doing this exposure—to learn whether or not bad things happen in this particular social situation. Try to be specific: What is it *exactly* that you're afraid will happen during the exposure?

PATIENT: Other people will be angry at me. They'll think I'm stupid.

THERAPIST: All right, so those are the negative outcomes that concern you. I want you to think of this exposure as an experiment that allows you to test whether or not other people get angry at you, and think you're stupid, for asking them for the time. Sound good?

PATIENT: Okay.

THERAPIST: We should also consider the possibility that at least one person might actually be upset with you, or say mean things to you. If this happens, you will be able to see if this is really as terrible as you anticipate. So, this experiment will allow you to learn two things: (1) *whether or not* other people get angry at you and think you're stupid when you ask them for the time, and (2) *if this actually happens,* how bad it really is. Does this make sense?

PATIENT: Yeah. Just like we did with my last exposure when I said "Hi" to people in the lobby.

THERAPIST: Exactly. And just like last time, in order for you to learn from the experiment, you have to be able to figure out what the outcome was. How did other people react to you? Did your predictions come true? Your job—and mine too since I'll be standing nearby—will be to try to figure out whether or not the people you speak to are angry with you or think you're stupid. Since we're not in the business of mind reading, how can we tell how they're reacting to you? What should we look for?

PATIENT: They might not stop because they're too busy. If they stop and tell me what time it is they might seem annoyed.

THERAPIST: What would it look like if they seemed annoyed?

PATIENT: They might frown, shake their head, roll their eyes—you know, look angry. Maybe they'll point to my watch or the clock and ask me why I couldn't figure out the time for myself.

THERAPIST: Great! We'll be on the lookout for those things. We'll watch their faces and body language, and see what kinds of things they say to you. We'll try to ignore what we *think* they're feeling about you, and focus instead on how they *behave* toward you. Sound good?

PATIENT: Yeah.

THERAPIST: One last thing. We've discussed your tendency to focus on yourself when you're feeling anxious in social situations. You pay attention to your voice and whether or not you're sounding awkward or unintelligent, and you pay attention to your hands to see if they're shaking. Can you see a problem if you do that during this exposure?

PATIENT: Well, it's hard to notice how other people are reacting if I'm so focused on myself.

THERAPIST: Right. The only way for you to learn from this exposure is to notice how other people are reacting to you. That means you need to make eye contact with them as you speak, listen to what they say, and pay attention to their facial expressions and body language. That way, you'll be able to tell whether or not they were angry with you or thought you were stupid. Are you ready to begin?

IMPLEMENTING RESPONSE PREVENTION

The lives of socially anxious persons are often dominated by avoidance. Exposure therapy is effective to the extent that patients are able to implement the cognitive and behavioral skills learned during exposure sessions into their daily lives. This requires patients to gradually fade their avoidance behaviors, as well as the numerous in-situation safety behaviors they use in social contexts. Some safety behaviors, such as avoiding eye contact, are often used in *every* social context. Their continued presence may hamper clinical improvement by interfering with corrective learning during all exposure tasks conducted prior to their elimination.

Safety behaviors designed to reduce social anxiety are often subtle and may not be discernable to the therapist or in some cases even to the patient. Examples include avoiding eye contact, speaking softly, wearing baggy clothing, rehearsing what is to be said, and deflecting conversation topics away from oneself. Even apparent acts of conscientiousness and kindness, such as arriving early for therapy sessions, offering compliments, or failing to be assertive when one has been slighted, may be veiled attempts to prevent negative evaluation. Therapists should be on the lookout for subtle safety behaviors and discuss them with the patient. Given the interpersonal nature of many safety behaviors, therapists should also be aware of the patient's use of them in therapist–patient interactions. When they occur, the therapist should highlight the suspected safety behaviors and reinforce successful efforts to resist them. Consider the example of a 44-year-old patient with social phobia who habitually arrived 15 minutes early for therapy sessions. After discussing this safety behavior with the therapist, the patient arrived 5 minutes late for the subsequent session, an act praised by the therapist (but not encouraged to become a habit!).

HINTS, TIPS, AND POTENTIAL PITFALLS
Comorbid Depression

Depression often co-occurs with social anxiety and can intensify concerns about being rejected, decrease motivation, and impair learning during exposure (Wilson & Rapee, 2005). When patients present with both social anxiety and depression, the therapist should carefully consider which problem to address first. If depression appears to be the result of the patient's social anxiety, the therapist should consider targeting the social fears first. Hofmann and Otto (2008) recommend several strategies for conducting exposure therapy for patients with both of these problems. For example, exposure tasks should be devised that provide an opportunity for fun, such as seeing a movie with a friend. Therapists should consider prescribing nonsocial activities that might promote feelings of well-being (i.e., behavioral activation), such as physical exercise. Additional cognitive restructuring may be required to assist patients who have difficulty processing the outcome of exposure tasks or acknowledging their progress in therapy.

Social Skills Deficits

Individuals with social phobia tend to appraise their social performance skills overly negatively, often doubting their ability to create desired impressions and meet the perceived expectations of others. However, there is little evidence that most persons with social phobia have bona fide social skills *deficits* (Stravynski & Amado, 2001), and their occasionally unskilled social behavior may be a product of the negative cognitions, physiological arousal, and safety behaviors associated with social anxiety. Accordingly, exposure therapy does not typically include techniques for directly modifying social skills as a matter of course. Such techniques are usually considered unnecessary given that exposure tasks provide patients with frequent opportunities to practice their social skills, and by the end of treatment most patients perceive themselves as having improved interpersonal and performance skills.

In some cases, however, socially anxious individuals do exhibit deficits in their communication skills. Habitual avoidance of interpersonal interactions and use of in-situation safety behaviors may deprive especially fearful individuals from the opportunity to practice basic social skills such as making eye contact, maintaining a conversation, and exhibiting appropriate body language. In such instances, the default assumption is that the patient likely has the capacity to exhibit appropriate social behaviors, but is inhibited from practicing and applying them because of his or her social anxiety. For such individuals, exposure tasks may be used both as a means to test feared predictions and to practice applying social skills. Prior to conducting exposure tasks, the patient may benefit from rehearsing the appropriate use of relevant social skills such as how to initiate a conversation, make appropriate eye contact, speak at an appropriate volume, manage body language (e.g., smiling), compromise, and make assertive comments.

Therapist Social Anxiety

In our experience, it is not uncommon for patients with social phobia to ask their therapist to model exposure tasks. Such requests may be motivated by fear or hesitancy to conduct an exposure. In other cases, patients find it helpful to have the therapist model how they are supposed to behave during a social interaction. As such, therapists must be both willing and able to perform exposure tasks with manageable levels of anxiety. In our work with many socially anxious individuals, we have engaged in social mishaps while modeling exposures, such as mumbling unintelligibly during conversations with strangers, spilling drinks, dropping coins on the floor in crowded malls, posing bizarre questions to others (e.g., asking for a map and directions to the current location), and dressing in unusual and conspicuous ways. Such exposures are somewhat embarrassing and sometimes anxiety-provoking, but our willingness to conduct them, and our ability to do so while appearing outwardly calm, has facilitated treatment on numerous occasions. Social anxiety is common, even among therapists, and not all treatment providers are prepared to engage in such behaviors. Thus, we propose that therapists tackle some of their own social concerns via exposure prior to treating patients with social phobia. Doing so may avoid awkward conversations in which the therapist has to explain why the patient needs to engage in behaviors that the therapist him- or herself is unwilling to perform.

CASE ILLUSTRATION

Maria was a 24-year-old medical student who, after being teased and taunted throughout her childhood, suffered from severe, generalized social phobia. She had developed a lifestyle characterized by social isolation and avoidance of interpersonal interactions, including attending a university where the classes were large and she could remain relatively unnoticed. An excellent student, Maria was admitted to a small medical school where she found it impossible to remain anonymous. Professors frequently called upon her to answer questions and classmates socialized often and invited her to accompany them. Toward the end of her first semester, she took a medical leave of absence and sought treatment for her social anxiety.

Information gathered during the functional assessment revealed that Maria was afraid others would notice her visible symptoms of anxiety, particularly sweating. She believed that others paid close attention to her, would easily notice these "imperfections," and would mock and ridicule her as a result, or think that she was incompetent. Maria employed a range of safety behaviors, including wearing loose-fitting clothing to mask sweating; excessively rehearsing her speech; avoiding eye contact; and avoiding as many social and interpersonal situations as possible. Fortunately, Maria was highly intelligent and clearly understood the cognitive-behavioral model of social anxiety presented by the therapist at the end of her first session. She was highly motivated for treatment and wanted to return to her classes as soon as possible.

Following the first and second sessions Maria completed daily self-monitoring forms to assist her in understanding the connection between her exaggerated beliefs, body sensations, anxious feelings, and safety behaviors. A clear pattern emerged in which anxiety-related body sensations prompted her to predict negative evaluation, which in turn resulted in escalating anxiety, use of safety behaviors, and ultimately in the conviction that she had narrowly escaped ridicule once again. Maria was encouraged to consider the evidence from her own experience regarding the accuracy of her feared predictions, and she reported that others had actually *not* overtly mocked or ridiculed her since high school (although she attributed this to her avoidance and use of safety behaviors). Exposure was described as an opportunity for Maria to learn whether the reactions she expected from others based on her early life experiences were still occurring.

The second half of the third session was spent creating an exposure hierarchy. Items were generated on the basis of the functional assessment as well as the therapist's suggestions about how to target the social cost of appearing foolish. At the same time, a list was generated of safety behaviors to eliminate. Maria was encouraged to begin fading them on her own and was informed that once exposures began she would need to try to eliminate them, to the extent possible, from her daily life. The final exposure hierarchy was as follows:

Description of the exposure task	SUDS
Making eye contact with strangers	50
Eating lunch alone in crowded restaurant	60
Asking strangers for the time	70
Having conversations with strangers	80
Dropping change in crowded place	90
Making foolish statements to strangers	95
Having others notice her sweaty armpits	100

The first exposure took place during the fourth session. Maria and the therapist simply walked around the hospital lobby. She was encouraged to hold her head up and make eye contact with others. She was surprised to note that others seemed to be paying her little attention, and those who did make eye contact with her often smiled. Daily homework assignments for the upcoming week consisted of walking in shopping malls and crowded stores while making eye contact with others. During the following session, the therapist accompanied Maria to the food court of a local shopping center. Maria ordered lunch, sat by herself, and ate in the presence of several dozen people. Her anxiety habituated after approximately 25 minutes and she once again reported that few people seemed to take notice of her.

Session 6 involved exposure to asking people for the time in a busy hospital walkway. After successfully approaching four strangers, she reported minimal anxiety. The therapist, however, observed that she had chosen relatively "safe" people to approach (e.g., older women, people who appeared not to be in a hurry) and instructed her to continue the exposure by approaching people who seemed to be in a rush and might be irritated by having to stop and answer her question (e.g., doctors dressed in scrubs). During the following session, the therapist accompanied Maria to three different hospital waiting rooms. She was asked to approach individuals sitting by themselves and initiate a conversation by discussing the weather. Although initially quite anxious, her SUDS had decreased to 20 following seven interactions. Maria noted that others had generally seemed pleased to talk with her; despite having stumbled in her speech on several occasions, she did not observe any obvious signs of criticism or rejection.

Maria and the therapist spent the following session dropping a large handful of coins in a crowded hospital lobby. The therapist offered to model the exposure for Maria, who was initially quite anxious and reluctant to conduct the task. After observing that several people helped pick up coins dropped by the therapist, Maria agreed to attempt the task on her own. She dropped coins on six occasions, in six different places, during the next hour. In each case, others helped her pick up the coins and not a single person overtly mocked or ridiculed her. Other people noticed and stared, of course, which permitted Maria to test the severity of acting foolishly and being the center of attention. Her anxiety habituated following the fourth exposure and by the last trial she reported enjoying the task and having to suppress laughter.

The final two exposure sessions involved Maria deliberately acting in a foolish manner during social interactions. In session 9, the therapist accompanied Maria to a shopping mall and modeled two interactions in which he asked a store employee for items that were obviously not in the store. Maria subsequently conducted five exposures in which she asked restaurant employees in the food court how much it cost to order baklava (none served this dessert). For the final exposure session, Maria wore a tight, gray T-shirt and doused her armpits with water from a restroom sink. She and the therapist traveled to the hospital lobby where she initially walked alone for 10 minutes and later asked strangers for the time and initiated several brief conversations. Her SUDS decreased from 90 to 10 after 50 minutes of exposure. At this point, she reported being confident that others were generally unconcerned with her and were unlikely to notice, or seemingly to care very much about, her social behavior. She also reported that acting in a foolish manner wasn't all that bad, and was even "kind of fun." Treatment was terminated following the next session, and Maria returned to medical school shortly thereafter.

ADDITIONAL RESOURCES

Heimberg, R., Liebowitz, M., Hope, D., & Schneier, F. (Eds.). (1995). *Social phobia: Diagnosis, assessment, and treatment.* New York: Guilford Press.

Hofmann, S. G., & Otto, M. W. (2008). *Cognitive behavioral therapy for social anxiety disorder.* New York: Routledge.

Hope, D., Heimberg, R., & Turk, C. (2008). *Managing social anxiety: A cognitive-behavioral therapy approach* [therapist guide]. New York: Oxford University Press.

Kearny, C. (2004). *Social anxiety and social phobia in youth: Characteristics, assessment, and psychological treatment.* New York: Springer.

10

Unwanted Intrusive Thoughts

CLINICAL PRESENTATION

For some individuals, anxiety and fear are provoked by negative, senseless, bizarre, or repugnant unwanted intrusive thoughts (UITs) that may take the form of ideas, images, doubts, and urges that persist despite efforts to avoid, control, or neutralize them (see Table 10.1). A clear example of these is *obsessions* as defined in the DSM diagnostic criteria for OCD. Obsessions primarily (but not exclusively) concern violence, sex, religion, mistakes, and the possibility of being responsible for causing (or not preventing) harm. Table 10.2 provides examples of obsessional thoughts in these various categories. Another example of UITs is the uncontrollable worry and doubt over unlikely disasters often observed in people with GAD. Examples of common worries are listed at the bottom of Table 10.2. Memories of traumatic events represented another type of anxiety-provoking UITs, which we discuss in Chapter 13.

Whereas worries usually involve catastrophic thoughts about low-probability events that have a basis in real-life circumstances (e.g., being fired from one's job, relationship troubles, financial woes), the content of obsessions is usually uncharacteristic of the individual's normal tendencies and might represent the complete antithesis of his or her moral or ethical standing (e.g., an impulse to behave violently or to yell profanities). In the case of obsessions, the individual fears the presence, significance, and consequences of having the UIT (e.g., "I might act on the thought"; "I'm an immoral person for thinking this"; "I must be crazy because of my senseless thoughts") and concludes that he or she must take action to control or dismiss the thought, or prevent feared disastrous consequences that could result (e.g., Rachman, 1997, 1998; Salkovskis, 1996).

In the effort to prevent feared consequences of UITs or to reduce the

TABLE 10.1. Quick Reference Overview: Anxiety-Provoking Intrusive Thoughts, Images, Worries, and Doubts

Fear-evoking stimuli
- Obsessional thoughts, images, and doubts
- Uncontrollable worries and doubts

Prototypical examples
- Thoughts of stabbing a loved one
- Blasphemous or sacrilegious thoughts
- Thoughts of unwanted or inappropriate sex acts
- Worry about losing one's job, a relative's health, or incurring financial loss

Safety behaviors
- Mental neutralizing or undoing
- Thought suppression
- Checking, reassurance seeking, analyzing the purpose of thoughts
- Worrying as a problem-solving strategy

DSM-IV-TR diagnostic categories
- OCD
- GAD

Treatment overview
- Typical length: 14–20 sessions
- Begin with assessment and psychoeducation
- Use cognitive therapy techniques to challenge beliefs about thoughts and worries
- Begin exposure by session 3 or 4
- Implement response prevention along with exposure

Obstacles
- Elusive mental rituals
- Exposures with therapist could provide reassurance
- Naturally brief situational exposures
- Conflicts with religious faith
- Fears of negative consequences that cannot be known

thought itself and its associated discomfort, individuals with UITs may resort to various sorts of safety behaviors, including mental rituals (e.g., replacing "bad" thoughts with "good" ones), praying, checking, and seeking reassurance. They might also repeat simple behaviors (e.g., going through a doorway, flipping a light switch) while trying to dismiss the thought until the activity can be completed without the UIT. Those with persistent doubts and worries may also use distraction or reassurance-seeking strategies to reduce their distress (e.g., calling someone on the phone, checking). However, some individuals with GAD use worry as a coping mechanism—that is, as a way of trying to analyze or solve the problem (Borkovec & Roemer,

TABLE 10.2. Examples of Obsessional Thoughts, Images, Doubts, Worries, and Impulses

Theme	Examples
Harm and violence	• Thought of drowning the baby in the bathtub • Thoughts of pushing an innocent bystander into traffic • Images of loved ones in awful accidents • Impulse to hit someone with a wine bottle • Doubt about a hit-and-run car accident • Thoughts of loved ones dying • Thought of opening the emergency exit of an airplane • Thought of harassing or murdering a loved one • Doubt that one mistakenly poisoned someone else • Thought of attacking a family member or pet in their sleep
Sexual	• Thoughts of having sex with a relative • Urge to stare at a woman's chest • Impulse to touch a baby's genitals • Doubt about one's true sexual preference ("Am I gay?") • Unwanted image of having sex with a stranger
Religious	• Thought of desecrating a place of worship • Impulse to curse God • Doubt about whether one's religious faith is "strong enough" • Images of burning in hell and punishment from God • Thought that God is very upset with you • Doubt about whether one has committed a sin • Blasphemous thoughts (e.g., "God is dead") • Sacrilegious images (e.g., Jesus masturbating) • Doubt about whether one acted immorally
Mistakes	• Doubt whether important paperwork was completed properly • Thought of causing a house fire because you left a light or appliance on or running • Thought of causing a burglary because you left the door unlocked • Doubt whether you sufficiently warned people of a hazard • Doubt that maybe you offended someone by mistake
Miscellaneous worrisome thoughts	• A loved one getting injured or in an accident • Losing one's job and becoming very poor • Losing one's good health • "What if my romantic partner breaks up with me?"

1995; Davey, Tallis, & Capuzzo, 1996). They may believe that worrying helps prevent negative outcomes or prepare for the worst-case scenario (Freeston, Rheaume, Letarte, Dugas, & Ladouceur, 1994).

Often, UITs are triggered by stimuli in the environment, such as knives, curse words, certain people, and situations. Avoidance of such cues is therefore common. For example, one man complained of unwanted sexual thoughts about Jesus. He believed it was immoral to have such blasphemous thoughts and that he would be punished if he did so. Thus, he tried to control or stop the thoughts by thinking about positive spiritual things (e.g., picturing a large cross), avoiding religious icons that triggered the thoughts, and repeating prayers for forgiveness. He also refrained from telling anyone else about his thoughts.

Because the safety behaviors used by individuals with UITs are often covert (e.g., mental rituals, thought suppression), as opposed to overt (e.g., washing or checking), some clinicians label this problem "pure obsessions" (e.g., Baer, 1994), which implies that *only* obsessional thoughts are present. Yet, as we have discussed, safety behaviors are nearly always present as well. It is just that the types of safety behaviors used to neutralize UITs can be difficult to detect because they might be very subtle or take place only in the person's mind. This highlights the importance of careful assessment for such phenomena (as we discuss later in this chapter). Moreover, even experienced clinicians sometimes find it a challenge to distinguish the anxiety-*provoking* intrusive thoughts and worries from the anxiety-*reducing* mental rituals and worrying that serves as distraction or as a coping mechanism.

BASIS FOR EXPOSURE THERAPY

Theoretical Considerations

Current cognitive-behavioral models of obsessional problems (e.g., Rachman, 1997, 1998; Salkovskis, 1996) are very useful for understanding UITs. Numerous studies have documented that nearly everyone in the general population experiences negative, unwanted thoughts, ideas, doubts, or images (e.g., Rachman & de Silva, 1978; Salkovskis & Harrison, 1984). Moreover, the thoughts of healthy individuals concern the same topics experienced by individuals with clinical obsessions and worries. Thus, clinically severe UITs are thought to originate from normal intrusive negative thoughts. Specifically, normal intrusions are thought to develop into clinically severe problems when a person misinterprets such thoughts as very significant or threatening.

To illustrate, consider the unwanted idea of stabbing a loved one in his or her sleep. Most people experiencing such an intrusion would regard it as a meaningless cognitive event with no harm-related implications (i.e., "mental noise"). Yet such an intrusion can develop into a clinical obsession if the person appraises it as having serious consequences (e.g., "This thought means I'm a dangerous person who must take extra precautions to make sure I don't hurt anyone"). Such appraisals evoke distress and motivate the person to try to suppress or remove the unwanted thought (e.g., by replacing it with a "good" thought), and to attempt to prevent harmful events associated with the intrusion (e.g., by sleeping in a different room or by hiding the knives). Thus the "problem" is not the UIT, but the *undue importance* that the individual places on such thoughts.

Safety behaviors such as avoidance of external cues, cognitive avoidance (i.e., thought suppression), mental rituals, checking, trying to analyze the meaning of the thought, and reassurance seeking are conceptualized as efforts to reduce anxiety, prevent feared consequences, or control or neutralize the UIT itself. Yet because these behaviors sometimes engender an immediate reduction in anxiety and a temporary reprieve from the UIT, they become habitual. Unfortunately, however, these behaviors prevent the person from learning that his or her UITs are not dangerous or significant and that safety behaviors are unnecessary to prevent feared catastrophes. Safety behaviors also increase the frequency of intrusive thoughts by serving as reminders, thereby triggering their reoccurrence. Attempts at distracting oneself from an unwanted thought, for example, often paradoxically increase the frequency of intrusions. Seeking reassurance and analyzing the implication of thoughts leads also to greater preoccupation with possible negative consequences. Thus, the very strategies used by the person in response to the UITs end up backfiring in different ways, thereby completing a vicious cycle.

Implications for Exposure Therapy

Since UITs are fundamentally normal and harmless intrusive thoughts, treatment must incorporate exposure to such thoughts as well as their triggering stimuli. The aim, therefore, is not to remove the UIT per se, but to weaken the connection between such thoughts and anxiety by helping the patient (1) consider UITs as senseless mental noise rather than as significant and threatening, and (2) learn to manage acceptable levels of uncertainty, risk, and doubt associated with the UITs. Response prevention must entail dropping safety behaviors so that the patient can learn that such responses are not necessary for preventing feared consequences or reducing anxiety.

FUNCTIONAL ASSESSMENT

Table 10.3 includes a summary of the information likely to be obtained from a functional assessment of UITs. Next, we discuss the assessment of each parameter in detail.

TABLE 10.3. Functional Assessment of Intrusive Thoughts at a Glance

Parameter	Common examples
Fear cues	
External situations and stimuli	Objects, situations, people in the environment that serve as reminders of intrusive thoughts and worries
Internal cues	Sensations associated with anxious or sexual arousal, the physical "urge" to act
Intrusive thoughts	Repugnant or distressing intrusive thoughts, images, impulses, doubts, and worries regarding violence, sex, immorality, sacrilege, mistakes, accidents, health, and harm to self or others
Feared consequences	Fear of acting on the intrusive thought. Fear that the thought's presence means it is realistic. Fear that thinking will make it so. Fear that thinking the thought reveals some deep-seated negative trait about oneself. Fear that others would be shocked or horrified if they knew about the content or frequency of the thoughts.
Safety behaviors	
Avoidance patterns	Situations and stimuli that trigger intrusive thoughts or worries (e.g., horror movies, cemeteries, certain words and sounds)
In-situation safety behaviors	Trying to "undo," "cancel," or suppress thoughts (i.e., neutralizing), rituals (overt or covert), reassurance seeking, analyzing, distraction, worrying as a coping strategy
Beliefs about safety behaviors	Safety behaviors are necessary to prevent feared consequence(s) from occurring; anxiety-provoking thoughts must be neutralized or completely eliminated; worry is useful in preparing for, preventing, and/or coping with feared outcomes

Fear Cues

External Situations and Stimuli

UITs are often triggered by stimuli in the environment. For example, seeing a police officer's gun might cue a violent thought. Learning about an incoming ice storm might trigger worries about a loved one getting into a car accident on the way home from work. Other common external triggers include horror movies, funerals, sexual or erotic stimuli, specific people, words (e.g., *murder*), numbers (e.g., *13*), and religious icons. One OCD patient with UITs about the devil was afraid of anything related to the Tampa Bay *Devil Rays* baseball team. He even avoided items associated with the city of Tampa (e.g., postcards). A heterosexual woman with obsessional doubts that she was becoming a lesbian was afraid of lingerie stores (e.g., Victoria's Secret) because of the possibility of seeing attractive women and experiencing thoughts such as "She has a nice figure." Still another patient's unwanted thoughts of harming his newborn daughter were evoked by holding the child or bathing her in the bathtub.

UITs concerning harm and mistakes might be triggered by routine activities such as leaving the house ("What if I left an appliance on and a fire starts?") or turning off a light switch ("What if I only *imagined* turning it off?"). Other possible cues include driving (fear of hitting pedestrians), seeing one's boss ("What if I get fired?"), discarding junk mail (fear of throwing away something important), going to work ("What if I made a mistake and I get in trouble?"), seeing broken glass (thoughts about being responsible for injury), or completing paperwork (thoughts of mistakes). For one patient who worked as a teacher, grading her students' papers provoked worries that she might assign a bad grade by mistake and "ruin a child's life." Most individuals are aware of the external triggers that provoke their UITs.

Internal Cues

UITs can be accompanied by distressing physical responses—for example, some individuals experience what seem like *urges* to act on their violent intrusions. One man with UITs of strangling his father reported the feeling of his hands being drawn to the elderly man's neck. Another individual interpreted his escalating feelings of anxious arousal as an indication that he was about to give in to the unwanted urge to drive his car off the road. A different type of internal cue that sometimes occurs along with unwanted sexual intrusions is the perceived feeling of sexual arousal. Some individuals report the unwanted feeling of a "sexual rush" or the beginning of an erection (in men) that accompanies unacceptable sexual thoughts.

From the therapist's perspective, these sensations are not cause for alarm: in and of themselves, they do not indicate the *desire* to act. Rather, they're best considered as innocuous responses to which the patient is hypervigilant. To patients, however, these sensations are often quite alarming: they may be interpreted as confirmation that the unwanted intrusive thought is significant or dangerous. It is best to normalize such experiences and inquire about them in a direct and dispassionate way—for example, "Sometimes when people have unwanted sexual obsessions, they actually have sexual *feelings* along with their thoughts. For example, you get a feeling in your penis when an unwanted image of molesting your child comes to mind. That might seem very scary—tell me about your experiences with these kinds of feelings."

Feared Consequences

As alluded to earlier in this chapter, UITs are often catastrophically misap-praised as personally significant or as signs of some deeply rooted personal failing. Thus, someone with UITs of violence, sex, or blasphemy might fear that he or she is (or is *becoming*) someone he or she is not (and would not want to become)—for example, a cruel, deviant, perverted, depraved, evil, or immoral *person*. He or she might fear punishment from God for think-ing "immoral" thoughts, or be concerned that he or she will impulsively act on his or her sexual or violent intrusions and impulses. For example, "If I don't control my thoughts about incest, I will lose control and rape my brother." Others fear that their intrusive unwanted thoughts about some-thing unpleasant mean that deep down they really *want* something awful to happen (e.g., "Thinking about molesting children means I want to molest a child").

For some people, the consequences of UITs are that bad things will hap-pen to *others*—for example, the fear that merely *thinking* about an awful event (e.g., images of one's grandchildren dying in a car accident) could cause the corresponding events to occur. Often, the individual feels a sense of personal responsibility to prevent the feared catastrophes from occurring, even those over which the person has little control. For example, one man feared he was personally responsible for the space shuttle *Challenger* explo-sion in 1986 owing to his failure to perform a ritual (counting to a certain number) after having an unwanted premonition of an explosion.

Often, the *uncertainty* regarding the meaning, significance, and out-come of negative UITs is very anxiety-provoking, for example, not knowing whether UITs about worshipping the devil will lead to eternal damnation. Doubts about whether one is "completely heterosexual" or "definitely in love" with his or her spouse or partner might trigger distress over not being able to definitively confirm (i.e., with 100% certainty) such things. Interest-ingly, for most people with problems tolerating uncertainty, the UITs con-cern circumstances that cannot really be objectively confirmed (e.g., going to heaven or hell). In these instances, the lack of a guarantee is a feared con-sequence in and of itself. Finally, some individuals fear that the anxiety (and the fight–flight response) associated with UITs will continue indefinitely or spiral "out of control" once triggered.

In Chapter 4, we discussed methods of assessing feared consequences, yet there are a number of self-report (paper-and-pencil) questionnaires that have been developed to assess fears and beliefs associated with UITs in par-ticular. These include the Interpretations of Intrusions Inventory (Obsessive–Compulsive Cognitions Working Group, 2005) and the Thought–Action

Fusion Scale (Shafran, Thordarson, & Rachmen, 1996). For patients with religious obsessions, the Penn Inventory of Scrupulosity (Abramowitz, Huppert, Cohen, Tolin, & Cahill, 2002) assesses the fear of committing sins and catastrophic beliefs about divine punishment.

Safety Behaviors

Avoidance Patterns

In an effort to prevent their feared consequences, individuals with anxiety-provoking UITs typically try to avoid situations and stimuli that serve as reminders of their intrusions—for example, knives, certain people, places of worship, religious icons, cemeteries, sexual cues, cue words, movies, and shows. They may avoid situations in which they fear acting on unwanted impulses, such as driving on a busy street, bathing a child, or using a knife while standing near a loved one.

Individuals with doubts about harm or mistakes may avoid situations and activities in which they perceive that they could be responsible for causing or preventing harm. The clinician should use knowledge of situational triggers and the UITs themselves to guide the assessment of avoidance behavior, as this is usually intuitive. Specific examples include driving, using the oven, writing bank checks, and being in charge of locking up the house (e.g., the last person to go to bed or to leave the house). Some avoidance is subtler, such as not driving near school busses for fear of hitting children. One patient avoided listening to music or watching television while she wrote or typed on the computer because she was afraid that the distraction would lead to mistakenly writing obscenities. Another tried to avoid exposure to all obscene words or gestures for fear that he might use them inappropriately.

In-Situation Safety Behaviors

Therapists should assess for the presence of *neutralizing*, defined as "undoing" the unwanted intrusive thought. The purpose of neutralizing behavior, which is often subtle and covert, is to put matters right—to reduce the moral discomfort associated with a repugnant UIT or impulse and/or to reduce the likelihood or severity of a feared consequence (Rachman & Shafran, 1998). Examples include trying to suppress or dismiss the thought, saying a prayer, repeating a safe phrase or number, or "canceling out" the unacceptable thought with a "good" thought. When neutralizing strategies are repeated to excess, they become mental rituals. It is important for the clinician to keep in mind the distinction between recurring UITs (i.e., obsessions) and recurring mental strategies intended as neutralizing responses (i.e., mental rituals).

Mental rituals can be assessed by asking questions such as, "Sometimes people with obsessional thoughts use mental strategies such as repeating special 'safe' words, phrases, prayers, or images to themselves to 'cancel out' their obsessions. Can you tell me about your experiences with these kinds of strategies?" Some patients mentally review their behavior or analyze particular events over and over to reassure themselves of the invalidity of their UITs (e.g., trying to reason through whether or not they are likely to act on an unwanted thought). A variation is "testing," wherein the person tries to collect some sort of evidence that feared consequences of UITs are improbable. For example, one heterosexual woman with UITs that she was becoming a lesbian repeatedly looked at men while focusing attention on her internal state to make sure she could still feel sexually aroused.

Patients with distressing thoughts and doubts may engage in overt rituals as well, such as repeating routine activities. For example, one man had to put his clothes on the "correct way," otherwise he feared his thoughts of family members dying would come true. Often he would dress and undress multiple times because he didn't feel the ritual had been done properly, or the thought was still present in his mind. The link between repeating rituals and fears of disasters is not always intuitive and may seem magical or superstitious. Other examples include having to tap a certain number of times or to go through doorways the "correct" way in response to having a UIT. In some instances, the number of times the ritual can (or can't) be performed is determined by lucky or unlucky numbers (e.g., even numbers, multiples of 5). We have also observed patients who perform washing rituals to "wash their UITs away" as if feeling contaminated by them (moral contamination). Thus, it is therefore important to assess for a range of possible safety behaviors by asking questions such as, "What else do you do when these unwanted thoughts come to mind?" and "how do you deal with these thoughts?"

Compulsive checking and reassurance-seeking rituals are the chief methods of relieving anxiety and uncertainty over intrusive doubts. Checking is typically related to the patient's feared consequences (e.g., being responsible for harm) and may occur in the home (locks, appliances) and elsewhere (driving, at work). Clarify the frequency and duration of checking rituals and inquire about whether the checking involves visual inspection, touching whatever is being checked (e.g., to make *certain* the light switch is in the off position), or the involvement of other people. Other examples include checking that someone has not been hurt (e.g., watching the news), checking for mistakes (e.g., in paperwork or e-mail messages), and checking that one did not do anything awful or egregious (e.g., "Did I use a racial slur in conversation?").

Reassurance seeking, which can be thought of as "interpersonal checking," is also a common method of reducing distress over disturbing UITs, specifically those that provoke doubt and uncertainty. Patients may repeatedly ask questions of others (e.g., "Do you think I am a good enough Christian?"), look up information on the Internet (e.g., about whether people with OCD kill their children), and repeatedly seek out advice from different "experts" to gain a guarantee regarding the likelihood of feared consequences. Some individuals confess their obsessional thoughts to others as a way of gauging their response or to warn them of the presence of such thoughts. Reassurance-seeking behavior can be subtle or overt and should be assessed very carefully. Some individuals do not recognize that it is even related to their problem with UITs.

Some individuals use worrying as a safety behavior. Used in this way, worry might function to distract the person from his or her feared consequences. It might serve as a way of further analyzing the situation to either determine the likelihood of a "worst-case scenario" or to come up with a solution in case the worst possible consequences do occur.

Beliefs about Safety Behaviors

People with UITs often become quite attached to their safety behaviors. Not only might such behaviors provide a temporary respite from UITs and anxiety, but they become viewed as the *reason that* feared consequences have not materialized. Other types of positive beliefs about safety behaviors include viewing worry as helpful with analytical thinking, helping to prepare for the worst-case outcome, and minimizing the impact of negative events should they occur (e.g., Freeston et al., 1994).

In some cases, the connection between a safety behavior and the consequence it is intended to prevent is obvious, as when the person who fears hitting a pedestrian avoids driving. In other cases, however, patients have idiosyncratic and often illogical beliefs about the manner in which safety behaviors prevent disaster. For example, one woman believed that repeatedly counting to 18 prevented her son from suffering a fatal car accident. Assessment of beliefs about safety behaviors, including *how* they are perceived to prevent harm, can prove useful when implementing exposure and response prevention. Cognitive therapy may be used to assist patients in more accurately appraising the degree to which their safety behaviors actually prevent feared consequences (which are unlikely to begin with). Exposures can also be framed as experiments that test the power of certain safety behaviors; in the example above, the woman who repeatedly counted was able to learn that this behavior was in fact unnecessary to prevent a car accident.

PRESENTING THE RATIONALE
FOR EXPOSURE THERAPY

Although the general conceptual model of anxiety problems that we presented in Part I applies to the case of intrusive thoughts, ideas, images, and doubts, it may be a challenge for the patient (and perhaps even the therapist) to apply this model to fears of intrusive *thoughts*. Thus, when helping the patient to understand his or her problems with UITs, the therapist should draw from the information presented earlier in this chapter in the section on theoretical considerations. Specifically, we recommend the following approach:

• Begin by normalizing the experience of UITs. Explain that research shows that over 90% of the population experiences the exact same kinds of unwanted, unpleasant intrusive thoughts, doubts, impulses, images, and concerns. Sometimes these thoughts come from "out of the blue," although they may also be triggered by specific situations.

• Have the patient read over (and then discuss) Figure 10.1, which is a list of intrusive thoughts reported by people *without* clinically severe obsessional or worry-related problems (i.e., OCD or GAD). Help him or her make a connection between his or her UITs and those reported by healthy people. The therapist might also disclose some of his or her own UITs to reinforce this point.

• Clarify the implication of normal intrusive thoughts: there is nothing strange, immoral, or otherwise *bad* about thinking UITs, or about the person who thinks them.

• Explain that people with obsessional and worry-related problems experience their intrusive thoughts and doubts more *frequently* and more *intensely* because they appraise these thoughts as overly significant.

• Explain how problems with UITs involve a vicious cycle that includes misinterpreting the meaning and importance of normal intrusive thoughts and doubts, leading to anxiety. To reduce anxiety, the person tries to control or get rid of the thought, seek reassurance, or prevent any feared consequences associated with the thought. Yet these strategies lead to greater preoccupation with the intrusive thought.

• Review the conceptual model presented in Figure 10.2. Then illustrate the vicious cycle using specific examples from the patient's repertoire of thoughts, interpretations, and safety behaviors.

• To further demonstrate the futility of trying to control intrusive thoughts, ask the person to try *not* to think of a white bear. (What's the first thought that comes to mind?) Explain that the white bear thought represents the person's UIT.

• Discuss exposure therapy as a way of reversing the vicious cycle. Instead of running away from intrusive thoughts and anxiety, the patient will practice *confronting* them. Explain exposure as a way of gradually

FIGURE 10.1. Actual intrusive thoughts reported by people without anxiety problems.

- Thought of jumping off the bridge into the highway below
- Thought of running car off the road or onto oncoming traffic
- Thought of poking something into my eyes
- Impulse to jump onto the tracks as the train comes into the station
- Image of hurting or killing a loved one
- Idea of doing something mean toward an elderly person or a small baby
- Thought of wishing that a person would die
- Impulse to run over a pedestrian who walks too slow
- Impulse to slap someone who talks too much
- Thought of something going terribly wrong because of my error
- Thought of having an accident while driving with children
- Thought of accidentally hitting someone with my car
- Image of loved one being injured or killed
- Thought of receiving news of a close relative's death
- Idea that other people might think that I am guilty of stealing
- Thought of being poked in eye by an umbrella
- Thought of being trapped in a car under water
- Thought of catching diseases from various places such as a toilet
- Thought of dirt that is always on my hand
- Thought of contracting a disease from contact with person
- Urge to insult friend for no apparent reason

- Image of screaming at my relatives
- Impulse to say something nasty or inappropriate to someone
- Impulse to do something shameful or terrible
- Thought that I left door unlocked
- Thought of my house getting broken into while I'm not home
- Thought that I left appliance on and cause a fire
- Thought of sexually molesting young children
- Thought of poking the baby's soft spot
- Thought that my house burned and I lost everything I own
- Thought that I have left car unlocked
- Thought that is contrary to my moral and religious beliefs
- Hoping someone doesn't succeed
- Thoughts of smashing a table full of crafts made of glass
- Thoughts of acts of violence in sex
- Sexual impulse toward attractive females
- Thought of "unnatural" sexual acts
- Image of a penis
- Image of grandparents having sex
- Thought about objects not arranged perfectly
- Thought that God is upset with me

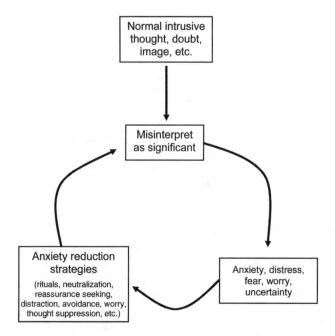

FIGURE 10.2. Cognitive-behavioral conceptual model of the vicious cycle that maintains obsessions and worries.

helping the patient confront distressing thoughts and trigger situations that are not objectively dangerous.

• Instead of trying to neutralize or cancel out the intrusive thoughts, he or she will use response prevention, the purpose of which is to teach the patient that safety behaviors are not necessary for anxiety reduction or to prevent feared disasters.

• Provide examples from the patient's repertoire of possible exposure and response prevention exercises and discuss the process of habituation as illustrated in Chapter 5.

DEVELOPING THE EXPOSURE HIERARCHY

It can be helpful to think of problems with UITs as similar to a "phobia of thoughts." Thus, the exposure hierarchy should incorporate primary imaginal exposures in which the individual repeatedly thinks the fear-provoking UIT, as well as *in vivo* exposure to situations and stimuli that evoke these intrusions. For example, if the unwanted thought to yell curse words is evoked by visiting libraries (i.e., where one is supposed to be quiet), exposure should involve going to a library and thinking of curse words without engaging in any avoidance or safety behaviors. The aim of this exercise is not to desensitize patients to the idea of acting inappropriately, but to help the sufferer learn that *thinking about* acting inappropriately is not what causes inappropriate behavior, and therefore avoidance and safety behaviors are unnecessary. Table 10.4 includes suggestions for imaginal and situational exposures for various common types of intrusive thoughts and doubts.

Written narratives and recorded audio describing anxiety-evoking scenes are the best methods of systematically exposing individuals to distressing UITs. This promotes habituation to the intrusion and modifies erroneous beliefs about the importance of, and need to control, them. Examples of imaginal exposure for violent obsessions include confronting progressively more disturbing images of killing loved ones in a blood bath. Situational exposures might include handling potential weapons such as knives (perhaps beside a sleeping baby or spouse), viewing violent movies, reading books about violence, or saying and writing words associated with violence (e.g., the patient writes *murder* on an index card and keeps it in her pocket).

Sexual UITs

For individuals with unacceptable homosexual intrusions, imaginal exposure might include images of engaging in homosexual behavior. Situational exposure might involve viewing homoerotic literature or pornography and visiting a gay bar. Similarly, for someone with unwanted sexual thoughts about animals, children, or incest, imaginal exposure should involve thoughts of such activities. Ideas for situational exposure include interacting with animals, watching children on playgrounds, seeing one's child naked, glancing at (or *noticing*) relatives' crotches, and the like.

Religious UITs

Religious obsessions present challenges for exposure therapists since the individual's religious and social environment may reinforce beliefs about the significance of such thoughts. Hierarchy items might include situations that provoke intrusive thoughts that may be *perceived* as blasphemous or immoral, but which are not necessarily condemned by religious authorities. For example, a person who is afraid of experiencing blasphemous thoughts while reading the Bible should read the Bible and purposely think the unwanted thoughts (e.g., "God doesn't exist"). Other examples

TABLE 10.4. Examples of Exposure Exercises for Different Types of Intrusive Thoughts and Doubts

Type of intrusion	Situational exposure stimuli	Imaginal exposures
Harming or killing loved ones	Knives, guns, other potential weapons, potential victims, "planning" to kill someone, write a story about killing, cemeteries, funeral homes, morgues	Vivid images of killing loves ones; doubts about whether thinking leads to acting; ideas of being a violent person
Thoughts of harming someone with a car	Driving—gradually move from easier situations to more difficult ones (e.g., bumpy roads, crowded with pedestrians), varying the level of distraction (e.g., radio, passenger)	Images or doubts of hitting someone, the person is injured on the road and it's the patient's responsibility, the police show up with an arrest warrant for vehicular homicide and leaving the scene of an accident
Blasphemy and sacrilege	Religious icons, places of worship, religious authority figures, situations in which sin or violation is *possible*	Blasphemous thoughts, doubts about whether God is angry, doubts about whether a sin or violation has been committed
Homosexuality	Homoerotica, gay people, textbook images of genitalia, locations frequented by gay people, pictures of models (e.g., magazines), words (*gay, penis*, etc.), opportunities to observe members of the same sex (e.g., gym, pool)	Images of engaging in homosexual behavior, doubts about sexual preference, thoughts of "coming out" to one's family
Sexual molestation and incest	People who are the target of the thoughts (e.g., children, relatives), pictures of these people, schoolyards	Thoughts, stories, and images of sexual contact with family members or children
Making mistakes at work	Make a small clerical error on purpose, work with loud music	Thoughts and doubts about the consequences of an error
Relative having a car accident	Relative goes out for a drive and doesn't come home on time	Worrisome thoughts and doubts about accidents, going to the emergency room, death, etc.

include reading books about atheism, reading satanic literature, and viewing religious icons that evoke unwanted intrusions (e.g., a statue of the Virgin Mary). We've worked with individuals who conducted exposure to UITs such as images of Jesus masturbating on the cross and of desecrating places of worship. The nature of these exposures requires that the treatment rationale be clearly explicated to the patient. If this is misunderstood, or the therapist is perceived as insensitive, the patient may view therapy as an assault on his or her religion. We explain to devoutly religious patients that although exposure might seem impious, its intent is to increase one's *faith* that God understands what's in the patient's heart and that intrusive thoughts (or other feared sins) are not intentional acts of blasphemy or sacrilege.

Intrusive Doubts

Exposure for intrusive doubts about responsibility for harm and mistakes should involve (1) confronting situations in which the patient fears becoming responsible for harm, (2) imagining the feared consequences, and (3) refraining from safety behaviors. If the individual is afraid of fires, exposure can involve leaving lights and appliances on while departing the home. Alternatively, switches can be turned off rapidly and without checking. Fears that one will cause bad luck can be addressed by having the patient do whatever he or she fears might cause bad luck—for example, by writing phrases such as "I wish Mom would get cancer." If patients are afraid of harming pedestrians while driving, they can drive in crowded places without checking the rearview mirror. Obsessions about making mistakes with paperwork can be confronted by working very quickly without rechecking for accuracy (perhaps with distractions as well). Each of these situational exposures should be followed by secondary imaginal exposure to being responsible for the feared consequences (or not knowing for sure whether the consequences will occur). This prolongs the exposure, facilitates habituation to the feeling of uncertainty, and helps the patient learn that he or she can manage uncertainty.

Worries

Exposure for persistent worries about situations and events that are remote either in probability or severity (e.g., losing one's job and being "out on the street") can be conducted using imaginal exposure in which the worrisome doubts, images, or thoughts are confronted. A hierarchy of gradually more distressing scenes can be generated for this purpose.

CONDUCTING EXPOSURE THERAPY SESSIONS

An important technique in the treatment of anxiety-provoking obsessions and worries is primary imaginal exposure using a digital voice recorder, loop cassette tape, or written scripts describing the distressing intrusions. When intrusions are triggered by specific external stimuli, these should be incorporated as situational exposures as well. For example, a patient who avoids knives for fear of thinking about killing her newborn infant might practice holding or using a knife (situational exposure) and purposely thinking about infanticide (primary imaginal exposure). The following is an example of how such an exercise might be introduced:

> THERAPIST: We've talked about your intrusive, distressing images of stabbing your baby, Ashley. You said these images often come to mind when you are with Ashley and you see a knife or anything sharp; and that you try to push the thoughts away or resist them; but that this doesn't work because the thoughts keep returning. So, as we have also talked about, today I'm going to help you learn a new and more helpful strategy for dealing with these thoughts. Do you remember what this strategy involves?
>
> PATIENT: Yes, you said I would have to purposely confront the bad thoughts.
>
> THERAPIST: That's right. It is actually helpful to practice having these kinds of thoughts on purpose repeatedly, and not engaging in any avoidance or reassurance seeking. When you practice this, you'll at first experience anxiety, but in time you'll find that your anxiety will diminish even if you don't push the thought away. As we have talked about, anxiety will naturally subside if you give it enough time. In the end, you'll weaken the connection between the upsetting images and anxiety. Do you see what I mean?
>
> PATIENT: Okay, I'm willing to give this a try since nothing else I've done to get rid of the anxiety has worked.

The therapist and patient worked together to come up with a script based on an earlier functional assessment. The patient read the script into a digital voice recorder (which can be purchased at most office supply stores for under $100):

> "Ashley is only 2 months old. I love her so much. She's so sweet and innocent. She's small and cuddly. I've been extra careful not to let anything happen to her. She's a wonderful little baby. But as much as I love her, I can't resist acting on my thoughts of murdering her, which seem to

always come to mind when I see a knife. ... I lose my self-control, take a knife from the drawer. I hold Ashley like I'm going to feed her, but instead I grab the knife and start slicing her neck. At first she screams and kicks in pain, but then there's no more noise. It's just blood gushing everywhere. ... I'm sitting there with her lifeless body on my lap and blood covering both of us. What have I done? Our precious baby—I've killed her! I wish I could rewind time, but I can't. What have I done? What have I done? My husband will be home in an hour. What will he do? How will I tell my friends and family that I murdered my child!?"

THERAPIST: Okay, great job. I know that was hard for you. How are you doing?

PATIENT: Oh, gosh. I'm very anxious right now. My SUDS is about 95.

THERAPIST: Okay. I know this is difficult. Your job is to try to make friends with this distressing thought. Allow it to hang out in your brain. Remember the anxiety will come down, but you have to give it time. Meanwhile, just allow yourself to think about the distressing idea. Remember, do not try to push it away. Work on accepting it as a distressing but senseless intrusive thought.

The patient then practiced listening to the intrusive thought using the digital voice recorder until her discomfort subsided to 50% of its initial level. She was reminded to engage the thought, keep a vivid mental image, and allow herself to experience the anxiety that it provoked, rather than distract or avoid thinking about it. Some patients do not report the characteristic reduction in SUDS, yet still appear as if they are no longer anxious (e.g., reduction in muscle tension, change in facial expression). We help patients draw the analogy between imaginal exposure and watching a scary movie. When we watch a horror film for the first time we might feel very scared. But if one were to watch the movie 100 times, it would become much less frightening. The habituation that occurs during imaginal exposure works in much the same way.

The distressing thought or image can be described by either the patient or the therapist, and there are pros and cons to consider regarding this choice. An advantage of having the patient take the lead is that he or she knows the UITs best and can therefore produce a scenario that best matches the intrusive thought or image as it is experienced. A disadvantage, however, is that the patient might avoid including the most distressing material in the exposure. Thus, the therapist must make sure the scene incorporates the patient's *worst* fears. Another consideration is that a self-generated script might seem more like "thinking" to the patient—especially if the patient is listening to his or her own voice on a tape recorder. If the patient is too fearful of creating the exposure script him- or herself, the therapist might create an initial script with the goal being for the patient to eventually do this him- or herself.

Depending on the specific content of the UIT, some exposures can be conducted completely in the clinic; examples include confronting knives, writing "unlucky" numbers, and completing important paperwork while being distracted. In other cases, it is necessary to conduct the situational exposure *outside* the office. Examples include accompanying the patient to his or her home to practice bathing a child, driving to confront fears of hitting pedestrians, and going to a funeral.

IMPLEMENTING RESPONSE PREVENTION

All safety behaviors—overt and covert—performed in response to UITs should be targeted in response prevention. Of special concern are mental rituals: urges to mentally cancel, review, replace, neutralize, analyze the meaning of, or suppress UITs. Special prayers in response to blasphemous or violent images should be ended. Patients with sexual obsessions must stop reviewing their sexual history or closely monitoring their body for signs of sexual arousal from unwanted stimuli (a covert form of reassurance seeking). Those patients who engage in worrying as a safety behavior must be helped to engage in the UIT, rather than use cognitive avoidance or "problem-solving" strategies.

Overt safety behaviors that serve to reduce uncertainty or the perceived probability of disastrous consequences should also be targeted. Examples include checking, asking for assurance, picking up hazards from the ground, reporting potential hazards to others, retracing steps, counting, making lists, and confessing. If checking involves simply *looking* (e.g., staring at a light switch or lock to make sure it's off or locked), the frequently checked objects can be covered or masked (e.g., with a piece of paper) to obscure them from view. For patients afraid of making mistakes, paperwork can be checked once (briefly), but without the use of spelling- or grammar-checking software. Seeking information or advice that has already been given should also be halted.

When ritualistic prayers, worrying, distraction, and other mental neutralizing strategies are difficult to stop all together, the patient can, as a preliminary step, be helped to purposely perform these safety behaviors *incorrectly*, or in a way that leads to feeling uncertain about feared consequences. Examples include praying "incorrectly" (or to the wrong deity), counting incorrectly or to the wrong number, and purposely "remembering" actions incorrectly. Family and friends should be instructed not to respond to requests for assurance, but instead to help the patient get through the temporary anxiety (e.g., "I know how hard it is for you, but your anxiety will go down if you stick it out. What can I do to help you get through this?"). Family members must also refrain from performing safety behaviors by proxy. Further information regarding family support is covered in Chapter 18.

HINTS, TIPS, AND POTENTIAL PITFALLS

Model Confidence with Imaginal Exposure

The therapist should exude confidence and remain calm and collected when discussing distressing, repugnant, worrisome, and otherwise objectionable thoughts, images, and doubts, and when suggesting (and implementing) exposure to these stimuli. Demonstrating conviction that such thoughts are ordinary and innocuous, and that exposure is likely to be helpful, increases the odds that the patient will agree to confront these stimuli and buy into the treatment rationale. A therapist's willingness to self-disclose his or her own UITs can be useful in this regard. On the other hand, if patients sense that the therapist is put off, offended, or shocked by UITs, they may be reluctant to fully engage in exposure.

Pay Close Attention to Mental Rituals

Mental rituals tend to occur along with UITs, and a common mistake *for both the patient and the therapist* is to confuse UITs (e.g., obsessions) with mental rituals (i.e., compulsions)—after all, both are cognitive in nature and therefore quite intangible. This highlights the importance of making sure it is understood that UITs are *involuntary* thoughts that *provoke* anxiety and mental rituals are *deliberate* thoughts that *reduce* anxiety.

Because of their elusive nature, some mental rituals can be difficult for the patient to resist. The therapist, therefore, should continually assess the patient's success with response prevention since the persistence of mental rituals will attenuate treatment effectiveness by impeding habituation. Because thinking UITs is incompatible with neutralizing them with mental rituals, the best form of response prevention for mental rituals is more exposure to the UIT (i.e., "Think the unpleasant UIT instead of the mental ritual"). Imaginal exposure can therefore be used as both exposure *and* response prevention. As a back-up plan, mental rituals that cannot be resisted may be performed incorrectly.

Pay Attention to the Perception of Responsibility

As is sometimes the case with exposure to other types of fears, the therapist's (or anyone's) presence during exposure to UITs can invalidate the exercise if the patient is able to transfer responsibility for any feared negative outcomes to the therapist (e.g., "The therapist wouldn't let me kill my son"). It is therefore wise to directly ask patients about whether your presence makes the exposure "easier" and whether performing the exposure without supervision would be more "realistic." For example, a patient with obsessional thoughts of harming her cat was afraid she would lose control and act on these thoughts. When this patient and her therapist conducted an exposure to holding a knife up to the cat, the patient said that she didn't feel anxious because she believed the therapist wouldn't let her murder the pet. Therefore, the therapist left the room so that the patient felt fully responsible for the feared outcome and could see that her anxiety declined despite having no one to stop her from acting on her UIT.

Use Imaginal Exposure to Prolong Naturally Brief Situational Exposures

Some situational exposures for UITs and doubts will necessarily be brief and will exclude the repetition of the same task within a single session. For example, locking the door and leaving the house takes only a few seconds, but repeating this activity (or prolonging it) would equate to de facto checking and reassurance seeking that the door is locked. Thus, instead of repeating such exercises multiple times during a single exposure session, the situational exposure should be followed by procedures to help the patient confront UITs and uncertainty associated with not checking. Secondary imaginal exposure to the feared consequences is the best way to accomplish this goal. Thus, the patient would leave the house and then imagine *not* having locked the door, which leads to a burglary. The patient also practices response prevention so that he or she learns to manage obsessional doubts and uncertainty without performing safety behaviors.

When Fears Concern Negative Consequences That Cannot Be Known

Some individuals present with UITs with feared disastrous consequences that won't occur for many years to come—for example, the fear of going to hell *when one dies* for thinking blasphemous thoughts. Others have obsessive doubts about matters that simply cannot ever be known. For example, "What if someone repeated my dirty joke to a child and I'm responsible for their 'corruption'?" or "What if the cumulative effect of my many brief exposures to cleaning products is that I will gradually become brain-damaged?" In such instances, exposure exercises should be designed to weaken the anxiety associated with *uncertainty*. Situational exposure exercises can incorporate situations and stimuli that arouse feelings of uncertainty; and imaginal exposure should focus on *not knowing for sure* whether the feared consequence will happen. Such exercises will facilitate habituation to, and help decatastrophize, feelings of uncertainty.

Exposure and Response Prevention with Religious Patients

Conducting exposure and response prevention with devoutly religious patients presents unique challenges. Differences between normal and pathological religious practice must be clarified and patients should understand that the purpose of exposure treatment is to restore normal religiosity. Patients with religious obsessions often hold catastrophic views of God as petulant, easily angered, and vengeful, which is inconsistent with most religious doctrine. According to most religions, people have not sinned unless they (2) intentionally decide to do things they know are evil (e.g., murder someone) and (1) remain remorseless. Therefore, *unwanted* thoughts, ideas, or images do not count as violations. The therapist can also point out to religious patients that if God created the human mind, then God understands that people sometimes have thoughts that are contrary to their true beliefs. The case should be made that exposure therapy will help the patient become a more faithful follower of his or her religion since it will help him or her to trust that God understands this. Thus, confronting blasphemous or "immoral" UITs as exposure exercises should be acceptable if the aim is to reduce suffering and if God already understands that these thoughts are not what is in the person's heart. However, the patient must learn how to have *faith* that God understands this. The implication here is that safety behaviors, such as reassurance seeking, praying, and asking for forgiveness, are unnecessary and must be dropped. God doesn't require such apologies or prayer in this case.

We often use the following metaphor to convey this message:

"Imagine you are pet sitting for a neighbor who has provided detailed instructions for how to take care of her dog: feed Spot at 8:00, take him for a walk at 10:00, feed him again at 12:00, play with him at 2:00, feed him dinner at 5:00, and so on. Now, suppose your neighbor keeps calling you (from her vacation) several times each day to remind you to do each of these activities and to make sure her dog is okay! How would you feel? Wouldn't this get on your nerves? How much does your neighbor really trust you if she keeps calling you like this? What does it say about how much faith she must have in you? Now, imagine that you are God in this scenario, and your neighbor is you. Do you see the parallel? Does God need to be reminded so many times of something God already knows? Wouldn't this get on God's nerves? What does this mean about your own faith?"

Informing patients that for centuries theologians have prescribed strategies similar to exposure and response prevention for people with religious obsessions is another way to encourage religious individuals with UITs to undertake exposure. Indeed, training manuals for pastoral counselors specifically recommend suggesting to people with scrupulosity that they purposely act *contrary* to their scruples (Ciarrocchi, 1995). Specific guidelines include (1) emulating conscientious people even if doing so might violate the religious rule in question, (2) allowing oneself to purposely evoke "impure" thoughts, and (3) disavowing oneself of repetitive confessions and redundant prayer (Jones & Adleman, 1959). Ciarrocchi's (1995) self-help book on scrupulosity (*The Doubting Disease: Help for Scrupulosity and Religious Compulsions*) presents an excellent discussion of this topic and is a useful resource for helping strictly religious patients who are highly ambivalent about engaging in exposure therapy.

Many religious patients will ask to consult with a religious authority (e.g., priest, rabbi) to seek assurance that it is allowable to do certain exposure exercises that are perceived as violating religious rules. We suggest allowing only a single consultation (only if absolutely necessary) and only if the patient agrees that the authority's suggestions will be followed without the pursuit of further advice or second opinions, which would constitute reassurance seeking. If exposure can be conducted by relying on what religious authorities have *previously* told the patient, this is ideal.

Deciding on the specific situations for exposure is also a delicate issue. Instructions to flagrantly violate religious laws are neither appropriate nor necessary to reduce problems with sacrilegious UITs. Exposure should entail situations that evoke doubts and uncertainty about sin, but that are not actual violations. As an analogous situation, consider a patient with OCD who has an obsession that that her food might be contaminated with urine. Her pathological anxiety involves uncertainty over whether or not her food is contaminated, not what to do when there is urine on food. Therefore, rather than actually putting urine on her food, exposure would involve taking risks such as eating meals in bathrooms. Accordingly, exposure for scrupulosity should evoke *uncertainty*, without subjecting the patient to blatant religious violations.

Very religious patients who suffer from unacceptable thoughts may also need help differentiating between healthy religious behaviors, on the one hand, and safety behaviors that masquerade as religious observance, on the other. Whereas the former need not be targeted in the response prevention component of treatment, if the latter persist, treatment cannot be maximally helpful. We urge therapists to show respect and understanding for patients' religious beliefs even if such beliefs are not shared. The patient, however, should be helped to see that some of their "religious" behavior is actually part of what maintains the problem with UITs. Whereas it will be perceived as an assault on religion to simply insist that the patient stop what might be perceived as important religious observances, a suggested approach is to have a dialogue that helps the *patient* make this point, as in the following example:

> THERAPIST: It sounds like you often turn to prayers for managing your obsessions. In other words, to get rid of your unwanted sexual thoughts.
>
> PATIENT: Yes. God is the only one who can save me from all my immoral thoughts and make them go away.
>
> THERAPIST: And what effects do the prayers have on the obsessions? Does praying make the thoughts go away?
>
> PATIENT: Well, if they worked, I wouldn't be *here*.
>
> THERAPIST: What do you mean? Tell me more about that.
>
> PATIENT: Even though I'm always praying to stop the thoughts, I'm still having them as much as ever. I think that lately they've even become worse, if anything.
>
> THERAPIST: Interesting. So what you're saying is that despite all your prayers, the obsessions have intensified. What do you think that says about praying as a strategy for managing obsessional thoughts?
>
> PATIENT: Hmm. (*Thinks to himself.*) I never looked at it *that* way before.
>
> THERAPIST: I know that prayer is important for you, and that it makes you feel closer to God. But since you are telling me that praying *about the obsessions* hasn't worked very well, would you consider learning a different strategy when it comes to dealing with these thoughts?
>
> PATIENT: Well, my pastor did say that I pray too much about the wrong things. Maybe he was right.

We also suggest allowing the patient to help with sorting out which religious behaviors could be labeled as safety behaviors and which as part of healthy religious practice. Religious behavior motivated by obsessional thoughts is not technically "religious." Such behavior is "fear-based" rather than "faith-based." Therefore, effective treatment will help the patient practice his or her religion in a more healthy way (without obsessive fear). The assistance of family members and religious authorities who can reinforce the distinction between healthy and unhealthy religious practice may be necessary for implementing response prevention for such patients.

CASE ILLUSTRATION

Matt was a 45-year-old devoutly religious (Catholic) man with OCD whose obsessions focused on senseless doubts that he might have impregnated a former girlfriend (Sally), who *could* have ended up having an abortion, which is strictly outlawed in the Catholic faith. Although Matt and Sally never actually had sex, Matt reported that once while hugging and kissing Sally (while fully dressed), he had experienced an erection, which triggered the intrusive doubt. Matt fully recognized the senselessness of his obsessions and Sally had denied having any abortions. Still, he engaged in compulsive reassurance seeking to reduce the distress associated with his UITs. Matt feared that he would go to hell for not doing enough to stop Sally from having an abortion (if she in fact had even become pregnant from Matt, or aborted this pregnancy). Matt's rituals included persistently questioning Sally about whether she had had an abortion, trying to check her work attendance records during the period he suspected it might have occurred, and asking mutual acquaintances if they knew whether Sally had ever become pregnant or had an abortion. To be on the safe side, he also prayed to God for forgiveness just in case an abortion had actually occurred. Functional analysis revealed that Matt's obsessions were triggered by seeing babies, words such as *sex* and *abortion*, and by anything that reminded him of Sally. He was avoiding these triggers as much as was possible.

Matt's exposure hierarchy was as follows:

Description of the exposure task	SUDS
Pictures of babies	55
Words: abortion, sex, Sally	65
Pictures of Sally	70
Images of Sally being pregnant with Matt's baby	75
Images of Sally having an abortion	75
Idea that God is very angry at Matt	80
Ideas of going to hell for not preventing an abortion	90

Matt's response prevention plan was as follows:

- No asking questions for assurances
- No reviewing attendance records from Sally's workplace
- No praying for forgiveness regarding a possible abortion

During the first exposure session, Matt's therapist helped him view pictures of babies, which provoked worrisome doubts that Sally might have had an abortion. Matt allowed these doubts to sit in his mind without using cognitive avoidance strategies. He put pictures of babies around his house and his office so that exposure was continual. These exposures provoked moderate levels of distress for Matt, which he was able to handle well. He observed that his SUDS levels decreased more quickly with each planned exposure.

During the second session, Matt added exposure to the words *abortion*, *Sally*, and *sex*. He said these words and wrote them several times on sheets of paper that he kept in his wallet. Although distressed at needing to confront these words, Matt was able to manage the temporary anxiety that they triggered. Homework practice included repeating these exercises daily. After 4 days of constant exposure, the words provoked only minimal anxiety.

At session 3, Matt viewed pictures of Sally and allowed himself to wonder whether she was pregnant with his baby. He conducted a secondary imaginal exposure to these doubts and images as well. Because Matt understood the rationale for exposure, he was willing to face these distressing stimuli despite his heightened level of anxiety. He also had the benefit of successes with his earlier exposures.

During the fourth session, Matt completed a primary imaginal exposure to images of Sally having an abortion. He practiced confronting these images between sessions 4 and 5. At session 5, he confronted ideas that God was very upset with him for not doing enough to prevent Sally from having an abortion. This particular thought evoked a great deal of distress at first. Matt, however, chose to persist with his work, and after practicing with this thought for 1 week, he felt more confident that such thoughts were "just mental noise."

Next, he moved on to imaginal exposure to thoughts and images of being "damned to hell" for not preventing the abortion. This exposure focused on the uncertainty associated with heaven and hell, eternal damnation, and judgment. These exposures also provoked intense distress at first, yet Matt was able to recollect his experiences with previous exposure exercises and recognize that these particular exercises weren't likely to be any different. Through exposure, Matt learned that although he couldn't know for sure what would happen to him when he died, he could manage the uncertainty.

ADDITIONAL RESOURCES

Abramowitz, J. S. (2006). *Understanding and treating obsessive–compulsive disorder: A cognitive-behavioral approach*. Mahwah, NJ: Erlbaum.

Abramowitz, J. S. (2008). Scrupulosity. In J. S. Abramowitz, D. McKay, & S. Taylor (Eds.), *Clinical handbook of obsessive–compulsive disorder and related problems* (pp. 156–172). Baltimore: Johns Hopkins University Press.

Abramowitz, J. S., & Nelson, C. A. (2007). Doubting and checking concerns. In M. M. Antony, C. Purdon, & L. Summerfeldt (Eds.), *Psychological treatment of obsessive–compulsive disorder: Fundamentals and beyond* (pp. 169–186). Washington, DC: American Psychological Association Press.

Clark, D. A. (2004). *Cognitive-behavioral therapy for OCD*. New York: Guilford Press.

Freeston, M. H., & Ladouceur, R. (1999). Exposure and response prevention for obsessive thoughts. *Cognitive and Behavioral Practice, 6*, 362–383.

Purdon, C. (2008). Unacceptable obsessional thoughts and covert rituals. In J. Abramowitz, D. McKay, & S. Taylor (Eds.), *Clinical handbook of obsessive–compulsive disorder and related problems* (pp. 61–77). Baltimore: Johns Hopkins University Press.

Rachman, S. (2003). *The treatment of obsessions*. Oxford: Oxford University Press.

Rachman, S. (2007). Treating religious, sexual, and aggressive obsessions. In M. M. Antony, C. Purdon, & L. Summerfeldt (Eds.), *Psychological treatment of obsessive–compulsive disorder: Fundamentals and beyond* (pp. 209–230). Washington, DC: American Psychological Association Press.

11

Bodily Cues
and Health Concerns

CLINICAL PRESENTATION

Concerns about bodily changes and sensations, overall health, and having a disease are common among anxious individuals. In some cases, patients misinterpret the presence of generally harmless somatic cues (e.g., a rash) as a sign of a terrible disease (e.g., skin *cancer*). Other individuals may believe that the presence of heart palpitations and shortness of breath indicates an impending heart attack. Among those with health-related concerns, presenting complaints typically focus on bodily signs or symptoms and their exaggerated feared consequences. Clinical health anxiety is excessive (i.e., more intense, frequent, and long-lasting) relative to the "normal" health-related concerns that most people experience and which can be adaptive in instances when a health risk is actually present.

Health concerns are central to a number of DSM diagnoses, including panic disorder (with or without agoraphobia), hypochondriasis, and a number of specific phobias (e.g., illness phobia). These diagnostic categories differ principally on three dimensions: (1) focus on immediate versus long-term feared health outcomes, (2) preoccupation with arousal-related (i.e., anxiety-related) versus non-arousal-related bodily cues, and (3) the belief that one either *currently* has or will *eventually* acquire a deadly disease. Generally speaking, hypochondriasis is characterized by the misinterpretation of non-arousal-related somatic cues (e.g., stomach pain) as indicating the presence of a terrible disease (e.g., cancer). Individuals with panic disorder and agoraphobia, on the other hand, typically worry that panic attacks themselves (i.e., the experience of intense arousal-related body sensations) indicate an imminent medical catastrophe such as death by suffocation. Illness phobia is marked by the concern that one will eventually acquire a deadly disease. Similarly, health concerns can be a prominent feature of OCD (i.e., the fear of contamination; see Chapter 12). Despite the separation of these diagnoses in the DSM, individuals often present with symptoms that cut across these categories. For example, one patient misinterpreted dizziness as signifying both an impending loss of consciousness and the presence of a brain tumor, and vacillated between worrying about acquiring cancer and believing she already had it.

Patients with health-focused anxiety often present with physical complaints and initially seek treatment in medical settings. They may repeatedly visit doctors, seek second opinions and additional medical tests, search health-related websites and medical texts, and solicit reassurance from others about somatic cues that have already been appropriately evaluated and judged to be benign (Olatunji et al., 2009). By the time they are referred to mental health professionals they may feel frustrated by what they perceive to be a persistent failure of treatment providers to identify a physical cause of their symptoms. Not surprisingly, they may express extreme skepticism when told that their problem is primarily psychological. Over time, these individuals often experience severe distress and substantial functional impairment (e.g., Katon & Walker, 1998; Leon, Portera, & Weissman, 1995). Table 11.1 provides a brief overview of the conceptualization and treatment of health-related anxiety.

BASIS FOR EXPOSURE THERAPY

Theoretical Considerations

A cognitive-behavioral account of health-focused anxiety begins with the observation that the bodily signs and symptoms feared by anxious individuals—dizziness, shortness of breath, aches and pains, fatigue, and so on—are ubiquitous and generally benign. Put another way, people have "noisy bodies." Whereas most individuals are relatively unconcerned with this somatic "noise," those with health-focused anxiety believe such bodily signs and symptoms have dire implications for their health—for example, that a headache signifies an impending stroke, that chest pain means the onset of a heart attack, and that nausea indicates the presence of a serious illness (Deacon & Abramowitz, 2008).

Individuals with such beliefs pay close attention to their bodies in order to detect feared somatic cues and prevent a possible health catastrophe (Schmidt et al., 1997). This "body vigilance," however, ensures that indi-

TABLE 11.1. Quick Reference Overview: Somatic Cues and Health Concerns

Fear-evoking stimuli

- Bodily signs and symptoms
- Public places from which it would be difficult or embarrassing to escape
- Potential sources of disease
- Information about diseases

Prototypical examples

- Heart palpitations, sweating, dizziness, shortness of breath, headache, fatigue, numbness
- Moles, skin blemishes, lumps, aches and pains
- Media reports about diseases

Safety behaviors

- Avoidance of physical activities or situations where a panic attack may occur
- Relaxation strategies, distraction, and prescription medication
- Excessive checking of one's body and medical information
- Seeking reassurance from family/friends and physicians
- Carrying safety aids such as cell phone, water bottle, medications

DSM-IV-TR diagnostic categories

- Panic disorder with or without agoraphobia
- Hypochondriasis
- Specific Phobia, Other Type (e.g., "Illness Phobia")

Treatment overview

- Typical length: 12 individual therapy sessions
- Begin with assessment and psychoeducation
- Use cognitive therapy techniques to challenge beliefs about the dangerousness of feared somatic cues
- Begin interoceptive exposure by session 3 or 4
- Begin situational exposure by session 6 or 7
- Combine imaginal and situational exposure
- Implement response prevention along with exposure

Obstacles

- Patient must recognize problem as psychological, not medical
- Patient may fear social consequences of somatic symptoms
- Sensitivity to context effects

viduals who fear particular nondangerous bodily signs become exquisitely sensitive to them and are therefore especially likely to notice them. Because of their mistaken beliefs about the meaning of bodily sensations, health-anxious individuals quickly respond to somatic cues by engaging in safety behaviors with the goal of preventing feared health catastrophes. Such behaviors come in many forms and include seeking reassurance from physicians, searching the Internet for health information, practicing relaxation exercises, seeking the presence of a "safe person," escaping from anxiety-provoking environments, and taking prescription antianxiety medication (i.e., benzodiazepines such as Xanax or Ativan). Patients also frequently avoid potential sources of disease, refrain from engaging in arousal-inducing activities (e.g., exercising), and excessively check their body for possible danger signs and symptoms. In agoraphobia, this avoidance extends to all places in which the person fears that anxiety or panic may occur, or in which help may not be immediately available (e.g., large crowds, rural areas). In the most severe instances, individuals with agoraphobia cannot leave home at all for fear of a panic attack. As discussed in Chapter 3, these maladaptive attempts to cope with anxiety paradoxically maintain (and even exacerbate) the problem, as the individual is unable to learn that the feared bodily cues are harmless.

Implications for Exposure Therapy

Based on the above framework, the primary goal of exposure therapy is to assist individuals in learning that the bodily cues they fear are (1) tolerable and (2) unlikely to lead to the feared catastrophic health consequences. Treatment proceeds by helping the patient intentionally experience the feared bodily cues and refrain from the use of safety behaviors. By doing so, he or she learns that the prolonged experience of feared body sensations does not lead to health catastrophes. The health-anxious person also gains experience tolerating the ambiguity and uncertainty associated with unexplained bodily sensations. That is, although the sensations are *most likely* just innocuous body noise, one cannot immediately obtain a *guarantee* that they do not represent something more serious. Lastly, patients learn to accept the *presence* of uncomfortable feelings, which is essential given that body sensations such as heart palpitations, shortness of breath, and unexplained aches and pains are normal and unavoidable (although they may be a nuisance). Individuals who strive to completely eliminate these experiences, or who demand an explanation for every bodily perturbation, are fighting a losing battle.

Depending on an individual's particular fears, treatment may incorporate a combination of interoceptive, situational, and imaginal exposure to address feared body sensations, external stimuli, and imagined health consequences, respectively. For people who fear that intense arousal-related body sensations will lead to immediate health catastrophes, exposure therapy may be able to completely disconfirm these maladaptive beliefs. For those who fear longer term or more gradual diseases such as AIDS or Alzheimer's disease, exposure may be more useful in helping them learn to tolerate the uncertainty associated with *not knowing for sure* whether such feared consequences will eventually occur. The above discussion, of course, assumes that the patient has been appropriately examined and deemed medically healthy.

FUNCTIONAL ASSESSMENT

Table 11.2 includes a summary of the information likely to be obtained from a functional assessment of health-related anxiety. Next, we discuss the assessment of each parameter in detail. It also is necessary to begin this assessment with a review of the patient's actual medial history to rule out actual organic illnesses.

Fear Cues

External Situations and Stimuli

Health concerns may be triggered by a wide variety of external stimuli. For patients with panic attacks who fear arousal-related body sensations, anxiety may be elicited by any situation or object with the potential to produce feared sensations. Examples might include strenuous physical activities, spicy foods, scary movies, amusement park rides, caffeine, and places where escape might be difficult (e.g., elevators) or embarrassing (e.g., crowded restaurants) in the event of anxiety symptoms. Other sorts of health anxiety may be triggered by media reports, television programs, books, and movies featuring specific diseases. Appointments with treatment providers may also be a source of great apprehension for individuals who fear the bad news they might receive.

Internal Cues

Arousal-related sensations most commonly feared by patients with panic attacks include heart palpitations, chest pain or pressure, shortness of breath, dizziness, sweating, feeling of choking, chills or hot flushes, trembling or shaking, nausea, numbness or tingling, and feeling detached from oneself or one's surroundings. These symptoms may be exacerbated when the individual becomes anxious, is under stress, or ingests a stimulant such as caffeine. Bodily signs and symptoms not generally exacerbated by the fight-or-flight response include musculoskeletal pain, fatigue, and skin anomalies (lumps, rashes, moles). Some patients exhibit a circumscribed fear of a particular sensation, like the 42-year-old man who presented with the sole concern

TABLE 11.2. Functional Assessment of Bodily Cues and Health Concerns at a Glance

Parameter	Common examples
Fear cues	
External situations and stimuli	Situations, environments, objects, and other stimuli that elicit feared body sensations or concerns about acquiring/having a disease
Internal cues	Arousal-related body sensations, body signs and symptoms
Intrusive thoughts	Recurrent thoughts and images of one's own death
Feared consequences	Imminent physical or mental health catastrophe, serious illness, or death due to a deadly disease
Safety behaviors	
Avoidance patterns	Situations and stimuli that elicit feared body sensations; situations and stimuli associated with the acquisition or reminder of feared diseases
In-situation safety behaviors	Arousal-reduction strategies, relying on a "safe person," carrying safety aids, body checking, searching for health information, excessive and unnecessary health care utilization
Beliefs about safety behaviors	Safety behaviors are necessary to prevent escalating body sensations from resulting in a health catastrophe; checking is useful in detecting a serious disease

that his perceived difficulty swallowing (despite no medical findings) meant that his throat was closing in, which would cause him to suffocate. More often, patients fear *multiple* internal cues and worry about the occurrence of *multiple* health catastrophes.

Intrusive Thoughts

Intrusive thoughts may also be part of the symptom presentation for patients who worry about the consequences of having a deadly disease. For such individuals, intrusive thoughts and images may involve themes of experiencing debilitating medical symptoms, death, and being alone for all eternity after life has ended (i.e., eternal consciousness).

Feared Consequences

Patients with health-focused concerns typically fear the occurrence of a physical or mental catastrophe. Such catastrophes tend to be either immediate or longer term in nature. Patients with panic attacks tend to be concerned with *imminent* health problems such as heart attacks, suffocation, stroke, vomiting, loss of control, or loss of consciousness, with the ultimate fear often (but not always) being death. Other concerns include permanent insanity, permanent disconnection from reality, and being negatively evaluated by others for publicly exhibiting anxiety symptoms. Individuals with other forms of health anxiety are often concerned about death or severe impairment due to a *progressive or long-term* problem (e.g., amyotrophic lateral sclerosis [ALS], Alzheimer's disease, cancer).

Safety Behaviors

Avoidance Patterns

Patients with health-focused anxiety tend to avoid situations and stimuli that might elicit their feared body sensations. Such avoidance ranges from staying off of amusement park rides to not leaving one's home altogether. Individuals with recurrent panic attacks may try to avoid the experience of physiological arousal at all costs by evading a broad range of activities that could induce such a state (e.g., sex, exercise, excitement, caffeine). Those who fear having a specific disease often avoid stimuli that serve as reminders, including people with the disease. Some patients avoid hospitals and medical examinations out of concern that their worst fears will be confirmed. One patient, a 68-year-old woman with a history of breast cancer in her mid-40s, had avoided seeing her physician for more than a decade out of fear that she might receive news that her breast cancer had recurred. The idiosyncratic nature of avoidance patterns among individuals with health-focused anxiety highlights the need for careful understanding (through functional assessment) of the links between avoidance patterns and the feared consequences they are designed to prevent.

In-Situation Safety Behaviors

Individuals worried about the consequences of bodily signs and symptoms often develop a wide repertoire of strategies for managing their health concerns. Frequent body checking and scanning, and searching for information about feared symptoms and diseases, may be used to monitor one's health and detect the presence of a possible threat (e.g., quickening pulse, skin lump, scratchy throat). Using relaxation techniques, soliciting reassurance from trusted persons, self-distracting, seeking medical attention, and escaping from anxiety-provoking situations are often used to reduce escalating bodily sensations and feelings of anxiety. Patients may carry safety aids on their person, such as benzodiazepine medication, a cell phone, a water bottle, and snack foods to be used "just in case." To minimize the negative social consequences of appearing anxious in the presence of others, some individuals avoid making eye contact, minimize or refrain from conversation, keep their hands in their pockets, and leave social situations at the first sign of anxiety.

Beliefs about Safety Behaviors

Patients who fear imminent health catastrophes may believe their safety behaviors are capable of preventing disaster. In some cases, as with a 51-year-old man who believed sitting down and breathing deeply during panic attacks had prevented heart attacks on numerous occasions, individuals believe their safety behaviors are specifically responsible for their continued survival. It is often clinically useful to assess exactly how patients believe their safety behaviors prevent feared health consequences from occurring. For example, those who fear passing out during a panic attack often report that relaxation techniques are effective in preventing this outcome. Individuals with health-focused anxiety also typically report that body checking and searching for health information seems useful in detecting potential health problems—a notion that may be critically examined by reviewing the patient's medical history and patterns of health care utilization.

PRESENTING THE RATIONALE
FOR EXPOSURE THERAPY

The therapist should begin by making sure that the patient understands the connections between thoughts, feelings, and behaviors, and how they maintain health anxiety. Once the patient understands his or her problems in terms of this model, the rationale for exposure becomes self-evident: exposure therapy offers a way out of this vicious cycle by helping the patient learn what happens when feared internal and external stimuli are confronted without the use of safety behaviors. Specifically, he or she learns that the catastrophic consequences are either unlikely, or in the case of less severe outcomes such as embarrassment or a panic attack, are usually manageable and short-lived. He or she also learns to better manage the everyday uncertainty that most people have (but don't dwell on) regarding their own unexplained bodily sensations. All of this bolsters coping self-efficacy by demonstrating that the individual possesses the internal resources to successfully manage anxiety symptoms and navigate anxiety-provoking situations and physical sensations. Moreover, by assisting patients in overcoming their fears and abandoning avoidance behaviors, exposure produces improvements in quality of life and functioning in occupational, social, and other spheres.

In addition to presenting this rationale, it is often helpful to present some didactic information about the physiology of anxiety and the normalcy of internal and external bodily "noise." Abramowitz and Braddock (2008), for example, include a set of handouts for this purpose. This information provides possible alternate (less catastrophic) explanations for bodily sensations, and provides a foundation for exposure therapy. The therapist, however, must use such information cautiously so that it does not turn into a form of reassurance seeking.

Situational Exposure

For someone with agoraphobia, exposure might involve walking through a rural area unaccompanied and without a cell phone or visiting a crowded stadium, movie theater, or shopping mall. Such exposures can teach patients that they need not fear the anxiety and panic that occurs in such situations. For patients with hypochondriasis, situational exposure may be useful in (1) demonstrating that anxiety gradually declines in the presence of fear cues such as hospitals, sick people, and reminders of illnesses (i.e., habituation), and (2) helping the patient learn to tolerate not being absolutely certain about whether longer term illnesses will occur.

Interoceptive Exposure

Interoceptive exposure is the most powerful intervention for patients who fear arousal-related body sensations. Habitual attempts to minimize and avoid sensations such as dizziness, breathlessness, and heart palpitations contribute to the false notion that these feelings are unmanageable and dangerous if they are not kept in check. Through experiencing these sensations in an intense, systematic, and prolonged manner without attempting to minimize or escape from them, patients learn that the catastrophes they fear are either unlikely to occur, or are indeed manageable and transient (e.g., intense autonomic arousal, being negatively evaluated by others). This technique also demonstrates to the patient that intense fear eventually decreases even while experiencing very strong body sensations. The knowledge that previously feared sensations are temporary and harmless allows patients to better accept and tolerate such feelings when they naturally occur. In the following dialogue a therapist presents interoceptive exposures to a patient.

> THERAPIST: Now that we have identified that you are afraid of certain body sensations which are not as harmful as you think, we can

focus on helping you see that these feelings and sensations are actually safe, and that they don't signal some major medical problem.

PATIENT: Okay, but it is hard to imagine how we could do that.

THERAPIST: Sure. Let me explain a helpful way to understand this. Because you are afraid of feeling dizzy, breathless, and having a racing heart, you're always trying to avoid these feelings. But although avoiding makes you feel safer for the time being, you never really give yourself the chance to see what happens if you let the uncomfortable body sensations just run their course. That is, you never get the chance to learn that they are temporary and not harmful. Do you follow that?

PATIENT: Yes, I think I understand.

THERAPIST: Good! So if we do something to purposely provoke these body symptoms inside you, and you don't try to fight them, make them go away, or do anything else to make yourself feel safer, then you will be able to learn that you can manage these feelings, that they are temporary, and that they are not harmful. When you repeat this kind of exercise over and over, you will get better at tolerating these sensations, and you'll feel much better about them. Do you see what I mean?

PATIENT: I think so.

Imaginal Exposure

Patients who experience anxiety-provoking intrusive thoughts about the consequences of suffering from a serious disease may benefit from imaginal exposure, which involves using voice recordings and written narratives to confront the fearful thoughts and images. The process of vividly thinking about, for example, suffering through painful chemotherapy and eventually dying from cancer may initially appear quite scary to an individual with health anxiety. However, with repeated and prolonged imaginal exposure to such imagery, the patient's anxiety will gradually habituate, thereby weakening the connection between the images and fear. We find it helpful to compare the process of imaginal exposure to watching a scary movie over and over. As with anxiety-provoking imaginal exposure scenarios, even the most frightening horror movie eventually becomes boring when viewed repeatedly.

DEVELOPING THE EXPOSURE HIERARCHY

Information gathered during the functional assessment is used to guide the selection of items for the exposure hierarchy. The therapist should consider both the types of feared stimuli (internal and external) and the feared consequences identified by the patient. Candidate items for the exposure hierarchy thus include feared situations, body sensations, and other stimuli volunteered by the patient, as well as tasks generated by the therapist that target the patient's feared consequences. Most patients with health-focused anxiety fear places, objects, or activities associated with disease or feared body sensations. Accordingly, situational exposure tasks will be part of the fear hierarchy for most individuals. Imaginal exposure exercises should be used for patients who fear intrusive thoughts and images with themes related to suffering from a terrible disease.

Interoceptive exposure tasks should be used for patients who fear arousal-related body sensations. Items are typically selected for the fear hierarchy following an interoceptive exposure assessment. This assessment involves having the patient participate in a number of brief exercises, each of which induces a unique set of arousal-related body sensations. The goal is to identify exercises that successfully re-create the patient's feared sensations. The anxiety-provoking exercises from the interoceptive exposure assessment are then added to the patient's fear hierarchy.

Table 11.3 describes the exercises we use when conducting an interoceptive exposure assessment. A number of easily procured supplies are necessary, including a stopwatch or watch with a second hand, thin (cocktail-size) straws, and a swivel chair. The room should have an open space large enough to allow the patient to run in place, spin while standing or sitting in a swivel chair, and do push-ups.

The patient should be informed that the goal of the interoceptive exposure assessment is to identify exercises that re-create *feared* body sensations. Patients are encouraged to participate in the exercises fully and intensely and not to try to minimize their sensations. For each exercise in Table 11.3, the therapist begins by describing and modeling the task for the patient. We find it useful to conduct the exercises together with the patient when working with highly anxious individuals. Following each exercise, patients are asked to (1) identify and rate the intensity of each body sensation they experienced, (2) rate their overall level of anxiety, and (3) rate the similarity of the sensations induced by the exercise to the feared symptoms experienced in daily life (e.g., a panic attack). The assessment also provides an opportunity to determine the feared consequences of specific bodily sensations.

Therapists can often predict which exercises will induce anxiety for patients who fear certain types of body sensations. Cardiac symptoms are elicited by running in place and holding ones' breath. Spinning and head shaking produce dizziness. Shortness of breath and choking sensations are induced by straw breathing, breath holding, and rapid swallowing. Feelings of unreality, shakiness, numbness and tingling, and lightheadedness commonly occur during hyperventilation. Table 11.4 lists sample expo-

TABLE 11.3. Exercises for the Interoceptive Exposure Assessment

Exercise	Description and duration	Body sensations typically induced
Shake head from side to side	Rotate head from shoulder to shoulder at rate of two or more rotations per second; 30 seconds	Dizziness, lightheadedness
Place head between legs	Place head between legs while sitting in chair; 30 seconds	Head rush, dizziness, lightheadedness
Run in place	Jog at rapid pace, keep knees high; 60 seconds	Palpitations, chest pain, breathlessness, sweating
Hold breath	Pinch nose and hold breath for as long as possible, take quick breath and repeat; at least 60 seconds, minimum of two trials	Breathlessness, palpitations, chest pain, choking
Swallow quickly	Without drinking water, swallow as quickly as possible 10 consecutive times	Throat tightness, choking
Spin	While sitting or standing, spin at rate of one rotation per 2 seconds; 60 seconds	Dizziness, lightheadedness, nausea, depersonalization/ derealization
Push-ups	Either hold push-up position or repeat push-ups, depending on level of strength; 60 seconds	Muscle tension, chest pain/tightness, sweating, palpitations
Breathe through straw	Using small cocktail-size straw, pinch nose and breathe as long as possible, take quick breath and repeat; at least 60 seconds, minimum of two trials	Breathlessness, palpitations, choking
Hyperventilate	Take rapid and deep breaths at rate of one breath every 2 seconds; 60 seconds	Dizziness, lightheadedness, palpitations, sweating, depersonalization/ derealization, numbness, tingling

sure exercises for different types of common health concerns. Although we focus on interoceptive exposure in this chapter, it is often beneficial to combine these exercises with situational and imaginal exposures. That is, after patients have successfully completed interoceptive tasks in the office, they can be encouraged to practice them in feared situations. Examples include ingesting caffeine prior to going to a theater, jogging alone in a rural area, and wearing a turtleneck and heavy coat while riding in a crowded elevator.

TABLE 11.4. Examples of Exposure Exercises for Different Types of Health Concerns

Type of health concern	Exposure stimuli
Heart attack	Vigorous exercise (e.g., running, walking up stairs), push-ups, heat-inducing activities (exercise, sauna, sitting in hot car, eating spicy foods), holding breath, high-dose caffeine ingestion
Fainting/loss of consciousness	Spinning, hyperventilation, shaking head from side to side, heat-inducing activities
Suffocation	Straw breathing, holding breath, swallowing quickly, wearing turtleneck or scarf, vigorous exercise, heat-inducing activities, riding crowded elevator
Loss of control, insanity, and concerns related to depersonalization/ derealization	Prolonged hyperventilation, staring at oneself in a mirror, staring at small dot on wall, sitting in a dark room with strobe light, staring at moving spiral, stimulus deprivation (standing in dark room, wearing blindfold and sound-proof headphones), staring at fluorescent lights
Vomiting	Spinning (chair or standing), eliciting gag response with tongue depressor, overeating, physical exercise after overeating, drinking alcohol
Embarrassment/negative evaluation	Simulating anxiety symptoms in presence of others by shaking hands, grabbing chest (as if having chest pains), stating that one is anxious and/or having a panic attack, stuttering, sweating, or committing social mishaps
Having a specific disease	Reading about the feared disease (via medical websites, books/pamphlets), watching movies depicting the disease, visiting disease-specific unit of hospital, exposure to stimuli associated with acquisition of the disease (provided actual risk is acceptable), engaging in physical activity that produces symptoms similar to disease, imaginal exposure to having the disease and worst-case scenario occurring (including death)

CONDUCTING EXPOSURE THERAPY SESSIONS

Interoceptive exposure is typically conducted prior to situational or imaginal exposure because learning not to fear anxiety-related body sensations helps the patient approach later exposure tasks without being frightened of their own anxiety response. If the patient is primarily afraid of the feelings associated with anxiety itself, interoceptive exposure alone may be sufficient, although as mentioned, it still might be important to confront feared sensations in varied situations and contexts. A relatively small number of exercises, usually no more than five or six, should be selected for the fear hierarchy, given that most exercises will induce comparable body sensations and target similar core fears. Habituation tends to occur rapidly during interoceptive exposure exercises—usually within 10–20 minutes.

The patient's predicted negative outcome of the exposure (e.g., "I will faint") should be specified prior to conducting the exercise so that the task can serve to disconfirm these predictions. It is advisable to acknowledge the possibility that mildly aversive but harmless negative outcomes such as dizziness, nausea, or embarrassment *could* occur with some exercises such as spinning (although even these are highly unlikely). By doing so, the therapist frames the exposure as a test of both the *probability* and the *cost* of feared outcomes, and prepares the patient for this low-probability (yet tolerable) outcome.

There are two commonly used methods of conducting interoceptive exposure exercises. One is to break the task into a series of brief trials. For example, hyperventilation may be conducted in three consecutive minute-long trials, each separated by a short rest period during which the patient is encouraged to relax and allow his or her body sensations to return to baseline (e.g., Barlow & Craske, 2007). A second method is to conduct the exercises in a continuous manner, taking short breaks at regular intervals only to collect SUDS ratings. Although research has yet to compare these approaches, we advocate the latter. In prolonged exposures, patients are able to learn that the consequences they fear are unlikely to occur even while experiencing prolonged and intense body sensations.

After the patient has made some progress with interoceptive exposures it may be necessary to combine these exercises with situational or imaginal exposures. For example, hyperventilating in crowded areas, large department stores, hospital waiting areas, and while driving. The aim of such combined exposures is to help the patient generalize his or her learning to different contexts. Regardless of the task, patients are encouraged to remain in the situation until their anxiety has habituated substantially. Some patients with panic attacks fear the social consequences of appearing anxious; situational exposures similar to those recommended for individuals with social phobia (see Chapter 9) should be used in such instances. If such social fears are not adequately targeted in exposure therapy, individuals with these concerns may continue to appraise arousal-related body sensations as threatening and fail to fully benefit from treatment (Hicks et al., 2005).

Imaginal exposure for health anxiety is typically conducted using scenarios in which the patient is suffering a feared illness or dying a terrible death. Scenarios that amplify uncertainty associated with *whether or not* the person currently has, or will acquire, a disease can also be useful. The following is an example of an imaginal exposure narrative from a 46-year-old patient with hypochondriasis:

> "I am trying to sleep, but as I lie in bed I notice a slight pain beginning in my throat. I am not sure if it's just nothing or if it's pain from a developing throat tumor. I wonder whether my breathing has become more shallow, and then I feel a little short of breath. I think about my own death. I think about my daughter's college graduation and how I will miss out on such wonderful events. Then I start to think that I should call the doctor to make sure it's *not* something serious. As I lay there the pain gets worse and I think I feel a growth pushing on my neck. I am in doubt. What if this is the real thing???"

The process of vividly thinking about developing an illness may initially appear quite scary to an individual with health anxiety. However, with repeated and prolonged imaginal exposure to such imagery, the patient's anxiety will gradually habituate, thereby weakening the connection between the images and fear.

IMPLEMENTING RESPONSE PREVENTION

Once the exposure phase of therapy begins, patients are helped to begin eliminating their safety behaviors and signals. Given that patients with health anxiety often attribute their very survival to certain safety behaviors, some actions and signals (e.g., carrying antianxiety medication) will be especially difficult for them to resist. The process of fading safety behaviors may therefore proceed gradually, with the most difficult-to-eliminate behaviors being worked on during in-session exposures. For example, a woman with agoraphobia practiced leaving her medication locked in the therapist's office while she conducted exposure to walking increasingly longer distances from the clinic building. During exposure tasks, simply *having access* to safety cues such as medication, medical devices, food, and drink may function in much the same manner as actually engaging in a safety behavior. In fact, mere access to safety aids was shown to interfere with the effectiveness of exposure therapy regardless of whether or not the safety aids were actually utilized (Powers, Smits, & Telch, 2004). Simply knowing that such items are available during an exposure task may cause patients to attribute their success to knowing that they *could* use the safety aid if it became necessary. The therapist should therefore be aware of this possibility and attempt to gradually remove access to relevant safety aids (including the therapist's own presence) during exposure tasks.

HINTS, TIPS, AND POTENTIAL PITFALLS

Therapist Reservations about Interoceptive Exposure

Despite its demonstrated effectiveness, interoceptive exposure is rarely used in clinical practice (Freiheit, Vye, Swan, & Cady, 2004). Although lack of training is surely a culprit, we suspect that many therapists also have reservations about using this technique. The practices of spinning a patient in a swivel chair to induce dizziness and walking up and down a stairwell with a patient concerned about having a heart attack may seem far removed from the context of the typical therapy session. Untrained therapists may view such exercises as awkward, embarrassing, and as perhaps crossing therapeutic boundaries. Additionally, they may worry that interoceptive exposure exercises, such as prolonged hyperventilation, are unreasonably aversive and may even lead to the very negative outcomes (e.g., passing out) that patients fear. We recommend that novice exposure therapists practice interoceptive exposure exercises themselves prior to using them with their patients as there is no better way to gain insight into how patients will experience these tasks. Therapists who realize that interoceptive exposure exercises, despite their discomfort, are actually safe, tolerable, and helpful will be most likely to have success using this technique.

Patient Views the Problem as Medical, Not Psychological

Some patients with intense health anxiety believe their problem is primarily *medical* and are thus skeptical about the value of *psychological* treatment. Exposure therapists must be sensitive to this view and take steps to avoid conveying the idea that the somatic symptoms of anxious patients are "all in their heads." Obviously, willingness to regard one's problem as at least partially psychological in nature is a prerequisite for successful participation in exposure therapy. This may require the use of motivational interviewing strategies as presented in health anxiety treatment resources authored by Abramowitz and Braddock (2008) and Taylor and Asmundson (2004). Motivational interviewing is a therapeutic style that aims to promote behavior change by helping patients to explore and resolve their ambivalence (Miller & Rollnick, 2002)

CASE ILLUSTRATION

Lisa was a 28-year-old waitress who began experiencing daily unexpected panic attacks 3 months prior to her evaluation. She was extremely distressed by her symptoms and sought treatment in the emergency room on five occasions during this time. Moreover, she was only able to travel outside of her home when accompanied by her mother, with whom she lived. Although her doctors tried to reassure her that she had nothing to worry about, Lisa remained concerned that her rapid heart rate and shortness of breath meant that she was "running out of air" and suffocating. As a result, she developed a repertoire of in-situation safety behaviors to prevent such an outcome, including sitting down, breathing deeply, drinking water, seeking reassurance from her mother and medical professionals, and taking benzodiazepine medication (alprazolam). She also avoided physical exertion and situations where she might be unable to obtain immediate medical assistance (e.g., driving alone, traveling more than a few miles away from the hospital).

During the first treatment session Lisa's therapist conducted a functional assessment and discussed an individualized cognitive-behavioral model of her panic disorder. She was provided with a handout describing the physical, mental, and behavioral effects of anxiety (e.g., Barlow & Craske, 2007) and instructed to review this material between sessions. During the second session, the therapist reviewed the nature of the fight-or-flight response and emphasized the adaptive and harmless (yet uncomfortable) nature of the accompanying body sensations. For homework, Lisa was asked to self-monitor the body sensations, negative automatic thoughts, and safety behaviors that occurred during her panic attacks so that she could understand the connections between these symptoms.

Session 3 involved cognitive restructuring. The therapist assisted Lisa in examining the evidence regarding the probability of suffocation due to a panic attack. Lisa acknowledged that she was unlikely to suffocate during a panic attack and she expressed willingness to proceed with exposure despite concerns about the dangerousness of her panic symptoms. Accordingly, the next session consisted of the interoceptive exposure assessment. Lisa completed the nine exercises listed in Table 11.3 and experienced at least moderate anxiety during four of them. These exercises were rank-ordered by their distress level and formed the interoceptive exposure portion of her fear hierarchy as shown below.

Description of the exposure task	SUDS
Interoceptive exposures	
Running in place	50
Spinning in chair	55
Swallowing rapidly	70
Hyperventilation	80
Situational exposures	
Driving	90
Walking alone outside of town	95

Session 5 began with exposure to running in place. Lisa ran in the therapist's office for a series of consecutive minute-long trials, each separated by a short break during which she provided a SUDS rating. Despite experiencing an intense and varied array of body sensations (heightened by her lack of physical conditioning), Lisa's anxiety decreased from 80 to 20 after 14 trials. Next, Lisa sat in a swivel chair and was spun by the therapist for 12 trials, each lasting 1 minute. As before, her anxiety habituated from a peak of 80 to 20. The therapist emphasized the difference between *feeling* uncomfortable and actually *being* in danger (which she acknowledged was very unlikely). Lisa was given the homework assignment of completing on her own each of the interoceptive exposure exercises that she had practiced in the session, until habituation, on a daily basis. She was also encouraged to eliminate, to the extent possible, her avoidance and in-session safety behaviors and to use "accurate thinking" as her primary coping strategy.

Lisa arrived for session 6 in good spirits owing to the fact that she hadn't experienced any panic attacks during the past week. The first interoceptive exposure, swallowing quickly, required only four trials before Lisa reported being unafraid and requested to move on to the next item on the hierarchy. The remainder of the session was spent conducting a hyperventilation exposure. As before, this was conducted in a series of minute-long trials followed by a 15-second break during which Lisa provided a SUDS rating. Lisa's SUDS rating peaked at 90 during the sixth trial, and she reported a 75% probability of suffocation. She was encouraged to stick with the exercise. After remaining constant for several trials, her anxiety gradually began to attenuate. After her SUDS had decreased to 50 Lisa was encouraged to hyperventilate even more intensely. Five trials later, following her reported SUDS of 30, she was asked to stand in the middle of the room and continue hyperventilating intensely. After four more trials, her SUDS had decreased to 10 and the exposure was terminated. As Lisa's SUDS decreased throughout the hyperventilation exposure, the therapist gradually shifted from encouraging Lisa to continue the exercise to suggesting she *bring on* the physical symptoms as much as possible and eventually to "see if you can make yourself suffocate." After the last interoceptive exposure trial, Lisa reported no concern that her intense and uncomfortable body sensations were dangerous (i.e., 0% probability of suffocation). She was instructed to complete the hyperventilation exposure until habituation on her own each day for the next week.

Session 7 began with an updated functional analysis of Lisa's symptoms. She was now panic-free for over 2 weeks and reported substantial decreases in body vigilance and concerns about the dangerousness of previously feared body sensations. However, she continued to prefer the presence of her mother, and avoided traveling more than a few miles from home. Lisa revealed lingering concerns about her ability to manage her anxiety and the possibility of a physical catastrophe, when alone or far removed from the possibility of immediate medical help. Accordingly, she agreed to conduct several situational exposures involving driving and walking alone outside of town.

The following session consisted of situational exposure to driving. The therapist accompanied Lisa to her car and asked her to drive several miles outside of town. Following 20 minutes of driving with the therapist, Lisa reported moderate but manageable anxiety. At this point, the therapist exited the car and asked Lisa to drive by herself for another 20 minutes. She did so, and then returned to pick up the therapist before heading back to the clinic. Lisa was then asked to complete several exposures involving driving alone out of town each day until the next session. The therapist also discussed the possibility of combining the two situational exposures, so that Lisa might drive to a nature trail 15 miles outside of town and go hiking by herself. She agreed to do so.

Lisa completed the assigned exposures and arrived for session 9 reporting no remaining concerns about panic attacks or being alone away from the safety of the hospital. She hadn't experienced a panic attack for 4 weeks and her quality of life had improved dramatically. The therapist reviewed relapse prevention strategies, including continued periodic exposures, elimination of her safety behaviors, and the development of a more active lifestyle that incorporated naturalistic exposures (e.g., regular physical exercise, more frequent travel). Lisa and the therapist agreed to terminate, and a follow-up session was scheduled for the following month. Lisa had remained panic-free by that time, as well.

ADDITIONAL RESOURCES

Abramowitz, J. S., & Braddock, A. E. (2008). *Psychological treatment of health anxiety and hypochondriasis: A biopsychosocial approach*. New York: Hogrefe.

Barlow, D., & Craske, M. G. (2007). *Mastery of your anxiety and panic* (4th ed.). New York: Oxford University Press.

Taylor, S. (2000). *Understanding and treating panic disorder: Cognitive behavioural approaches*. New York: Wiley.

Taylor, S., & Asmundson, G. J. G. (2004). *Treating health anxiety: A cognitive-behavioral approach*. New York: Guilford Press.

12

Contamination

CLINICAL PRESENTATION

The fear of contamination is one of the most common (and most well-rec-ognized) symptoms of OCD (e.g., Foa & Kozak, 1995). Individuals with such fears may report a variety of concerns including the fear of getting sick from using public restrooms, developing cancer from asbestos in the base-ment, mistakenly infecting others with a sexually transmitted disease (STD), or even gaining weight from contact with "germs" from an obese coworker. Such fears can become a near constant intrusion, given the seemingly ubiqui-tous nature of germs (which usually cannot be seen with the naked eye) and the ability of contamination to be easily "spread." For example, a man who wore his coat to the hospital may fear that the coat became contaminated with "cancer germs," and in turn contaminated the closet the coat is stored in, his wife's coat which it hangs next to, and even his wife who subsequently wore her coat. To reduce feelings of contamination, and the fear associated with becoming ill, individuals often avoid sources of the feared contaminants and engage in ritualistic washing, cleaning, and other forms of "decontami-nation" just in case of contact, or if avoidance is unsuccessful. Table 12.1 includes an overview of the conceptualization and exposure treatment of contamination-related fears. Table 12.2 provides examples of the variety of contamination-related fears and associated decontamination rituals.

BASIS FOR EXPOSURE THERAPY

Theoretical Considerations

Contamination fears fit neatly into the cognitive-behavioral framework for understanding the maintenance of anxiety as presented in Chapter 3. The vicious cycle begins when an individual confronts an object or situation

TABLE 12.1. Quick Reference Overview: Contamination Fears

Fear-evoking stimuli

- "Dirty" objects
- "Unclean" places
- "Undesirable" people

Prototypical examples

- Getting a disease from bathroom door handles
- Suffering brain damage from contact with chemicals
- Disgust with germs from dirty clothes

Safety behaviors

- Excessive hand washing
- Cleaning objects
- Avoidance of contaminated objects

DSM-IV-TR diagnostic categories

- OCD
- Specific phobia

Treatment overview

- Typical length 14–20 sessions
- Begin with assessment and psychoeducation
- Begin exposure by session 3 or 4
- Use cognitive therapy strategies to address overestimation of threat and intolerance of anxiety
- Implement response prevention along with exposure

Obstacles

- Therapist comfort level
- Anxiety reductions due to anticipated delayed washing
- Contracting illnesses during exposures

(e.g., bathroom, doorknob, dirty clothes) which he or she believes is likely to cause illness, perhaps due to the spread of germs. In some instances, individuals experience *disgust* rather than fear of illness. Regardless, the illness concerns or disgust provoke unacceptable levels of distress. To manage the distress, the person may try to avoid sources of perceived contamination, such as public bathrooms, contact with other people, certain areas of town, or, in extreme cases, remaining confined to the house or even to a specific room. When complete avoidance is not possible individuals may use barriers such as paper towels or their sleeves to open doors and turn off faucets. In situations where contact with a perceived contaminant can't be prevented, the individual may feel compelled to decontaminate him- or herself or his or her environment through ritualized hand washing, constantly spitting,

TABLE 12.2. Examples of Contamination Fears

Category	Examples
Germs	• Getting bird flu from spit particles in the air • Getting cold sores from touching money • Catching an STD from faucets in bathrooms • Getting sick from touching light switches • Unremitting disgust (or getting sick) from taking out the trash • Being dirty from reusing a bath towel • Catching a disease from elevator buttons • Getting food poisoning from a certain restaurant • Becoming very ill from contact with urine, feces, saliva, or blood
Chemicals	• Suffering brain damage by smelling fertilizer • Losing intelligence by breathing around cleaning products • Chemicals seeping into food and causing food poisoning • Developing cancer from using bug spray • Getting sick from taking vitamins • Smelling cigarette smoke, leading to a drug addiction
Other people	• Acquiring someone else's personality after touching him or her • Gaining weight from contact with an overweight coworker • Becoming homosexual after meeting a lesbian • Contracting AIDS from walking past a gay bar • Developing cancer from being around a cancer survivor
Harm to others	• Impregnating women by shaking their hands • Transmitting STDs through touching doorknobs • Bringing home an illness and infecting family • Giving parents cancer by touching them • Making a child ill by touching toys with dirty hands
Other	• Being dirty from touching own anus or putting hand in pants pocket • Losing running speed from being around fatty foods • Ruining computer keyboard by typing with smelly hands • Feeling dirty due to inadequate cleaning after using toilet • Fear that food on hands will damage everything one touches

showering multiple times a day, using elaborate wiping rituals after using the bathroom, or scouring the kitchen counter. They may also ask others for assurances of safety from contaminants. These "active avoidance" strategies serve the same anxiety-reduction purpose as passive avoidance of contamination cues—all are considered safety behaviors.

The cognitive-behavioral framework described in Chapter 3 can be applied to understand how contamination fears (and related behaviors) persist and even strengthen over time despite the fact that the feared contaminants do not pose nearly as great a danger as the individual believes. Specifically, every time an individual avoids perceived contamination, or removes it via decontamination, he or she misses out on a chance to learn that the feared contaminant does not pose a significant threat, and that his or her distress (fear or disgust) would have decreased naturally over time anyway. Thus corrective learning is never achieved, and the exaggerated beliefs regarding danger remain unchallenged. As cleansing rituals are relatively effective for immediately decreasing anxiety, this response is negatively reinforced, leading to more frequent cleaning, thus completing a self-perpetuating cycle.

Implications for Exposure Therapy

To short-circuit this vicious cycle, the link between "contaminated" stimuli and anxiety needs to be weakened by allowing the individual's distress to gradually subside despite feeling "contaminated." In addition, the connection between decontamination rituals and anxiety reduction needs to be weakened by preventing the use of safety behaviors in response to perceived contamination. Numerous studies support the overall effectiveness of exposure and response prevention for contamination symptoms (Abramowitz, Franklin, Schwartz, & Furr, 2003; Foa, Steketee, & Milby, 1980).

FUNCTIONAL ASSESSMENT

Table 12.3 contains a summary of the key parameters of the functional assessment of fears of contamination. We discuss the specifics of each parameter in the sections that follow. The stimuli that elicit contamination fears can be very idiosyncratic, circumscribed, and sometimes inconsistent with other behaviors of the individual. For instance, one child we evaluated feared contamination from food-related grease, although her bedroom was constantly dirty. Such apparent contradictions can be understood through a careful functional analysis of the sources of contamination, the feared consequences, and the means by which the contamination may spread and is dealt with.

Fear Cues

External Situations and Stimuli

Fears of contamination are most commonly cued by objects that many people feel are dirty or dangerous such as bathrooms, bodily waste and

TABLE 12.3 Functional Assessment of Contamination Fears at a Glance

Parameter	Common examples
Fear cues	
External situations and stimuli	Objects or places that are contaminated with germs or other undesirable qualities
Internal cues	Images of germs, doubts or feelings of being dirty, greasy, smelly, infected
Intrusive thoughts	Thoughts and images of germs, disease, or other undesirable qualities
Feared consequences	Fear of developing an illness that leads to impairment, death, or missing out on experiences. Fear of feeling dirty forever. Fear of spreading illness to others. Fear of ruining objects by soiling them
Safety behaviors	
Avoidance patterns	Not touching dirty items, or when necessary using a barrier; avoiding environments associated with feared contaminants
In-situation safety behaviors	Washing hands, changing clothes, wiping, rubbing, cleaning dishes, clothes, and other inanimate objects
Beliefs about safety behaviors	Safety behaviors are necessary to prevent illness or to decrease dirty feeling.

secretions, floors, dirt, trash cans, animals (e.g., insects), food residue, and chemicals or substances (e.g., insecticides, detergents, fertilizer). Items associated with diseases may also become triggers, such as needles or blood (AIDS), dead animals (rabies), and hospitals (cancer). Some stimuli become triggers because they are merely associated with, or have been in *contact* with, a feared contaminant. For example, someone concerned with a fear of herpes might be afraid of a certain baseball hat, the living room couch, or a drawer with a letter in it because these items were touched by an uncle who once had a cold sore on his lip. Alternatively, a patient afraid of contracting AIDS may avoid anything red because that is the color of blood, and AIDS can be transferred through contact with blood.

As we alluded to previously, many (but not all) individuals with contamination fears assume that contaminants are easily spread to nearby objects or surroundings (e.g., urine gets on the floor), thus secondary and tertiary triggers of contamination fears also need to be identified during functional assessment. For example, a woman with fears of bodily waste and secretions who felt her genitals and anus were contaminated also believed that her underwear, dirty laundry, and anything these items had contacted (e.g., the laundry basket) were equally contaminated. Another patient avoided a local restaurant owned by a gay couple due to his fear of AIDS. Moreover, his avoidance extended to the entire neighborhood, another area of town where the restaurant owners once lived, and another store where he had once seen this couple. Similarly, parts of an individual's own home, such as rooms and closets, may become contaminated from the presence (either past or present) of a "dirty" object. Other locations may be contaminated based on their inherent nature, such as hospitals with ill patients, work sites with toxic construction materials, or aisles in the grocery store where cleaning chemicals or insecticides are kept.

Internal Cues

Patients with contamination fears often report persistent images and doubts regarding germs and illness attributable to contact with the external cues described previously. Sometimes the doubts concern the possibility of contaminating others and thereby causing them harm (see the section on feared consequences). Rachman (1994) described a phenomenon known as *mental pollution*, a sense of internal dirtiness that may not be traceable to a particular source, but may be induced by events such as memories of traumatic events, unwanted unacceptable thoughts (e.g., images of molesting children), or humiliation.

Feared Consequences

Illness is a commonly feared outcome from contact with contaminants. Many patients describe a general fear of getting sick without specifying the illness or any long-term consequences; others focus on how illness would disrupt their routine. For example, one individual feared that germs would lead to a cough or cold that would harm her ability to sing in the choir. Other patients fear more specific and severe consequences such as contracting STDs, getting the H1N1 virus (i.e., swine flu), or developing a serious long-term or deadly illness (e.g., SARS). Other examples include the fear of brain damage from exposure to chemical odors, poisoning from rotten or spoiled food, and getting "high" (or losing brain cells) from contact with drugs in public places.

As mentioned above, some patients are primarily concerned with the fear of spreading contamination to unsuspecting strangers or loved ones who would become ill or even die as a result. For example, one postal worker feared that if his hands were contaminated with "urine germs," he would endanger entire neighborhoods by handling mail that would be brought inside homes and then touched by the entire family. One girl was afraid to touch her parents or brother for 3 hours after using the bathroom because of her fear of contaminating them.

A less common class of feared consequences involves taking on the characteristics, typically less desirable ones, of other people through being contaminated with their "germs"—for example, the fear that shaking hands with (or even using items that belong to) an obese person will lead to gaining weight. One patient feared losing her ability to play basketball, which she excelled at, if she breathed the air around less skilled players. Another man feared that if he touched items belonging to a visually impaired coworker he would lose his own sight.

Some patients may be unable to articulate any specific consequences of contamination. For these individuals, a sense of disgust (and perhaps the fear of vomiting) may be the main concern. Moreover, some fear spreading these disgusting contaminants to their possessions. For example, patients may go to great lengths to protect their most coveted books, electronics (e.g., cell phone), and accessories (e.g., hairbrush) from sources of contamination. Often these individuals report that spreading germs to a coveted item would "spoil" the item.

Safety Behaviors

Avoidance Patterns

Those with contamination concerns typically attempt to avoid contact with objects and situations perceived to be sources of feared contaminants. Some of the most common avoidance patterns include bathrooms (public or private), floors, shaking hands, going into rooms or buildings deemed "off limits," people associated with contamination, touching "dirty" parts of the body or dirty laundry, using chemical agents, touching items often touched by others (e.g., railings, doorknobs), and being in rooms with strong odors. To perform actions that cannot be avoided, such as opening a door or using a bathroom faucet, individuals may use a paper towel, sleeve, or gloves as a barrier. It is also important to assess whether individuals in the patient's life (e.g., parent, spouse or partner) are accommodating the contamination fears by avoiding feared situations for the patient.

In-Situation Safety Behaviors

The most common response to contact with germs is washing, particularly hand washing. Hand-washing rituals may range from frequent quick rinses or use of hand sanitizer to thorough and prolonged scrubbing of the hands, wrists, and forearms, as well as ritualized showering that can take hours at a time. Rather than regular strength soaps, patients may use stronger ("extra strength") disinfectant cleaning agents. Other self-care routines can also become safety behaviors, including excessive teeth brushing, grooming, and ritualized toileting routines. For instance, patients concerned with contamination from bodily excrement may use entire rolls of toilet paper to the point of stopping up the toilet or rubbing sores on their genitals or anal area. Patients may also change clothes frequently, such as after using the bathroom or upon returning home from a public place. Paradoxically, if the burden of a routine becomes too great, patients may avoid the activity altogether, such as a patient who stopped brushing his teeth because it took 30 minutes to do an "adequate" job.

In addition to cleaning themselves, patients may clean inanimate items such as kitchen counters and bathrooms, do extra loads of laundry, wash certain contaminated clothes separately from "clean" clothes (and then clean out the washing machine), wipe down items brought into the house (e.g., mail, groceries), and clean their shoes. These efforts might also include sanitizing cell phones, steering wheels, TV remote controllers, and video game controllers with baby wipes.

In addition to easily observable decontamination rituals, there are a host of more subtle safety behaviors that the therapist should assess for. If washing is not possible, individuals may remove germs by blowing or rubbing away the "germs." Other patients may spit or exhale forcefully to remove contamination from their mouth, lungs, or body. Mental rituals may also be used to decontaminate, such as saying the name of a "clean person" to remove the association with an undesirable one or repeating a phrase (e.g., "AIDS away") to remove illness-related contamination. Since these actions may be difficult for the therapist to detect, it is important to assess for them by asking questions such as, "Is there anything *else* you do to stop feeling dirty?" or "Is there anything that you say in your head or do with your hands to get rid of germs?" Finally, other people in the patient's life might be involved in performing safety behaviors for the affected individual.

Beliefs about Safety Behaviors

Washing, avoidance, and other safety behaviors are completed to remove or prevent contamination. In general, patients believe that safety behaviors reduce the chance of contracting or spreading disease. Alternatively, if they are not specifically afraid of illness, they believe that cleansing themselves through safety behaviors is the only method for reducing their sense of anxiety or disgust. These beliefs are maintained and strengthened by the fact that the safety behaviors are technically "effective" in reducing fear and disgust in the short term. Moreover, when no illness occurs, patients attribute this to the safety behavior rather than to the low probability of feared illnesses.

PRESENTING THE RATIONALE
FOR EXPOSURE THERAPY

It is important to set the stage for exposure therapy by making sure the patient understands how contamination fears are maintained by beliefs about feared consequences (i.e., the dangerousness of contaminants), and the use of avoidance and safety behaviors that are negatively reinforced. Exposure and response prevention then follow as logical techniques to disrupt this vicious cycle. The therapist might explain this cycle as follows:

> THERAPIST: Whenever you touch the clothes that you wore to the hospital you think you are being exposed to HIV and this makes you fearful. By washing your hands you believe you have removed the risk of HIV, and so your anxiety goes down. Does this make sense?

> PATIENT: Sure.

> THERAPIST: Okay. But unfortunately, because washing your hands makes you feel better *at the moment*, this tricks you into washing more and more. This is why your washing has become compulsive. Another problem with using washing to make you feel safer is that by washing your hands you prevent yourself from learning that it is actually very unlikely that you will get HIV from old clothes. You also never have the chance to see that even if you didn't wash, your anxiety about HIV would eventually decrease. Do you see what I mean?

> PATIENT: Yes ... I think so. Everyone tells me that, but it's hard to believe.

> THERAPIST: Sure. I can understand how you'd feel that way. You've never taken the chance to see what happens. So, the best way for you to learn is to take the "risk" and handle those clothes without washing afterward. I realize this seems difficult, but you'll see that it's a risk worth taking.

The therapist should also ensure that the patient has a good understanding of the relation between contamination cues, anxiety, and cleansing rituals by having him or her explain the conceptual model in his or her own words.

In addition, clarify that the goal of exposure therapy is *not* to prove defini-tively that there are no germs present (indeed germs are probably present everywhere). Instead the patient should learn from his or her own experi-ence that exposure to such "everyday" germs is generally not harmful and that avoidance and decontamination behaviors are not necessary to prevent feared consequences. As with other applications of exposure therapy, get-ting over fears of germs and contamination requires learning to live with acceptable levels of uncertainty. Ultimately, it is impossible to obtain abso-lute certainty regarding what constitutes a safe or dangerous level of contact with a feared contaminant.

DEVELOPING THE EXPOSURE HIERARCHY

Exposure hierarchies for contamination fears typically consist of a combi-nation of two elements: (1) touching things that are dirty and (2) spread-ing germs to places that are clean. Regardless of whether individuals are concerned with contaminating themselves or others, virtually all hier-archies should involve actual contact with "contaminated" items. For example, hierarchy items for a woman afraid of getting sick from touch-ing things often handled by others, may include touching doorknobs and magazines in the waiting room, using drinking fountains, and even using public restrooms. For those individuals afraid of spreading contamina-tion, the hierarchy will also need to include touching other people (and/or their possessions) as well as going into uncontaminated environments to spread the "germs." For example, a man afraid of infecting strangers with AIDS (despite a clean bill of health) might begin by "contaminating" (i.e., touching) items in the therapist's office, then items in the waiting room, the mouth pieces of public phones, and finally silverware at a public cafeteria. Imaging the feared consequences (e.g., being responsible for the spread of AIDS), via imaginal exposure would be a necessary hierarchy item as well.

The need to target the spread of contamination is not limited to indi-viduals with a fear of harming others. In an effort to find relief from their worries, some patients have a "safety zone," such as their bedroom, or cer-tain objects that they work hard to keep "clean." These patients may report that an exposure is not bothering them, yet they would have to wash their hands before entering a safety zone or handling certain objects. In such circumstances, it may be necessary to create a hierarchy that intersperses "contaminating" oneself, one's "safety zones," and one's protected objects. Table 12.4 provides additional examples of ideas and items for contamina-tion hierarchies.

CONDUCTING EXPOSURE THERAPY SESSIONS

Exposure sessions for contamination fears are spent encouraging the patient to become as thoroughly contaminated as possible with the "dirtiest" object they are ready to tolerate. The goal for each exposure task is for the patient to have full contact with the contaminant by spreading it all over his or her body. Thus, whereas touching the urinal flusher (for example) with the tip of one's finger is a potential starting point, it is not sufficient for learning that flushing the toilet is safe. Instead, the patient should fully grip the flusher with both hands, rub his hands in his clothes, hair, and face, and touch his fingers to his mouth or eat finger foods without washing first. Therapists might sometimes need to accompany patients on "field trips" to confront items that are not easily brought into the office (e.g., funeral homes, certain areas of town). If patients bring contaminated items to the session (e.g., a cloth that touched a container of Deet from a hardware store, or a napkin from a feared restaurant) it may reduce the need for such field trips.

Some patients with OCD have excessive and highly debilitating fears

TABLE 12.4 Examples of Exposure Exercises for Some Common Contamination Fears

Source of contamination	Exposure stimuli
Bathrooms	Touch doorknobs, faucets, toilet seat, urinal, floor; eat food off floor. As a first step, the patient might contaminate a paper towel with bathroom germs and practice touching the towel until ready to confront the actual item.
Urine, feces, other bodily fluids	Touch genitals after going to the bathroom without washing hands; touch toilet plunger, flusher, dirty underwear; contact with piece of tissue containing a small amount of urine, feces, blood, semen, etc.
Chemicals	Handle container, handle open container, use chemical as directed on container, contact with tissue containing small amount of chemical (if reasonably safe to do so)
Grease ruining possessions	Touch doorknobs, dirty silverware, apple, potato chips, pizza before using wallet, belt, new shoes, pencils, radio, telephone, TV remote control, computer keyboard
Making others ill with asbestos	Collect unknown fibers, touch them, spread them in public places, place on grill when cooking dinner

of contamination from substances that do pose potential danger, such as poisonous household chemicals and bodily fluids or wastes. Implementing exposure in such instances requires great care. Fortunately, when it comes to fears of toxic contaminants, many individuals (e.g., those with OCD) are simply fearful that they *might* have been exposed to dangerously high levels while engaging in routine and acceptable (i.e., safe) behavior and activities. For example, a woman with excessive fears of mercury poisoning from fluorescent light bulbs avoided rooms with such bulbs because of the fear that mercury might leak out, leading to irreversible neurotoxicity (mercury is a potent neurotoxin). Of course, this patient (or any other) need not douse herself with mercury (or any toxic chemical) during exposure. Rather, exposure exercises need only provoke the sense of uncertainty associated with such chemicals. For example, the patient described above can visit a hardware store where fluorescent bulbs are sold, touch the bulbs themselves, and change a bulb. Exposure for fears of other harmful chemicals, such as pesticides (often among the most toxic chemicals used around the house), may involve handling bottles of the chemicals and applying the chemicals as directed on the label (e.g., without engaging in excessive safety behaviors). At no point do patients need to come into direct contact with toxic chemicals.

Exposure to bodily fluids and wastes may be handled similarly, with the caveat that on a daily basis, most people come into contact with these substances (whether or not they realize it). Thus, in addition to using bathrooms and touching surfaces where such substances might be found (e.g., toilet seats, bathroom sink facets, one's own anus, genitals, or laundry), harmless spots or stains from actual urine, feces, blood, semen, sweat, mucous, and so forth can be obtained on a paper towel, which may be touched, carried around in the patient's pocket or used to contaminate other "safe" areas. For patients concerned with floor germs, entire exposure sessions may be conducted while seated on the floor (in an office or perhaps in a bathroom). For individuals who are fearful of spreading contamination, exposure might involve shaking hands with "innocent victims" or tainting objects by touching them. The aim of helping patients to repeatedly practice taking such "risks" is not to permanently alter their hygiene practices. Rather, the desired goal is belief change and tolerance of uncertainty about feared contaminants. That is, the patient learns that their feared consequences (i.e., illness, causing other to become ill) are far less likely than he or she had anticipated.

As mentioned, secondary imaginal exposure to feared consequences is often a useful adjunct to situational exposures to feared contaminants. If not knowing whether feared consequences will happen (or have already happened; e.g., "I could have poisoned someone without realizing it") is a source of anxiety, the scene should focus on *uncertainty* (i.e., not knowing the outcome). The following is an example for someone with a fear of contaminating others with "bathroom germs" causing them to become sick.

> "You went into a public restroom and touched the sink, toilet, door, and toilet paper dispenser. You were very concerned about germs from these items, which you can't really see or feel. Then, you went and shook hands with unsuspecting people—the clerk at the store, the parking lot attendant, and the doorman. You wonder whether you might have infected them with germs from the bathroom, which will make them very sick. You can just imagine these poor unsuspecting people becoming needlessly ill because of what you did. But you don't know for sure. Maybe they will get sick and maybe they won't. You don't know for sure. ...

IMPLEMENTING RESPONSE PREVENTION

The goal of response prevention for contamination fears is to keep the patient feeling contaminated at all times—so that exposure to feared contaminants never really ends. The following guidelines can be used, keeping in mind that patients might need to work toward them gradually.

• Limit washing of hands, face, and other body parts—even after using the bathroom, taking out the garbage, and before eating or handling food— to once per day (teeth may be brushed more often). Exceptions can be made if, *without close inspection*, one can see or smell undesirable and potentially dangerous substances (e.g., gasoline) on the hands. Swimming pools should also be avoided during treatment.

• Refrain from using any methods to remove or prevent contamination, such as using gloves, shirtsleeves, towelettes, or tissues. Also, avoid wiping hands on clothes or on other objects. Don't use gels or wipes in place of washing (throw these away to avoid the temptation!). If a patient is extremely fearful of urine or feces, he or she might wear gloves when he or she uses the bathroom to avoid contact with these items until they have been systematically confronted as exposure items.

• No washing or cleaning of inanimate objects, such as furniture or tools, and no extra loads of laundry or dishes. Patients are to wear clothes (and use dishes) at least once before washing them.

• One daily 10-minute shower is permitted each day (using a timer). This shower should be just enough to be hygienic and should not be turned into a ritual. The aim of showering during response prevention isn't to be *perfectly clean*, but to be *cleaner than when the patient started*. The person should use regular strength soap and wash each body part only once. When the shower is complete, the patient should immediately recontaminate with an item from the exposure hierarchy.

• Friends and family members are not to participate in washing or cleaning behaviors and should be encouraged to follow the same guidelines the patient is following (although this is the loved one's choice).

• Others are not to be asked for reassurance about whether something is safe or clean.

• "Clean" objects or environments should not be avoided just because one is feeling contaminated.

It is important to begin response prevention early in treatment, although a gradual approach is sometimes necessary. Although patients should be encouraged to resist all decontamination rituals, it is most critical that contamination associated with recent exposure items not be removed. For example, after a woman who fears contact with a certain coworker (who once had a cold sore) successfully completes an exposure to handling a memo written by that coworker, she should no longer perform decontamination rituals following exposure to items from this coworker. If she cannot resist the urge to decontaminate, the patient should be instructed to "recontaminate" after ritualizing by touching the exposure item again to reinstate feelings of distress.

HINTS, TIPS, AND POTENTIAL PITFALLS

Ground Exposures in Reality

Conducting exposure to contamination sometimes entails activities that people do not do intentionally or on a regular basis—for example, we have asked patients to lick their fingers immediately after touching a toilet seat. Since the goal of therapy is to help patients learn to manage ordinary risk and uncertainty, exposures should be rooted in typical experiences. For instance, it is not unusual for people to put down a toilet seat, use the bathroom, neglect to wash their hands, and subsequently chew on their finger nails or eat with their hands. *Thus, the difference between exposure exercises and common experiences is intent.* Grounding exposures in everyday actions also ensures that exposures are safe and appropriate to conduct. For instance, using one's hands to eat when they do not have any obvious signs of contamination is quite common, whereas one would be advised to wash if *without close inspection* he or she noticed dirt or other substances on his or her hands.

Readers may be surprised by some of the exposure and response prevention suggestions provided in this chapter. For example, "Isn't it dangerous not to wash after using the bathroom?" But, as alluded to above, lots of people don't wash their hands after using the bathroom, and yet remain healthy. In some cultures, such washing isn't even done at all. As for not washing before eating, people do this all the time as well—consider what often happens at ballgames and movies when people buy snacks. People, especially children, often touch garbage cans, floors, and other "dirty" objects without washing their hands. Even those who claim to keep to the highest standards of cleanliness (doctors, nurses, etc.) sometimes violate their own rules—often without even thinking about it. The only difference between what happens in day-to-day life and what happens during exposure therapy is that in treatment patients *purposely* confront feared contaminants and *deliberately* abstain from washing. It is possible (although not *probable*) that abiding by our response prevention guidelines will increase the chances of getting sick (we should note, however, that none of us can recall the onset of any serious illnesses to ourselves or patients during exposure therapy for contamination). Meanwhile, the long-term *benefits* of not washing very likely outweigh any short-term risks.

Manage Your Comfort Level

Providing treatment for contamination fears demands that the therapist also be exposed to stimuli that make many people cringe. ("You had the patient do what!?" is not an uncommon reaction from colleagues attending our case conferences.) Therefore, therapists need to be aware of their own comfort level with contamination to ensure that their reactions do not interfere with treatment. Modeling a manageable level of disgust prior to an exposure can be helpful. However, if the therapist is visibly very uncomfortable, this reaction will likely increase the patient's discomfort and impede habituation.

Prevent Delayed Washing

Some patients may initially express skepticism regarding exposure treatment because they already confront contamination daily without immediately washing. Typically, these patients are able to tolerate being dirty for some period of time because they know that they will be able to thoroughly cleanse themselves later that day. Yet, if patients approach exposure therapy with this mind-set, the intervention will be ineffective. Thus, if patients are not becoming anxious during exposures or are not making progress, the therapist should reassess for delayed washing and ensure that that the patient understands the importance of ending this behavior.

Contracting Illnesses

At times patients (and therapists) will develop colds or other minor illnesses during the period they are exposing themselves to various and sundry germs. Therefore it is important to frame negative consequences in terms of being *unlikely*, rather than *impossible*, and to discuss the severity of feared outcomes if they did occur. For instance, while going through treatment most patients can state that catching the occasional cold is not as bad as suffering from OCD.

CASE ILLUSTRATION

Susan was a 34-year-old mother of two with contamination-related OCD symptoms. She was specifically afraid of becoming ill from contact with dirty clothes, public areas, bathrooms, and trash cans, which she went to great lengths to avoid. For instance, she had stopped doing laundry and would leave garbage on the counter top in order to avoid touching the trash can. When she came in contact with "germs" she would wash her hands thoroughly (10 to 20 times a day), and often shower when she got home from work. When her children began to complain about her nagging them to wash their hands and change clothes after they returned from school, she decided to pursue treatment.

During the first session, Susan's therapist completed a comprehensive interview and discussed the rationale for exposure therapy. In the next session Susan and her therapist created the fear hierarchy shown below.

Description of the exposure task	SUDS
Door handles	20
Dirty clothes	50
Trash cans at home	60
Books and magazines in public places	70
Trash cans in public	90
Sidewalk and street germs	90
Public bathrooms	100

During the third session, Susan and the therapist touched the doorknob in the therapist's office. They made sure to thoroughly rub the handle to get their hands full of "handle germs." Next, they rubbed their hands on their pants, shirt, arms, face, and hair, and then licked their fingers. During this exercise Susan's SUDS peaked at 45 and decreased to 0 in approximately 25 minutes. At the end of the session, Susan reported that the experience was not as bad as she thought it was going to be, and that she was optimistic exposures would help her symptoms. She agreed to continue exposures with door handles in the days between this session and the next, and to contaminate other areas of her home with "door handle germs."

For session 4, Susan brought a basket of dirty clothes to the office. Initially she put the basket, without the clothes, in her lap and ran her hands around the outside. Once she became more comfortable, she rubbed her hands inside the basket along its sides and bottom. She then rubbed the germs all over herself just as she had done with the doorknob. When this was completed she placed the dirty clothes on her lap and rubbed them on her body, face, and tongue. During these exposures her anxiety rose to 70 and decreased to near 20 over the next half-hour. Susan agreed to complete similar exposures to dirty clothes and doorknobs over the following week, while also touching the dirty clothes to "clean" areas of her home.

At the beginning of session 5, Susan reported that doorknobs were no longer causing her any problems and that she felt much more comfortable with her own dirty clothes. During the session, Susan and the therapist conducted an exposure to a trash can Susan had bought from home following the same steps as they had with the laundry basket. At one point, Susan stated that she would not be able to eat dinner that night with trash-can germs on her hands. Thus, the therapist suggested that Susan eat some potato chips after dropping them in the empty trash can. After her anxiety decreased from 80 to 20, Susan felt she could eat without washing off the trash-can germs. In addition, she and her therapist agreed upon the following plan for response prevention: First, after exposure to an item, Susan would stop avoiding and washing after future contact with that item. Second, if Susan couldn't resist washing, she would "recontaminate" herself after the ritual with the contaminated item to which she was currently practicing exposure.

During the sixth session, Susan was feeling somewhat overwhelmed by OCD and other sources of stress in her life. She and therapist used this session to review and consolidate her progress by repeating previous exposures to the trash can from home and dirty clothes. Both items were much easier to touch than during the initial exposures. In the 8th through the 11th session Susan made steady progress completing exposures to progressively dirtier trash cans (office, waiting room, street corner), as well as items that had been handled by the public, such as library books and magazines from waiting rooms. She also worked on touching the faucets and flushers in public bathrooms. Following the 12th session, Susan was planning to visit a friend in the hospital and was concerned about the many potential sources of germs. To help her prepare, Susan and her therapist visited a hospital and Susan confronted hallways, trash cans, and wheelchairs.

At this point, Susan had experienced a marked decrease in her OCD symptoms. As new challenges arouse she was able to independently face them with her own exposure and response prevention plan, including swimming in a public pool and volunteering at her children's school without showering afterward. She and her therapist concluded that it was time to complete the final exposures that would make daily experiences with germs pale in comparison. Susan decided that if she could eat crackers off the floor of a public bathroom she could handle anything she might encounter in daily life. With initially moderate anxiety, Susan successfully completed this exposure.

Overall, Susan met with her therapist 17 times over approximately 3 months. The initial sessions occurred twice weekly to help her progress quickly. After she became more comfortable doing exposures and response prevention at home, she and her therapist agreed to decrease the frequency of sessions to once per week. Toward the end of treatment, the length of time between sessions was increased to 2 weeks, and then 1 month. Susan returned to see her therapist the next fall to discuss some work-related stress. At that time she was functioning well with little to no OCD symptoms.

ADDITIONAL RESOURCES

Abramowitz, J. S. (2006). *Understanding and treating obsessive–compulsive disorder: A cognitive-behavioral approach*. Mahwah, NJ: Erlbaum.

McKay, D., & Robbins, R. (2007). Contamination fears in OCD: Disgust and anxiety features. In J. Abramowitz, D. McKay, & S. Taylor (Eds.), *Clinical handbook of obsessive–compulsive disorder and related problems* (pp. 18–29). Baltimore: Johns Hopkins University Press.

Riggs, D. S., & Foa, E. B. (2007). Treating contamination concerns and compulsive washing. In M. M. Antony, C. Purdon, & L. Summerfeldt (Eds.), *Psychological treatment of obsessive–compulsive disorder: Fundamental and beyond* (pp. 149–168). Washington, DC: American Psychological Association.

13

The Aftermath of Trauma

CLINICAL PRESENTATION

Although most people who suffer or witness traumatic events do not suffer long-term psychological consequences, many develop the symptoms of PTSD in the wake of such an experience (e.g., Rothbaum, Foa, Riggs, Murdock, & Walsh, 1992). According to the DSM (American Psychiatric Association, 2000), a *traumatic event* is one in which a person's life or physical integrity is either threatened or perceived to be threatened and in which he or she experiences horror, terror, or helplessness. Although by this definition almost any negative event *could* become a trauma depending on how the experience is perceived, the most common examples include physical and sexual assault, being threatened with a deadly weapon, natural disasters (e.g., fire, tornado), motor vehicle accidents, and witnessing a close friend or loved one being seriously injured or killed.

Table 13.1 includes an overview of the cognitive-behavioral parameters and treatment of posttraumatic stress symptoms. For people who develop Acute Stress Disorder or PTSD, the aftermath of trauma is characterized by three domains of symptoms: (1) reexperiencing the event (e.g., intrusive trauma-related thoughts, nightmares), (2) avoidance (e.g., of reminders of the trauma, emotional numbness and detachment), and (3) hyperarousal (e.g., anxiety and fear, exaggerated startle response, hypervigilance, irritability; American Psychiatric Association, 2000). Individuals commonly respond to their increased anxiety about the world by using safety behaviors to manage perceived threats and control the symptoms of anxiety. Examples of safety behaviors in PTSD include excessively checking for signs of danger, sleeping with weapons, driving very slowly, and being accompanied by a "safe person." The degree of functional impairment among people with this type

TABLE 13.1. Quick Reference Overview: Trauma-Related Anxiety and Fear

Fear-evoking stimuli

• Thoughts and tangible reminders of the trauma, situations similar to the trauma

Prototypical examples

• Pictures of the attacker
• Anniversaries of the trauma
• Driving past the site of the trauma
• People associated with event
• News-related stories about the actual event or one similar to it

Safety behaviors

• Avoidance of reminders
• Avoidance of thinking about the experience
• Excessive checking for safety
• Being accompanied to places perceived as unsafe

DSM-IV-TR diagnostic categories

• PTSD, Acute stress disorder

Treatment overview

• Typical length: 12 individual therapy sessions
• Begin with assessment and psychoeducation
• Incorporate cognitive therapy to address mistaken beliefs underlying depression, guilt, and shame
• Begin situational exposure by session 3 or 4
• Begin imaginal exposure by session 4 or 5

Obstacles

• Persistent avoidance
• Realistic threats of additional traumatic events
• Extreme anxiety during exposure

of anxiety ranges from occasional intrusive memories of the trauma with intermittent avoidance to chronic anxiety, daily flashbacks, and avoidance of all reminders of the event, accompanied by severe social withdrawal.

BASIS FOR EXPOSURE THERAPY

Theoretical Considerations

Contemporary models of trauma-focused anxiety (e.g., Foa, Hembree, & Rothbaum, 2007; Foa & Riggs, 1993) begin with the notion that many of the symptoms of posttraumatic stress (i.e., reexperiencing, avoidance, and hyperarousal) are actually normal and natural sequelae of exposure to trauma. Typically, these symptoms dissipate over time as the person thinks about the event and routinely comes across reminders of it—that is, as he or she *processes* it. This occurs because processing the trauma and resuming one's normal routine fosters a healthy sense of self and maintains an adaptive view of the world as a generally safe place. As a result, the links between the trauma and the initial fear and shock it provoked are weakened. If, however, the trauma survivor consistently avoids reminders of the trauma, tries not to think about the event, and takes needless precautions to ensure safety in situations that are already objectively safe (e.g., installing extra locks on the front door or on internal doors), it interferes with adaptive processing of the traumatic event and hinders the natural reduction of the associated fear. As a result, thoughts, memories, images, and situations or stimuli that are objectively safe, yet which serve as reminders of the trauma, continue to activate fear responses and maladaptive beliefs, such as "the world is a dangerous and uncontrollable place."

Some theorists (e.g., Ehlers & Clark, 2000) highlight the importance of catastrophic misinterpretations of the posttraumatic symptoms themselves as indicating an ongoing threat (e.g., "Nightmares mean I am losing my mind"). Such misinterpretations intensify the distress related to these symptoms, resulting in efforts to suppress thoughts about the traumatic event or take additional excessive precautions (safety behaviors). Suppression attempts fail, however, because they paradoxically lead to *increased* trauma-focused thoughts, increased perceived threat, and increased use of safety behaviors, resulting in a self-perpetuating vicious cycle.

Implications for Exposure Therapy

The use of exposure therapy for trauma survivors follows from the conceptual framework described above. Treatment must help the patient to emotionally engage with objectively safe trauma-related stimuli, as well as with thoughts and memories (i.e., to *process* the experience). The patient must also drop safety behaviors and correct dysfunctional beliefs that maintain anxiety and fear. Processing can occur via confronting trauma-related thoughts, memories, and reminders, since this gives the patient the opportunity for anxiety to naturally decline (i.e., habituate) in the presence of such stimuli, and for the maladaptive cognitions that maintain the anxiety to be disconfirmed. Treatment therefore incorporates both situational and imaginal exposure. Situational exposure involves repeated and prolonged confrontation with safe or low-risk places, situations, activities, and objects that serve as reminders of the trauma and provoke excessive anxiety. Imaginal exposure involves confronting the memory of the traumatic event, that is, repeatedly visualizing or "reliving" the trauma from memory. Specifically, the patient is helped to vividly imagine the traumatic event and to describe it aloud, along with the thoughts and feelings that occurred during the event. Repeated exposure weakens the fear associated with such memories and teaches the patient that thinking about the trauma is not dangerous. Response prevention entails ending safety behaviors that prevent the natural extinction of anxiety.

FUNCTIONAL ASSESSMENT

Table 13.2 shows common examples of the various parameters of a functional assessment of posttraumatic stress symptoms. In the sections below we discuss the assessment of each parameter in detail.

Assessment of Traumatic Events

Functional assessment begins with collecting information about the major traumas in the patient's history. While some trauma survivors willingly describe their trauma history, others do not spontaneously disclose this information. Therefore, it may be helpful to probe with questions such as "Has anyone ever forced you to have unwanted sexual contact by threatening you?" A number of structured interviews have been developed for assessing traumas in more detail; for example, the Clinician Administered PTSD Scale (CAPS; Blake et al., 1995) includes both a self-report screener (the Life Events Checklist) and interview questions. Assessment should include questions about the patient's immediate and long-term response to the event(s), his or her feelings of helplessness, horror, and fear. We find it is best to ask about these emotions in an open-ended way (e.g., "Tell me about what the experience was like for you") rather than using closed-ended questions (e.g., "Were you afraid for your life?") so as to avoid leading the patient to give certain answers.

Fear Cues

External Situations and Stimuli

It is necessary to develop a list of the specific situations, objects, and places that provoke anxiety and distressing memories of the traumatic event so that these can be confronted during situational exposures. These stimuli will be highly specific to the individual's trauma, although common fear cues include the location of the traumatic event, people associated with it,

TABLE 13.2. Functional Assessment of Trauma Aftermath and Related Anxiety at a Glance

Parameter	Common examples
Traumatic events	Type of trauma, approximate date, initial reaction
Fear cues	
External situations and stimuli	Situations, places, people, objects, clothes, activities, times of day associated with the traumatic event
Internal cues	Posttraumatic stress symptoms such as heightened arousal and hypervigilance
Intrusive thoughts	Recurrent thoughts, images, and memories of the trauma that may appear as flashbacks and nightmares
Feared consequences	Being harmed (retraumatized), experiencing intense and long-lasting episodes of anxiety, being reminded of the trauma
Safety behaviors	
Avoidance patterns	Thoughts of the traumatic event, reminders of the event, activities unrelated to the event, but which are perceived as dangerous (e.g., going out at night), and social activities unrelated to the trauma
In-situation safety behaviors	Excessive checking for safety, keeping a weapon nearby at all times, keeping a "safety person" on hand at all times
Beliefs about safety behaviors	Avoidance and safety behaviors prevent intrusive thoughts about the trauma, keep one safer than they would otherwise be, and prevent harm from experiencing long-term anxiety

talking about the event, and seeing news reports or other tangible reminders (e.g., the clothes one was wearing, pictures). For those who have been in automobile accidents, anxiety may be triggered by driving, especially where the accident occurred under similar conditions (e.g., in the snow). Physical or sexual assault survivors might experience anxiety in crowds, with strangers, when going out alone, at night, when having physical or sexual contact with others, when seeing the name of the assailant, and when using public transportation. Those exposed to trauma in combat might be fearful of any reminders of the war, the military, and weapons. Aside from the assessment interview, asking the patient to self-monitor triggers that are encountered on a daily basis is an excellent way to obtain information about external fear cues.

Intrusive Thoughts

Recurrent unwanted thoughts, images, and memories of the traumatic event are part of the criteria of PTSD and are therefore likely to be present in patients with posttraumatic anxiety. Such intrusions might also take the form of nightmares or flashbacks, and regardless of form, provoke excessive anxiety and fear. The following is an example from a young woman who witnessed the death of her best friend in a car accident.

> "I get anxious when nighttime comes because whenever I try to go to sleep, all I can think of is the accident. It's like a horror movie. When I close my eyes, I see her slumped over the steering wheel and covered in blood. Her head is bleeding and her hair is all bloody. (*crying*) That's the most horrific part. And I can't get that image out of my mind. She was my best friend, but the only way I can picture her now is how she was killed."

Feared Consequences

Clinicians should assess for two domains of feared consequences in trauma survivors. The first concerns the fear of being retraumatized. Since many patients begin to view the world as unpredictable and unsafe after a trauma, they may feel especially vulnerable in situations they associate with their traumatic event. The second domain concerns fears of the posttrauma symptoms themselves. As described earlier, patients might fear that their intrusive thoughts and nightmares are a sign of "going crazy" (as opposed to being a normal response to traumatization). They might also show fears of the body sensations associated with hyperarousal (i.e., anxiety sensitivity; e.g., when my heart beats rapidly I fear I am having a heart attack). To the extent that these sensations are feared, the therapist might consider using interoceptive exposure to help the patient overcome the fear of such arousal-related body sensations (see Chapter 11) in addition to using the techniques described in this chapter.

Safety Behaviors

Avoidance Patterns

Patients often avoid reminders of their traumatic experience, such as the people they were with, clothes they were wearing, or type of cologne worn by an assailant, as well as news stories, television shows, and pictures of their, or similar, traumas. Such stimuli might not be perceived as intrinsically dangerous per se, yet they are avoided because they provoke distressing thoughts, images, and memories of the traumatic event which the patient is trying to avoid. Other situations may be avoided because the patient overestimates the likelihood of harm or danger. Examples include going out after dark, being in crowds, and being alone. Finally, trauma survivors may avoid activities such as socializing with friends, engaging in hobbies, exercising, sexual behavior, and religious worship whether or not they have a direct link to the trauma.

In-Situation Safety Behaviors

Trauma survivors may have both subtle and obvious safety behaviors that are meaningfully linked to their appraisal of threat (Ehlers & Clark, 2000). Common examples include substance use to control or reduce the experience of intense anxiety, distraction to take one's mind off of negative thoughts or situations, carrying or sleeping with weapons to ensure against being harmed, scanning the environment for signs of safety or danger, driving overcautiously (braking at green lights at intersections, continuous mirror checking) to guard against accidents, installing unnecessary extra door locks, staying close to exits in public places, and staying up very late to avoid nightmares. The person might also engage in elaborate checking behavior to determine whether it is safe to go out (e.g., asking others about the situation, making sure the assailant is out of town or in jail). As with other forms of anxiety, it is necessary to obtain a full list of safety behaviors so they can be targeted in response prevention.

Beliefs about Safety Behaviors

In general, patients who are trauma survivors use avoidance and in-situation safety behaviors to reduce the perceived likelihood of harm, to lower the likelihood of experiencing thoughts and memories of the traumatic event, and to control their distress and anxiety. The specific strategy used is based on the person's appraisal of danger. For example, one woman who was attacked by an ex-boyfriend believed that she was safe only if she knew this man was out of town. As a result, she called mutual friends to learn his whereabouts before leaving her home. Another individual believed that avoiding the street where he was mugged was necessary to prevent nightmares, which he believed were a sign that he was "losing his mind." This patient also routinely stayed up late and played soothing music in his room while he slept because he believed these behaviors prevented bad dreams.

PRESENTING THE RATIONALE
FOR EXPOSURE THERAPY

When presenting the treatment rationale to trauma survivors it is important to highlight that exposure aims to (1) reduce the need to avoid situations, thoughts, and memories that pose no more than acceptable risk; (2) reduce excessive anxiety that is triggered by feared situations, reminders, and memories; (3) disconfirm the belief that anxiety will continue forever if these stimuli are confronted; and (4) enhance the patient's sense of mastery over the traumatic experience. Situational exposure and imaginal exposure usually require separate rationales, and therefore are discussed separately on the following pages.

Situational Exposure

The rationale for confronting situations and stimuli associated with the trauma should include information about the detrimental effects of avoidance and the process of habituation that occurs during exposure. Exposure will enable the patient to think more freely about the trauma, experience normal memories of it, talk about it, reengage in activities and improve self-confidence, as well as confront reminders without intense and disruptive anxiety. It is also important to highlight that designing and implementing situational exposure will be a collaborative process and that the patient will never be forced to confront any situations that are realistically dangerous or that he or she can't handle.

When describing this process to patients it can be helpful to discuss how experiencing trauma naturally leads most everyone to begin to see the world as a more dangerous place and to view themselves as more vulnerable than they previously had, resulting in greater fear and anxiety. Responding to this fear with avoidance of situations, places, and activities may lead to feeling safer in the moment, but in the long run it prevents one from overcoming his or her fears. During treatment the therapist will help the patient gradually face situations and other stimuli that are realistically safe, but that have been avoided since the trauma. Through this process, the patient learns that he or she can handle the anxiety and that he or she will actually start to feel more comfortable again if he or she gives it enough time (i.e., habituation).

Imaginal Exposure

Some patients initially balk at the idea of imaginally reliving a traumatic experience in therapy. Thus, providing a convincing rationale for imaginal exposure is critical for establishing a trusting relationship with the patient and thereby fostering treatment adherence. One key point to convey is that reliving the memory helps the patient to fully make sense of the traumatic event—something that avoidance prevents. Another is that, via habituation, imaginal exposure weakens the connection between the trauma memory and intense anxiety. Specifically, this process teaches the patient that it is safe to think about the experience and that intense emotions such as fear and anger are temporary and have no negative long-term effects. By experiencing the temporary distress associated with the trauma memory, and allowing anxiety to recede on its own, he or she will learn to better manage anxiety and regain self-confidence. Finally, imaginal exposure reduces distressing flashbacks and nightmares. An example of how to convey this rationale can be found in Chapter 5 on page 97.

DEVELOPING THE EXPOSURE HIERARCHY

Guided by the functional assessment, the therapist and the patient generate a list (e.g., between five and 15 items long) of external fear cues such as those shown in Table 13.3. Items should be fairly specific and easily accessible for repeated exposure. Going "downtown," for example, is not specific enough. The therapist should determine, for example, what particular streets and time of day (or night) provoke the most anxiety, and use this information to specify the exposure task.

We recommend that hierarchy items be determined collaboratively with the patient to ensure that they are objectively safe and relevant to the individual's daily functioning. It may be helpful to inquire about normative behavior regarding situations that might be questionable—for example, finding out whether young women typically walk through a certain area of town unaccompanied. Realistically dangerous situations should not be included in the hierarchy; although if being accompanied by someone else would make the situation safer, this possibility can be considered. To illustrate, one woman who worked at a mall in a high-crime area had been mugged in the parking lot while walking to her car after work. In order to help her return to work, the therapist arranged for a mall security guard to escort the patient when walking through the parking lot during situational exposures. If there is any doubt about the realistic safety of a potential exposure item, it is best *not* to include it on the hierarchy, but rather to find a safer alternative.

CONDUCTING EXPOSURE THERAPY SESSIONS
Situational Exposure

Situational exposure should begin with confronting *moderately* distressing environments and stimuli before progressing to more fearful situations. The patient should remain in the situation until his or her level of distress

TABLE 13.3. Possible Exposure Hierarchy Items for Survivors of Different Types of Traumatic Experiences

Type of trauma	Possible exposure hierarchy items
Physical/sexual assault	• Going out alone (day, night) • Being alone at home (day, night) • Talking to strangers (same or opposite sex) • Visiting crowded areas (malls, stadiums, bus stations) • Physical or sexual contact with loved ones • Physical contact with a stranger (shaking hands, "high five") • Unfamiliar people with the same characteristics as the assailant (e.g., sex, height, weight, race) • Going out with friends at night • Being out in the open • Standing close to unfamiliar people
Assault or motor vehicle accident	• Using public transportation • Activities similar to the trauma situation (e.g., driving)
All	• Visiting the scene where the trauma took place • Reading or watching a show about a similar event • Tangible reminders of the trauma (e.g., words, names, pictures, clothes, scents, sounds)

decreases by at least 50%. Characteristics of the situations, such as the time of day and the people that are present, can be modified to achieve the desired level of anxiety during exposure. For one patient who was assaulted at night, driving by the street corner where the trauma occurred *during the daytime* evoked moderate discomfort (SUDS = 55), while driving there at night was extremely distressing (SUDS = 95). Table 13.4 shows an example of graduated exposure for a patient with fears of riding the subway after having been attacked there.

Some hierarchy items for posttraumatic anxiety can be confronted in an office, clinic, or hospital setting, such as speaking or making eye contact with strangers (e.g., men) or being alone amidst a large group of people (e.g., in a cafeteria). When situational exposure items cannot be confronted in the session, time should be spent discussing and planning such exposures as homework practice. We recommend that if at all possible, the therapist assist and supervise situational exposures during the treatment sessions. This might require field trips as we have previously discussed.

Imaginal Exposure

Imaginal exposure sessions may last from 60 to 90 minutes. The therapist should begin by making sure the patient understands the key points of the

TABLE 13.4. A Gradual Approach to Situational Exposure for a Patient Who Was Attacked on the Subway

1. Therapist accompanies patient to the subway station to walk around together.
2. Therapist accompanies patient to subway station and stays in a specific area while the patient walks around alone.
3. Therapist and patient ride subway together.
4. Therapist waits at station while patient rides the subway to a different station and then returns.
5. Therapist drives patient to subway station and stays in parking lot while patient walks around the station and takes the subway alone.
6. Patient goes to station alone and rides the subway and then calls the therapist who is waiting by a telephone.
7. Patient goes to subway station alone and doesn't tell or call the therapist.

treatment rationale. The process of imaginal exposure is then described in detail to the patient. The patient is then asked to recall his or her memories of the trauma while seated comfortably in the therapist's office with eyes closed to prevent distraction. He or she must try to *relive* the experience from start to finish by vividly recalling even the most distressing and horrific images, memories, and thoughts. This entails describing the experience in the *present tense* and in the *first person* (e.g., "Now I'm swerving to try to avoid the oncoming car"). The patient is encouraged to incorporate even seemingly minute details such as the clothes someone was wearing, facial expressions, and objects noticed in the background. A sample from one scene described by a patient who was surprised by a burglar in his own home appears below.

> "As I walked into the living room, I noticed that the window had been broken. Then I saw a shadow and the man jumped out at me holding a baseball bat. He was wearing a navy blue shirt and blue jeans. My heart started pounding immediately and I was terrified. He yelled, 'Get the f___ out of here!' and started walking and swinging the bat at me. I tried to jump out of the way, but I got hit in the side. He ran toward me and I ducked and rolled on the floor in pain. I wondered if he had a gun. Then I felt a blunt pain on my head and I figured I had been hit again with the bat. All I could think was that I was going to be killed right there in my own home."

The patient should feel in control of the process of remembering his or her trauma. Accordingly, the therapist should give permission to approach the memories slowly. If the patient remains reluctant to engage fully in imaginal exposure, discuss the rationale for exposure and remind him or her that the feared memories can be confronted gradually. For example, it is okay if during the first imaginal exposure the patient only includes sketchy details. In subsequent sessions, he or she should be encouraged to be more and more descriptive and the therapist can probe more deeply for thoughts and emotional reactions that accompanied the trauma.

Each imaginal exposure scene should last at least 15–30 minutes, and these are repeated twice and recorded (e.g., using a digital voice recorder) so that the patient can listen to the scenes between sessions. Every 5–10 minutes during the exercise the therapist should inquire about the patient's SUDS and ensure that the images remain vivid. As with other forms of exposure, expect that SUDS levels will initially increase and then gradually decline even as the patient continues to imaginally relive the trauma. If the patient's distress begins to increase to the point that he or she wants to stop the exposure, encourage him or her to let the anxiety just be there—to stay in the exposure and not push the memories away. Reminders that he or she is safe in the therapist's office can be helpful as well. Sensitivity and understanding also go a long way (e.g., "I know how hard this is for you—you're doing a great job"; "Stick with it; think of how great you'll feel when you've overcome this").

The therapist may also need to titrate the patient's emotional engagement with the scene by asking for more detail regarding what is happening and how the patient is feeling. If the patient is overwhelmed, the therapist can help him or her to decrease the detail and engagement. Help the patient notice when habituation is occurring and reinforce the success—for example, "Remember how anxious you were feeling when we started? You didn't even think you could face the memory. But you did a great job. I'm proud of you. I know how hard that was." As the patient becomes more and more comfortable with the imaginal exposure process, the therapist can help him or her focus specifically on those parts of the scene that provoke the most anxiety. These parts can then be repeated until habituation has occurred. Enough time should be left at the end of the session to review the exposure and discuss what was learned during the experience. The patient is then instructed to practice imaginal exposure using the recorded scenes once each day between sessions. It is important that he or she *not* conduct these practices right before going to bed as it may increase the risk of nightmares.

In general, it is critical that the patient feels comfortable and confident about the therapeutic relationship and trusts that the benefits of exposure outweigh the temporary distress and potential risks. To help establish a sound therapeutic relationship, the therapist should adopt a nonjudgmental attitude toward the patient; display a comfortable demeanor during exposures; demonstrate knowledge, expertise, and confidence about PTSD and its treatment; highlight the patient's personal resources and courage to seek treatment; and repeatedly normalize the patient's response to the trauma.

IMPLEMENTING RESPONSE PREVENTION

The therapist should also help the patient fade out the use of safety behaviors. This can be accomplished gradually and in conjunction with exposure. For example, during a driving exposure for a patient who had a traumatizing accident (he was broadsided at an intersection by someone who ran a red light) the therapist observed that the patient was driving well below the speed limit. Moreover, the patient would stop at all intersections, even when the traffic light was green (which ironically is very dangerous). Thus, during the exposure, the patient practiced gradually driving faster (up to the speed limit) and not stopping unless a stop sign or red light was present. It is important that patients understand the purpose of response prevention, which is to decrease the use of behaviors that aren't necessary in the first place, and therefore interfere with getting past the anxiety.

HINTS, TIPS, AND POTENTIAL PITFALLS

Persistent Avoidance

Patients may be unwilling to attend exposure therapy sessions. Therapists can address this by showing support, sensitivity, and conveying empathy regarding reluctance to confront painful memories. Elaboration of the basis and rationale for exposure might be necessary. We also recommend that therapists be directive in encouraging patients to attend treatment sessions, adhere to therapeutic instructions, learn new skills, and practice them between sessions. In the end, though, many therapists—including the authors—find themselves allowing trauma survivors more leeway with adherence to treatment techniques than they might for patients with other types of anxiety problems.

Realistic Threats with Situational Exposure

Because the fears of people who experience traumatic events are often strongly rooted in reality, it is important to carefully assess the degree to which the patient's perception of threat is realistic when developing the situational exposure hierarchy and when assigning homework exposure. It goes without saying that patients should never be asked to put themselves in situations where they are likely to encounter danger. Instead, it is incumbent upon the therapist to differentiate situations *perceived* to be dangerous from those that pose actual threat. This is especially relevant in cases of physical or sexual assaults in which the trauma was either deliberately caused by another person or perpetrated in a realistically dangerous situation (e.g., high-crime neighborhoods). Retraumatization is particularly a concern when patients are involved in legal action against an assailant, such as serving a restraining order, working closely with the police, or confronting the individual in court, which may intensify his or her perception of danger and level of fear and avoidance.

Extreme Anxiety/Distress during Imaginal Exposure

Some patients experience extreme emotional reactions during imaginal exposure to reliving their trauma. They may fear that the images will be in their mind forever or cause irreparable damage. Crying during this exercise is common, especially when the technique is first used. In addition patients may use subtle avoidance techniques such as becoming quiet and failing to recount the most horrific images. We have observed patients who turn their head to avoid very upsetting thoughts and images, such as that of an oncoming car just before a crash, an assailant's face or outstretched arm, or the thought of a gun being pointed at them. If this occurs, the therapist can ask for details about what is happening in the patient's imagery and, despite the distress, encourage him or her to *confront*, rather than *avoid*, the distressing images. It may be useful to treat the image as if it were a DVD movie that can be "paused" or played back in slow motion so that the patient can focus on the image and express his or her thoughts, feelings, and physical reactions in detail. The patient should be reminded to allow him- or herself to express all of his or her feelings, regardless of whether they involve anger, sadness, guilt, shame or fear.

Other patients become overly engaged in the imaginal exposure scene and report feeling overwhelmed or "out of control." Here, it may be helpful to remind them that they are in a safe environment within the therapy office, and that what they are reliving is only a painful *memory* (not an actual experience). We often explain that during imaginal exposure it is important to "keep one foot in the past (i.e., in the memory of the trauma) and the other foot in the present (i.e., in the therapy session)." Another way to help with grounding the patient is to have him or her keep his or her eyes open while reliving the trauma memory (looking at the floor or perhaps a calming picture on the wall). A brief touch on the arm or hand can also serve this purpose, but it is important to ask permission to use touch before trying this.

CASE ILLUSTRATION

Evan was a 38-year-old prison guard who was referred for treatment by the department of corrections after he had been severely injured while at work approximately 2 years earlier. During a prison riot he was severely beaten and sustained injuries to his head, neck, chest, and arms, all the while feeling convinced that he would be killed. Evan was knocked unconscious during the riot and woke up in a ditch, a quarter-mile from the prison. He was finally found and taken to the hospital where he underwent several surgeries and remained in intensive care for several days. After a few months of recovery, Evan tried to return to work one day, but as he got closer to the prison he experienced intense anxiety and a panic attack and had to turn around and go home. After the riot, Evan stayed in the basement at home most of the time, began sleeping on the couch, and became detached from his wife and children. He believed he would not live to the age of 40. He also experienced recurrent nightmares about the riot, and sometimes had flashbacks during the day. An initial evaluation found that Evan was suffering from severe PTSD and major depressive disorder. He had been receiving medication treatment since shortly after being released from the hospital.

Evan accepted the recommendation for a course of exposure-based therapy, although he expressed worry about being able to engage in imaginal exposure. He reported that when a previous therapist had tried to get him to talk about the trauma, he had tried, but found it intensely upsetting. During the first and second treatment sessions, Evan's therapist provided information about normal reactions to traumatic events and reviewed the rationale for situational and imaginal exposure, emphasizing that avoidance of this painful memory, although very understandable, was preventing Evan from recovering and taking back his life. Evan's dysfunctional beliefs about his role in the riot (e.g., "I should have stopped it") and his PTSD symptoms (e.g., "I'm a weak person because I can't get over this") were discussed and challenged in light of the normal reactions to trauma.

Evan's situational exposure hierarchy was as follows:

Description of the exposure task	SUDS
Watching television shows and movies about prisons	55
Watching news clips about prison riots on the Internet	65
His prison guard uniform	70

Reading news clippings about the riot that Evan was involved in	77
Talking about the riot with his family and with friends who worked in the prison	85
Gradually approaching the prison where the riot occurred	90

During the third session, Evan and his therapist viewed a television show about life in prisons which did not contain any violence. Evan took the tape containing the show home with him to watch on his own, and also rented the movie *The Shawshank Redemption* (which is about life in a prison) to watch between sessions. At the fourth session, Evan viewed news clips from the Internet of actual prison riots. During these initial exposures, Evan's anxiety level increased at first, but soon leveled off and declined so that after an hour of watching this material, he was only minimally distressed. At the fifth session, Evan brought in his prison guard uniform, which was blood-stained and torn. Evan was able to look at the uniform and even put it on, despite fairly intense distress at first. After this appointment, sessions were used to plan situational exposure exercises which Evan confronted on his own as homework, often with the help of his wife, who was very supportive and eager to assist with treatment.

Beginning with the sixth session, Evan began imaginal exposure to his memories of the riot. His therapist began by reiterating the rationale for this technique, which Evan said that he understood and was willing to try. Then Evan described what he remembered of the trauma. The therapist encouraged him to include as many details as he could about the actual events, and his own thoughts and feelings during the riot. The session was recorded on a digital voice recorder for Evan to play back between sessions. Although Evan found imaginal exposure highly distressing, he was able to engage in the exercise. He listened to the recording each day between the sixth and seventh sessions and also conducted the assigned situational exposure. In subsequent sessions, Evan found it easier to complete the imaginal exposures and he was able to incorporate more and more detail of the trauma with each exposure. His peak SUDS ratings also decreased with each successive session.

As treatment progressed and Evan was confronting people and places associated with his traumatic event, he reported that his nightmares and flashbacks were decreasing. He was feeling better about himself, his relationships, and his future, and had moved back upstairs with his wife. After 16 treatment sessions, and daily exposure homework practice, Evan's avoidance and hyperarousal symptoms had almost completely subsided and he no longer met criteria for PTSD. While he did not go back to his job as a prison guard, he found a job as a security officer at a local university which he found very satisfying. Treatment was stopped after 20 sessions, with Evan feeling optimistic and virtually symptom-free.

ADDITIONAL RESOURCES

Foa, E. B., Hembree, E., & Rothbaum, B. O. (2007). *Prolonged exposure therapy for PTSD: Emotional processing of traumatic experiences.* New York: Oxford University Press.

Foa, E. B., & Rothbaum, B. O. (1998). *Treating the trauma of rape: Cognitive-behavioral therapy for PTSD.* New York: Guilford Press.

14

Blood-, Injection-, and Injury-Related Stimuli

CLINICAL PRESENTATION

The types of fears described in this chapter typically fall into the category of specific phobia, blood–injection–injury (BII) type (American Psychiatric Association, 2000). Individuals with this type of phobia may fear a range of stimuli including seeing blood, receiving injections, and undergoing dental and medical procedures. BII fears typically develop during childhood (Antony, Brown, & Barlow, 1997) and often arise following painful or otherwise traumatic experiences (Ost, 1991). Presenting complaints among fearful patients vary tremendously in their scope and potential for functional impairment. Some individuals are simply distressed by the sight of others' blood. In other cases, BII fears cause sufferers to avoid taking careers in medicine, becoming pregnant, and undergoing important medical procedures (Marks, 1988). In extreme cases, the avoidance can literally become a matter of life and death.

BII phobias are unique among the anxiety disorders in that sufferers sometimes faint upon exposure to fear cues. In fact, 56% of people with phobias of needles report a history of fainting during injections and about 70% with blood phobia have actually fainted at the sight of blood (Ost, 1992). Unlike most phobic people, BII fearful individuals often exhibit a "diphasic" response to BII stimuli. This response is characterized by an initial increase in arousal followed by a sharp decrease below baseline levels of arousal that may lead to fainting if the individual cannot leave the situation (Page, 1994). Individuals with a history of fainting may have developed a conditioned fear of fainting that exacerbates their anxiety upon subsequent exposure to blood, injections, and other medical stimuli. The propensity to experience disgust is also strongly associated with BII phobias (Olatunji & McKay, 2009) and because disgust reactions are associated with parasympathetic activity (i.e., decreased physiological arousal) they increase the risk of fainting upon exposure to BII stimuli (Page, 2003). Table 14.1 provides an overview of the conceptualization and treatment of BII fears.

TABLE 14.1. Quick Reference Overview: Blood, Injection, and Injury Fears

Fear-evoking stimuli

• Needles
• Blood, open wounds
• Medical or dental procedures

Prototypical examples

• Receiving an injection, having one's blood drawn
• Undergoing surgery
• Having a dental cleaning or a cavity filled
• Viewing a graphic medical procedure in a TV show or movie
• Observing a bleeding wound

Safety behaviors

• Avoiding dental and medical procedures or situations that might result in exposure to blood–injection–injury stimuli
• Reliance on a safe person during dental and medical procedures
• Distraction (e.g., looking away during an injection)

DSM-IV-TR diagnostic category

• Specific phobia, blood–injection–injury type

Treatment overview

• Typical length: 1–6 individual therapy sessions; may be conducted in a single 3–4 hour session
• Begin with assessment and psychoeducation
• Teach applied tension if patient faints upon exposure to fear cues
• Begin situational exposure by session 2

Obstacles

• Having a traumatic experience during exposure
• Pain sensitivity

BASIS FOR EXPOSURE THERAPY

Theoretical Considerations

Individuals may fear BII stimuli for a variety of reasons. Some patients overestimate the probability of being directly harmed by the stimulus—for example, being contaminated by blood or needles, or being injured or dying during a medical procedure. In other cases, patients expect that the pain experienced during medical or dental procedures will be extreme and intolerable, possibly even leading to a loss of behavioral or mental control (e.g., unrestrained screaming, becoming psychotic). Patients with BII phobias may also react to stimuli such as needles, blood, and open wounds with strong feelings of disgust. For individuals with a history of fainting, BII stimuli may be feared because of their capacity to elicit this reaction (or bodily sensations associated with fainting) and the potential negative consequences individuals believe may accompany fainting (e.g., injury, medical catastrophe). In our own research, the experience of pain, disgust, and the fear of fainting each appear to be strong contributors to the fear of needles (Deacon & Abramowitz, 2006c).

Because exposure to BII stimuli is only an occasional occurrence for most people, patients with this type of phobia tend not to exhibit the large repertoire of daily rituals and in-situation safety behaviors observed with other sorts of problems with anxiety and fear. By far, the most salient safety behavior associated with this type of fear is avoidance. Individuals tend to avoid exposure to feared BII stimuli at every possible opportunity. Even when forced to confront feared situations (e.g., receiving a required immunization), many individuals will distract themselves in an attempt to avoid looking at the feared stimulus. Avoidant individuals may go for years (or even decades) without having injections or dental and medical procedures. Unfortunately, such avoidance often comes at the price of their health and quality of life. It also maintains maladaptive beliefs about (1) the dangerousness of feared stimuli themselves, (2) the extreme emotional reactions they elicit, and (3) the patient's inability to tolerate such reactions.

Implications for Exposure Therapy

This understanding of BII fears suggests that exposure therapy must provide corrective information regarding the specific maladaptive beliefs and feared emotional reactions that underlie the patient's phobia. Through repeated and prolonged exposure to feared situations without the use of in-situation safety behaviors, patients learn that BII stimuli are unlikely to cause them harm. Some may learn that their intense anxiety or disgust reaction upon exposure to blood, injury, and related stimuli gradually fades to manageable levels during prolonged exposure, while others may discover that the actual pain experienced during medical procedures is substantially less intense and more manageable than what they anticipated. Lastly, individuals with a propensity to faint upon exposure to BII stimuli may learn that the use of applied tension (a technique we describe later in this chapter—see Hints, Tips, and Pitfalls Section) during exposure to feared stimuli effectively prevents fainting.

It is important to note that BII phobia patients' feared consequences often contain a grain of truth. Dental and medical procedures *can* be painful. *Some* individuals do faint during exposure to BII stimuli, even when the exposure consists of something as innocuous as overhearing others discuss a medical procedure. Patients with severe BII fears *may have* actually "lost control" (e.g., screamed, been physically restrained, or experienced a dissociative episode) during prior medical procedures. Therapists should keep in mind the possibility that their patients' safety behaviors might actually be adaptive. For example, averting eye contact from the needle during a blood draw may actually prevent fainting for some individuals. A careful functional analysis can reveal the extent to which the patients' safety behaviors are logically connected to prevention of their feared consequences. Here again, BII phobias are somewhat unique among the types of fears described in this book in that exposure therapy may, as described below, involve equipping the patient with strategies designed to prevent the actual occurrence of their feared consequences.

FUNCTIONAL ASSESSMENT

In Table 14.2 we present examples of the various parameters of a functional assessment of BII fears. Each parameter is discussed in detail in the next sections.

Fear Cues

External Situations and Stimuli

Anxiety, disgust, pain, and fainting may be triggered by a variety of external stimuli. Visiting a dentist or doctor, and undergoing dental and medical procedures, are obvious examples. Other external triggers include receiving a blood draw or injection, seeing blood, and witnessing wounds, injuries, or mutilation (e.g., roadkill). Importantly, individuals may also react with anxiety, disgust, or losing consciousness by observing others' exposure to external BII stimuli (e.g., watching a family member receive an injection). It is not uncommon for individuals to fear the sight of others' blood but be unconcerned with their own. In some cases, simply talking about BII

TABLE 14.2. Functional Assessment of Blood, Injection, and Injury Fears at a Glance

Parameter	Common examples
Fear cues	
External situations and stimuli	Undergoing dental or medical procedures; situations or activities that might involve exposure to needles, blood, or injuries
Internal cues	Body sensations associated with anxiety and/or fainting (e.g., heart palpitations, dizziness, nausea, weakness, sweating)
Feared consequences	Aversive and intolerable feelings of pain, fear, or disgust; losing control or going crazy; fainting; getting contaminated or sick; injury or death
Safety behaviors	
Avoidance patterns	Situations or activities that might involve immediate exposure to blood–injection–injury stimuli; sustained engagement in activities that might involve future exposure to blood–injection–injury stimuli
In-situation safety behaviors	Distraction, breathing and relaxation techniques, reassurance seeking, reliance on a safe person, withholding information about symptoms to avoid health care procedures
Beliefs about safety behaviors	Prevent physical or mental catastrophe, prevent the experience of intolerable feelings, prevent fainting

stimuli, hearing others discuss these stimuli, or even thinking about such topics (e.g., imagining a surgical procedure) may elicit fainting and other unwanted emotional reactions.

Internal Cues

Physiological sensations associated with fainting (e.g., heart palpitations, dizziness, nausea, weakness, sweating, hot flushes, chills) may trigger anxiety among patients who associate these sensations with the possibility of losing consciousness. Internal sensations of pain are also a source of concern for many individuals.

Feared Consequences

The feared consequences of exposure to BII stimuli are heterogeneous and depend on the individual. Anticipation of intense physical pain and its possible consequences (e.g., losing control, going crazy) are prominent concerns for patients who fear dental and medical procedures. Some individuals believe that contact with blood and needles will result in contamination and the acquisition of a serious illness. The fear of fainting is a common concern among those with BII phobias and as discussed is often realistic given the high incidence of fainting in this population. Lastly, many sufferers report prominent and aversive feelings of disgust upon exposure to BII stimuli such as blood, wounds, and needles. High levels of disgust may not necessarily be associated with a specific threat appraisal. To illustrate, one patient with a blood phobia denied any concerns about the dangerousness of blood per se and reported that his distress and avoidance was motivated by the observation that "blood is just gross."

Safety Behaviors

Avoidance Patterns

Patients with BII phobias avoid situations that might involve exposure to feared stimuli, either at present or at some point in the future. Situations that are *guaranteed* to involve direct exposure to BII stimuli, such as receiving injections, cleaning a child's bloody knee after a fall, undergoing medical procedures, and visiting the dentist are commonly avoided. Other situations in which BII stimuli *might* be encountered may also be avoided. Examples include watching TV programs or movies with medical themes, viewing or attending violent sports (e.g., boxing), and engaging in activities with a high potential for injury such as downhill skiing. Lastly, patients may avoid situations and activities that would entail *eventual* exposure to BII stimuli. We have seen patients who, in order to avoid receiving injections, opted not to join the military or who took birth control to avoid getting pregnant. Other patients have described their painful decision to forego a career in medicine owing to their propensity to faint at the sight of blood or their strong disgust reactions to wounds and mutilation.

In-Situation Safety Behaviors

On those occasions when patients with BII phobias face feared situations, they typically do so with the use of in-situation safety behaviors. A common strategy is to engage in actions intended to reduce anxious arousal such as controlled breathing, mental imagery, and distraction (e.g., avoiding eye contact with a needle, listening to music during a dental cleaning). Patients often view such actions as useful in minimizing anxiety and preventing a loss of behavioral or mental control. Arousal-reduction strategies may also be used to prevent fainting, but may ironically *increase* the probability of fainting by facilitating the decrease in blood pressure associated with this response (see below for further elaboration). Patients may excessively seek reassurance from loved ones and health care professionals that dental and medical procedures and safe and tolerable. Fearful individuals may also opt not to divulge symptoms to their health care providers in order to avoid undergoing unwanted procedures.

Beliefs about Safety Behaviors

Safety behaviors are believed to prevent harm by preventing or minimizing the experience of pain, anxiety, or disgust, and the secondary outcomes often associated with these unwanted feelings (e.g., losing control). Patients may also believe that their safety behaviors reduce the probability of being directly harmed by potentially dangerous dental or medical procedures. Lastly, patients who faint upon exposure to BII stimuli often believe that their safety behaviors help prevent fainting.

PRESENTING THE RATIONALE FOR EXPOSURE THERAPY

The information gathered during the functional assessment provides the basis for the rationale for exposure therapy. The patient needs to understand how his or her maladaptive appraisals of BII stimuli are maintaining the fear. Likewise, it is essential to convey the message that habitual avoidance and use of in-situation safety behaviors prevents the patient from assessing the actual dangerousness of exposure to blood, injections, dental procedures, and medical procedures. By confronting feared situations without the use of safety behaviors (i.e., exposure and response prevention) patients may acquire corrective information that disconfirms their maladaptive beliefs about being harmed and experiencing intolerable pain and emotional reactions. In this manner, exposure helps patients to learn that BII stimuli are rarely dangerous, and elicit levels of pain, disgust, or anxiety that are manageable and that decrease with time and repeated exposure. When applicable, exposure may also assist patients in learning that fainting in the presence of BII cues can be effectively prevented with the use of applied tension as we describe later in this chapter.

DEVELOPING THE EXPOSURE HIERARCHY

Selection of hierarchy items involves consideration of both the patient's feared stimuli and feared consequences. Exposure tasks for patients with BII fears typically consist of situational exposures involving varying degrees of contact with feared stimuli. For a patient who fears needles, a typical progression might consist of looking at pictures and video clips of needles and injections, holding a needle in one's hand, holding a needle against one's arm, observing others receiving injections, then finally receiving an injection or blood draw oneself. For one who fears the sight of blood, exposure tasks might involve viewing images and video clips depicting blood, holding a jar of blood from a raw steak, holding the steak, observing others prick their finger with a lancet and bleed, receiving a blood draw, and donating blood. For many patients, the exposure hierarchy will be relatively succinct and need not consist of more than five or six items. For this reason, exposure therapy for BII phobias may often be completed in a small number of sessions, or even a single 3- to 4-hour session. It is important that the hierarchy includes tasks that involve patients facing their worst fears, which often involve receiving important medical or dental procedures the patient has been avoiding. Table 14.3 lists example exposure exercises for patients who fear blood, needles, dental procedures, and medical procedures.

CONDUCTING EXPOSURE THERAPY SESSIONS

Exposures to BII stimuli should be conducted to test the patient's beliefs about potential negative outcomes such as being injured, experiencing intolerable pain, or fainting. In the event that no specific threat appraisal is connected to the task (e.g., "it's just disgusting"), the therapist may frame the exposure as providing corrective information about the habituation of anxiety, the tolerability of negative emotions, and the patient's ability to cope with exposure to the feared stimulus. Most therapeutic tasks may be conducted for an extended period until habituation has occurred. For individuals who experience prominent feelings of disgust, exposures may need to last longer than usual as this emotion tends to habituate more slowly than does fear (Olatunji, Smits, Connolly, Willems, & Lohr, 2007). Some exposure tasks are necessarily brief, such as pricking one's finger with a lancet and receiving an injection. In these cases, the task may be repeated several times until habituation occurs, or it can be described as an experiment that provides patients with an opportunity to put their beliefs about dreaded feared consequences to the test. Lastly, patients who faint upon exposure to BII stimuli may benefit from learning applied tension prior to beginning exposure tasks. As long as the risk of fainting remains unacceptably high,

TABLE 14.3. Examples of Exposure Exercises for Blood, Injection, and Injury Fears

Feared stimulus	Exposure stimuli
Blood	View pictures of blood and wounds, watch video clips and movies depicting blood and/or medical procedures, hold a jar containing animal blood, handle a bloody object (e.g., raw steak), place fake blood on body and pretend it's real, prick finger with lancet, observe another person receive a blood draw, have one's blood drawn, donate blood
Needles	View pictures of needles, watch video clips and movies depicting needles and injections, view and handle needles, press needle against one's skin, prick finger with lancet, observe another person receive an injection or blood draw, receive an injection (e.g., immunization shot) or blood draw, observe or receive acupuncture, donate blood
Dental procedures	View pictures of dental procedures, watch video clips and movies of dental procedures, listen to audio clips of dental sounds, view and handle dental tools, sit in dentist's waiting room, sit in dentist's chair, observe another person undergoing dental procedures, have teeth cleaned by dentist, undergo needed dental procedures
Medical procedures	View pictures of medical procedures, watch video clips and movies of medical procedures, view and handle medical tools, walk through a hospital, sit in doctor's office waiting room, sit on examination table, observe another person undergoing medical procedures, see doctor about minor symptoms without receiving a full physical exam, have blood pressure taken by a nurse, see doctor for physical examination, undergo needed medical procedures

the patient and therapist should take precautions to minimize the risk of injury (e.g., falling and hitting one's head) during exposures. The therapist may also wish to consider referring patients who faint for a medical evaluation, as fainting can pose a health hazard in rare cases.

IMPLEMENTING RESPONSE PREVENTION

Patients should be encouraged to begin fading their avoidance and in-situation safety behaviors at the outset of therapy, and to strive to eliminate them completely once exposure sessions begin. Because passive avoidance is the primary safety behavior for most people with BII phobias, the act of initiating exposure therapy is itself a form of response prevention. Individuals with a history of fainting likely use a variety of strategies to prevent this. For example, a 38-year-old woman ate protein bars, drank sugary drinks, used diaphragmatic breathing, and listened to music as a distraction when she felt faint. It is important that such actions be eliminated during exposure and replaced with more adaptive coping strategies, such as applied tension (see below).

HINTS, TIPS, AND POTENTIAL PITFALLS
Preventing Fainting with Applied Tension

Conducting exposure with BII-fearful patients who faint upon exposure to BII stimuli poses a unique challenge and requires modifications to standard exposure therapy. Specifically, the therapist should first instruct the patient in *applied tension*. This method involves tensing the body's major muscles to counteract the rapid decrease in blood pressure that accompanies the fainting response. Muscle tension was first tested during World War II as a method to help prevent fighter pilots from blacking out during high centrifugal force maneuvers. Beginning in the 1980s, psychologists began applying this technique with individuals suffering from BII phobias. Research has since demonstrated that a single session of exposure accompanied by instruction in applied tension is a highly effective treatment (Hellstrom, Fellenius, & Ost, 1996).

Applied tension is designed to be used at the first sign that one is becoming faint. Patients are encouraged to attend to their physiological reactions to BII stimuli and use applied tension on an as-needed basis. The procedure is straightforward and consists of tightly tensing the muscles in the legs, arms, and torso, as if one is striking a bodybuilder pose. The tension should be held until the individual experiences a warm sensation or "rush" in the head, usually for about 15 to 20 seconds, followed by a 30-second relaxation period (Antony & Watling, 2006). Patients who intend to use this procedure during injections should practice tensing their muscles while relaxing the arm in which the needle stick will occur. Patients may also need to be reminded to breathe normally while tensing. Antony and Watling recommend conducting five trials of applied tension to prevent fainting. These authors further recommend that patients initially practice using applied tension five times per day, away from contact with BII stimuli, to become skilled with the procedure and more effectively make use of it during exposure to BII stimuli. Once the patient is skilled in its use, applied tension may be used in conjunction with exposure tasks. In our experience, it is sometimes necessary for patients to use more than five applied tension trials during exposures. We recommend that patients continue to engage in applied tension trials until they are confident that fainting will not occur. Applied tension may also be used to recover more quickly in the event that a patient actually loses consciousness.

Managing Extreme Pain Sensitivity

Patients with needle phobias often express concern that the level of pain experienced during injections will be intolerable. For some individuals, this concern is exaggerated and the therapist may use exposure tasks to assist the patient in learning that injections elicit only mild and temporary pain (see the case example below for an illustration). However, some patients are exquisitely sensitive to the discomfort of needle sticks and experience such extreme pain that receiving an injection is a traumatic experience. One patient, a 26-year-old woman with a severe needle phobia, experienced a psychotic episode requiring hospitalization for 2 days after she received an epidural during the birth of her first (and only) child. For such individuals, simply being willing to receive an injection, regardless of their level of discomfort, may be the most realistic outcome. In these cases the therapist should consider taking steps to reduce the pain of needle sticks rather than attempt to restructure the patient's catastrophic beliefs about needle pain. This strategy may also be useful in the treatment of children with needle fears. A number of highly effective, evidence-based techniques exist for reducing injection pain, including the topical anesthetics lidocaine-prilocaine and amethocaine (EMLA; Lander, Weltman, & So, 2006). Therapists should work together with dental and medical professionals, most of whom are familiar with these and other strategies designed to reduce injection pain (Meit, Yasek, Shannon, Hickman, & Williams, 2004).

CASE ILLUSTRATION

Kate, a 28-year-old married woman who was 6 months pregnant with her first child requested urgent treatment for her fear of injections. Kate had managed to avoid contact with needles for over a decade but was facing the prospect of a medically necessary injection in 3 weeks time. Concerned that she would not be able to tolerate this procedure, she was highly motivated to overcome her fear as quickly as possible. The therapist discussed the possibility of conducting a single-session, exposure-based treatment the following week during which Kate would quickly progress through a brief fear hierarchy that would include facing her worst fear: receiving an injection. A treatment planning session for the purposes of functional analysis and hierarchy development would occur before the intensive exposure session. The patient consented to this approach in an effort to prepare for her upcoming medical procedure.

Functional assessment revealed that Kate was concerned about being contaminated by needles and developing a serious illness. She also feared that the pain of a needle stick would be unbearable and expressed concern about the possibility of passing out. Kate recalled having lost consciousness on several occasions while receiving injections during her adolescence. Avoidance was her primary safety behavior, and she had not received an injection for approximately 10 years. Toward the end of the treatment planning session, the therapist assisted Kate in constructing a fear hierarchy. Given the brief duration (4 hours) of the planned single-session exposure treatment, items were selected by considering the feasibility of completing them within this time frame. It was deemed important for Kate to actually receive an injection in order to prepare her for her upcoming procedure. The final exposure hierarchy was as follows:

Description of the exposure task	SUDS
Learning about needles from a phlebotomist	40
Pricking finger with lancet	80
Observing therapist receive a blood draw	85
Receiving a blood draw	95
Receiving an injection	100

Kate returned for her exposure therapy session the next week. The session began with a review of the rationale and procedures for exposure therapy. Next, the therapist instructed Kate in the use of applied tension to manage any faintness she might experience during the exposure tasks. She practiced tensing her muscles for several minutes and was encouraged to use this procedure during any subsequent exposure trials in which she noticed herself feeling faint.

The first exposure task involved meeting with Mary, an experienced and empathic phlebotomist, in the hospital's phlebotomy department. The therapist had arranged this meeting in advance. Mary showed Kate the tools of the trade and described how they are used. Kate learned about needle sterilization procedures and reported that this information greatly reduced her concerns about contamination. Mary demonstrated the procedure of drawing blood using a doll and, after initially high anxiety, Kate was able to approach the doll and closely observe the procedure.

Next, the therapist and patient returned to the therapy office to conduct an exposure involving pricking fingers with diabetic lancets that had been purchased from the hospital pharmacy. The purpose of this exposure was to provide Kate with corrective information about the degree of pain produced by needle sticks. She initially expressed misgivings about this task due to the expected experience of intolerable pain, but agreed to proceed when the therapist modeled the exposure and suggested they complete the task together. After the first trial, Kate reported being surprised that the sensation of pricking her finger, while uncomfortable, was manageable and far less painful than she anticipated. Following five additional finger sticks, her SUDS ratings had decreased from 90 to 20.

The next exposure necessitated a return visit to Mary in the phlebotomy department. The therapist was seated and Mary slowly placed a tourniquet on his arm and cleaned the inside of his elbow with an alcohol swab, explaining each action in detail for Kate's benefit. The therapist then received a blood draw, with two vials filled. Kate stood next to the therapist and was encouraged to closely observe the procedures and ask any questions that came to mind. After this procedure was finished, it was Kate's turn to receive a blood draw. She was visibly apprehensive during the procedure, and her fear continued to escalate as the tourniquet and alcohol swab were applied and the needle was produced. Nevertheless, Kate asked Mary to proceed with the blood draw, and Kate remained seated until the procedure was complete. The therapist offered verbal support and praise during the exposure and encouraged her to attend to the procedure and observe that it was minimally painful and harmless.

The final hierarchy item required Kate to receive an injection, which she considered to be somewhat worse than having her blood removed via venipuncture. Once again, Mary's assistance was recruited for this task, in this case to administer a flu vaccination. Kate's shoulder was swabbed with alcohol and the needle was injected into her shoulder muscle. The patient appeared somewhat less visibly anxious than with the venipuncture and again reported that the pain was far less than what she had expected. Her self-efficacy in coping with injections and in tolerating the associated discomfort was reinforced at every possible opportunity by the therapist. Despite her preparation in applied tension at the beginning of the session, Kate did not report feelings of faintness during any of the exposures and did not utilize this procedure.

Kate was in good spirits following the final exposure and reported a substantial improvement in her fear of injections. She described being less concerned about the possible negative consequences of injections and was more confident in her ability to tolerate them. Given the time constraints posed by her forthcoming pregnancy-related injection, the stated goal of therapy was to improve her fear of injections by a degree sufficient for her to be (1) willing to undergo this procedure, and (2) able to do so with a manageable level of anxiety and pain. Kate appeared confident this goal had been met, and therapy was tentatively terminated with an open invitation for Kate to return for additional sessions if she desired. Two weeks later, she contacted the therapist and happily reported that she was able to receive the injection with moderate levels of anxiety.

ADDITIONAL RESOURCE

Antony, M. M., & Watling, M. A. (2006). *Overcoming medical phobias: How to conquer fear of blood, needles, doctors, and dentists.* Oakland, CA: New Harbinger Publications.

Meit, S. S., Yasek, V., Shannon, K., Hickman, D., & Williams, D. (2004). Techniques for reducing anesthetic injection pain: An interdisciplinary survey of knowledge and application. *Journal of the American Dental Association, 135,* 1243–12530.

15

Incompleteness, Asymmetry, and "Not-Just-Right" Feelings

CLINICAL PRESENTATION

If a patient complains of the need to reorder, realign, repeat, or engage in other types of seemingly senseless and nonproductive ordering or arranging behaviors, there is a good chance that he or she has OCD. Such rituals are among the more "classic" signs and symptoms of this disorder. Yet, as we have seen, rituals like these are usually a response to anxiety or distress and serve to *reduce* anxiety in the moment. Thus, these symptoms are appropriate candidates for exposure therapy targeting the anxiety-provoking elements. This chapter addresses how to tailor exposure therapy for the types of distress-evoking phenomena that trigger ordering and arranging rituals: namely, feelings of "incompleteness," "asymmetry," and the sense that things are "not just right." Table 15.1 presents an overview of the conceptualization and exposure-based treatment of these symptoms.

Clinical observations and research studies suggest that the distress associated with asymmetry can result from a fear of either causing negative events or of initiating an unending sense of incompleteness. Although these subtypes may seem similar on a superficial level (i.e., they both involve a sense of incompleteness), the underlying functional properties are in fact quite distinct (e.g., Summerfeldt, 2004, 2008). In the first form of this problem, the distress associated with negative events derives from magical thinking that links the perceived asymmetry with disastrous events that can only be prevented through ordering and arranging rituals—for example, "If the books are not arranged perfectly on the shelf, I will have bad luck" or "The layout of

TABLE 15.1. Quick Reference Overview: Incompleteness, the Need for Symmetry and Exactness

Fear-evoking stimuli

- Things being out of order, asymmetrical, "unbalanced," or "incomplete"

Prototypical examples

- Touch something with the left hand but not the right hand
- Books arranged out of order on a shelf
- Asymmetry in a figure or environment (e.g., more objects on the left than on the right)
- Picture hanging crookedly on the wall
- Odd numbers
- Handwriting that doesn't look "just right"
- One shirt sleeve rolled up more than the other
- Presence of dirt on an otherwise pristine surface

Safety behaviors

- Ordering and arranging rituals
- Repeating rituals to "put things right"
- Mental ordering/arranging or avoidance (distraction)
- Situational avoidance (e.g., completing paperwork, writing bank checks)

DSM-IV-TR diagnostic category

- OCD

Treatment overview

- Typical length: 14–20 sessions
- Begin with assessment and psychoeducation
- Begin exposure by session 3 or 4
- Implement response prevention along with exposure

Obstacles

- Identifying feared consequences of the "incompleteness"

---

my desk needs to be 'balanced,' otherwise Mother's plane will crash." Functionally, this "harm-avoidant" symptom pattern is similar to that described in Chapter 10 on anxiety-provoking thoughts. Specifically, the person uses ordering rituals to neutralize unacceptable thoughts and images.

The other form of incompleteness involves ordering and arranging rituals that are performed merely for the sake of obtaining a sense of "completeness" or "correctness" in the environment. These actions are not executed to prevent harm or other external negative consequences from occurring, but rather just to reduce discomfort (Summerfeldt, 2008). Whereas the harm-avoidant symptom pattern described above is usually accompanied by feelings of anxious apprehension, this latter presentation involves a feeling of dissatisfaction, "unfinishedness," or the sense that things are "not just right." Because the harm-avoidant form of this problem is covered in Chapter 10, the latter manifestation of incompleteness, asymmetry, and inexactness is the focus of the present chapter.

BASIS FOR EXPOSURE THERAPY

Theoretical Considerations

Intrusive thoughts and ideas regarding symmetry, exactness, the need for perfection, and the sense that something is *not just right* are relatively common experiences in most adults (e.g., Rachman & de Silva, 1978). These thoughts are known to be associated with uneasiness or situational anxiety, particularly in disorganized environments (Radomsky & Rachman, 2004). Ordering and arranging behaviors performed in the context of this sense of *incompleteness* or *not-just-right* experiences are associated with the reduction in the associated distress (Radomsky & Rachman, 2004). The replacement of "disorder" with "order" and the subsequent resolution of feelings of discomfort can be conceptualized as negatively reinforcing, thus leading to the habitual use of ordering rituals to reduce this sort of discomfort. Unfortunately, escape from the distress associated with incompleteness prevents the natural extinction of the distress. In other words, by ritualizing and restoring "completeness" or order, the person never has an opportunity to learn that he or she can tolerate his or her feelings of discomfort and to recognize that they will eventually subside on their own. Thus, from an exposure therapy perspective, ordering and arranging rituals maintain the idea that imperfection, asymmetry, and disorderliness are intolerable and that the only way to reduce this distress is by removing the not-just-right feeling.

We have observed some patients who become concerned that their feelings of anxiety and incompleteness will stay with them indefinitely and perhaps lead to physical or emotional "breakdown" or a loss of control. For such individuals, rituals serve a dual role of reducing feelings of incompleteness and preventing these feared consequences. We have also had patients who report to us that their ordering and arranging behaviors serve to prevent negative evaluation due to a "messy home," for example. Such a presentation is similar to that observed in individuals with fears of social situations, as described in Chapter 9.

Implications for Exposure Therapy

The conceptual model outlined above leads to a logical and coherent rationale for the use of exposure and response prevention techniques. Namely, corrective learning can take place only if the patient experiences unpleasant thoughts, images, and affective experiences associated with "not-just-right" or "incompleteness-related" stimuli *and* resists the urge to escape from these feelings. If in doing so the negative affective state subsides and no disastrous consequences ensue, this will weaken the psychological links between incompleteness-related stimuli and anxiety, as well as the links between urges to perform arranging rituals and anxiety reduction. As we have seen in previous chapters, this line of reasoning leads to the use of exposure to cues that trigger thoughts, ideas, and feelings of incompleteness, asymmetry, and the like, along with response prevention that involves refraining from performing safety behaviors to escape from the exposure stimuli. The ultimate goal is for habituation of anxiety and distress to occur with repeated prolonged exposure practice in the absence of safety behaviors (i.e., escape behaviors).

FUNCTIONAL ASSESSMENT

Examples of the various parameters of a functional assessment of incompleteness symptoms appear in Table 15.2. The next sections of this chapter describe this assessment in detail.

Fear Cues

External Situations and Stimuli

The most common triggers of feelings of incompleteness are situations, objects, feelings, or numbers (e.g., odd numbers) that the patient associates with "asymmetry," "imbalance," or "disorderliness"—for example, having books arranged "out of order" on a bookshelf or using "messy" handwriting on an important form. One woman became distressed if she was touched or brushed on one side of her body (e.g., her *left*) but not the other (the *right*). In fact, simply hearing the word *left* without hearing the word *right* evoked feelings of "imbalance." Another individual became anxious over odd numbers, for example, on the odometer or when balancing the checkbook. This person experienced no sense of danger, just the idea that odd numbers weren't "right." Most individuals can readily describe the specific situations that trigger this discomfort for them.

Intrusive Thoughts

Although intrusive thoughts are generally not part of this symptom presentation, some individuals report persistent thoughts about incompleteness that are difficult to dismiss.

TABLE 15.2. Functional Assessment of Incompleteness, Asymmetry Feeling at a Glance

Parameter	Common examples
Fear cues	
External situations and stimuli	Situations, environments, objects, and other stimuli (e.g., odd numbers) that provoke a "not-just-right," "incomplete," "unbalanced," or "unfinished" feeling or sense (e.g., asymmetry)
Internal cues	Sensations associated with anxious arousal or feelings of incompleteness ("not-just-right" feelings)
Intrusive thoughts	Recurrent thoughts about incompleteness and the need for order or symmetry
Feared consequences	Feelings of incompleteness are intolerable and will persist indefinitely or lead to dangerous consequences (e.g., physical harm, loss of control, mental breakdown)
Safety behaviors	
Avoidance patterns	Situations that trigger feelings of incompleteness (e.g., getting dressed, entering certain rooms, completing paperwork)
In-situation safety behaviors	Ordering and arranging rituals to bring about symmetry, order, completeness
Beliefs about safety behaviors	Rituals and avoidance prevent the feelings of incompleteness from persisting forever. Rituals prevent an "overload" of anxiety, which could lead to bodily harm, loss of control/going crazy, or mental "breakdown"

Feared Consequences

As we mentioned at the beginning of this chapter, incompleteness can be accompanied by fears that an *external* disaster (e.g., bad luck, accidents) will befall oneself or others if a compulsive ritual is not performed to reinstate "completeness." However, this sort of magical thinking is less common than the fear that if they are allowed to continue, feelings of incompleteness, imbalance, imperfection, and so on, will persist indefinitely. With the latter presentation, it is intense and enduring psychological distress that is the primary feared consequence. Others, however, are also concerned that the feelings of incompleteness, and the like will increase to unmanageable levels and result in some sort of *internal* harm, such as a loss of psychological control or a medical emergency (similar to a panic attack). We find that this fear is often difficult for patients to articulate. Thus, functional assessment must carefully attend to the possibility that such concerns are present (as we address later in this chapter).

Safety Behaviors
Avoidance Patterns

Patients with incompleteness concerns may avoid odd numbers, certain rooms with asymmetry, or completing paperwork, knowing that these situations would evoke discomfort and urges to perform rituals. Individuals might avoid buying new items to prevent having to continually work on their upkeep. One particularly severe patient isolated herself as much as possible because of her persistent urges to mentally count letters in words and words in sentences that she read or heard (to make sure there were an even number of letters and words).

In-Situation Safety Behaviors

The most common safety behaviors are rituals aimed to achieve order, perfection, and balance, and to reduce incompleteness-related distress. Such rituals may involve ordering and arranging, counting, repeating actions an even number of times, and rewriting. One individual drove his car until the odometer was on an even number. Another repeatedly opened and closed her bedroom door until the handle audibly clicked in the "correct" manner. Mental rituals might also be present; for example, the patient with left–right concerns subvocally said the word *right* if she heard the word *left* (and vice versa). As mentioned, some patients mentally count letters in words (or words in sentences) or stare at certain points in space to establish symmetry. A thorough functional assessment should readily identify such behaviors.

Beliefs about Safety Behaviors

Individuals with these concerns typically believe that their safety behaviors are necessary to prevent the feared consequences described earlier in this chapter.

PRESENTING THE RATIONALE
FOR EXPOSURE THERAPY

Using the previously described conceptual framework as a guide, the therapist can provide a rationale for exposure therapy to the patient that is similar to the one included in the following dialogue:

THERAPIST: The treatment techniques we will be using to help you with your ordering and arranging problems are called exposure and response prevention. They are designed to weaken two connections involving these rituals. The first connection is between situations, such as seeing a picture hanging off-center, or having one shoe tied more tightly than the other, and *increased* distress. The second connection we need to weaken is the one between ordering and arranging rituals and anxiety *reduction*. Does that make sense?

PATIENT: I see what you mean.

THERAPIST: Great! In exposure therapy, we will gradually help you confront the situations that trigger your uncomfortable feelings of incompleteness, while also practicing resisting the rituals you're using to artificially reduce your distress—the response prevention component. I know this will be difficult for you, but when you practice exposure and response prevention you will have the opportunity to find out that your distress does not stay forever. In fact, it will dissipate on its own if you give it time. For now, because you're always doing rituals and avoiding, you don't have the chance to see this for yourself. We'll go gradually so you're not feeling overwhelmed, but in the end, treatment will require you to face these uncomfortable situations and stay exposed—without ritualizing—until you "get used" to the feelings of incompleteness, which will happen eventually. When you do this consistently, you'll see that these feelings provoke less and less distress for you.

DEVELOPING THE EXPOSURE HIERARCHY

When developing the exposure hierarchy for patients with incompleteness problems, the therapist and patient must come up with stimuli that provoke the same sense of incompleteness, imperfection, asymmetry, imbalance, and the like as those situations that provoke distress or avoidance in the patient's day-to-day life. Most patients do not have difficulty identifying such triggers or assigning SUDS ratings for hierarchy items related to incompleteness. While the particular situations will be patient-specific, some examples from our work are as follows:

- Tilting pictures unevenly in the office or the patient's home
- Putting items in the "wrong" place or arranging them asymmetrically
- Purposely using poor handwriting
- Arranging bookshelves or drawers out of order

- Putting smudges on tables, windows, or the computer screen
- Writing odd numbers on one's hand
- Performing actions an odd number of times (e.g., flick the light switch five times)

For some patients, it will be important that exposure be consistent or involve the entire environment. For example, desks at home *and at work* must be rearranged or asymmetrical, and friends or relatives may be enlisted to help with such tasks. For others, exposure to specific incompleteness-related stimuli (e.g., a smudge on the right side—but not the left side—of a window) might be sufficient.

CONDUCTING EXPOSURE THERAPY SESSIONS

For the most part, exposure for incompleteness concerns lends itself well to gradual progression up the hierarchy. Whenever possible, situations should first be confronted in the therapy session under the clinician's supervision, and then between sessions for homework practice. Patients typically show the characteristic within- and between-session habituation of incompleteness-related anxiety and distress when exposure and response prevention are performed correctly. The therapist also helps the patient develop a more realistic appraisal of these feelings that views them as uncomfortable, yet temporary and manageable. That is, instead of requiring an immediate response to prevent ever-increasing distress, the patient learns from exposure that the distress associated with the sense of incompleteness fades naturally over time, and so that rituals are therefore unnecessary. Imaginal exposure is typically not needed in the treatment of this presentation of incompleteness.

IMPLEMENTING RESPONSE PREVENTION

In addition to confronting their sense of inexactness, unevenness, imbalance, and general imperfection, patients with incompleteness concerns must refrain from rituals. As part of response prevention, objects may not be reordered, cleaned, or rearranged. Efforts to "balance things out" (e.g., by counting to an even number, by rearranging) must be resisted. For some patients, counting is performed mentally and feelings of symmetry or order are achieved visually (e.g., by looking or staring in specified ways), or with special bodily movements (e.g., by tapping), or through vocalizations (e.g., by repeating words or phrases). Because of their pervasiveness, abruptness, and subtlety, such rituals might seem automatic and difficult to stop. A strategy that is often helpful in such cases is for the patient to initially track such rituals using a handheld counter. This can help the patient identify the antecedents to performing the rituals. Next, he or she practices executing the ritual incorrectly (e.g., counting to the wrong number, staring the "wrong way"), so that performing the behavior does not relieve distress. This intermediate step makes it easier to end the ritual completely.

Oftentimes, especially at the beginning of response prevention, patients will reflexively perform a ritual before having time to resist it. At these times the patient can "undo" the effects of the rituals by restoring the imbalance or incompleteness (e.g., by brushing the object against only his left side) in order to complete an exposure. If this purposeful elicitation of the sense of incorrectness is not successful, the routine can at least serve as a mild consequence for ritualizing that may make it easier to resisting ritualizing in the future.

HINTS, TIPS, AND POTENTIAL PITFALLS

Evoking Distress in Sessions

For some patients, intentionally setting up disorder or unevenness in the office may not sufficiently evoke anxiety, distress, or a sense of incompleteness. Patients may report that their distress only occurs when something *spontaneously* seems "not just right" and that it does not bother them to *purposely* make things uneven. In these situations it is still advisable to proceed with contrived exposure therapy. Sometimes patients experience more distress than they expected. Other times, it can be helpful to have the patient participate in a natural activity during the session, such as working on a computer, writing checks, or walking around out of the office, and wait for the sense of incompleteness or unevenness to arise naturally. Finally, it can be helpful to describe exposures as similar to practicing for a team sport. Although the drills and even scrimmages during practice can never be the same as a real game, those exercises help build skills to improve performance during the game. Thus, although the patients may merely be walking through the steps of exposures and response prevention in the session, it may increase the likelihood that they can respond in a similar fashion when the symptoms occur.

Incompleteness in Non-Anxiety-Based Disorders

It is important to distinguish between incompleteness symptoms that are experienced as *unwanted* and *distressing* (such as those that occur in OCD) and those that are experienced as worthwhile, as observed in many people with obsessive–compulsive personality disorder (OCPD). In the former instance, patients with OCD emphasize how such problems interfere with their functioning and wish they didn't have to be bothered with them. In other words, people with OCD try to resist these symptoms. In contrast, those people with OCPD often view their perfectionism and ordering/arranging rituals as part of who they are (i.e., "ego syntonic"). They *strive* to attain perfection because they have imposed unrealistically high standards for themselves. Thus, they do not view their symptoms as problematic, nor do they resist urges to reorder or rearrange. In fact, such individuals typically balk when others urge them to give up such behaviors. This key difference in the function of seemingly similar behaviors is often overlooked by clinicians, but has significant treatment implications: whereas exposure therapy is likely to be of help to people who view their incompleteness symptoms as anxiety-provoking, this therapeutic approach will not reduce the symptoms of OCPD, which are viewed as helpful or necessary by the person. This highlights the importance of the functional assessment.

CASE ILLUSTRATION

Jill was a 36-year-old woman who had a diagnosis of OCD with primarily ordering and arranging rituals that were triggered by a sense of "imperfection" and "imbalance." Activities such as completing paperwork often took her hours because Jill had to painstakingly make sure that letters were formed correctly and "perfectly" to avoid the feeling of incompleteness. Items in the house had to be arranged in certain ways, and Jill had to ensure that such order was maintained. Her most pervasive symptoms focused on evenness in her environment in that she was bothered by left–right "imbalance." For example, if she used her *right* hand to open a door or to grab something (e.g., from the refrigerator), she felt an urge to repeat the same behavior using her *left* hand (and vice versa) to achieve balance. These symptoms limited Jill's ability to function to the point that on many days she was unable to leave her house.

Jill's exposure hierarchy was as follows:

Description of the exposure task	SUDS
Write letters (i.e., *ABC*) "imperfectly"	40
Write imperfectly in checkbook	55
Leave items in the family room "out of order"	67
Leave items in her own room "out of order"	75
Say, write, and hear the word *left* without the word *right*	75

| "Notice" left–right imbalance | 80 |
| Touch items on right (or left) side only | 85 |

Jill's response prevention plan involved the following:

- No rewriting rituals
- No ordering/arranging rituals
- No attempts to achieve left–right balance visually, verbally, motorically, or otherwise

During the first and second exposure sessions, Jill practiced writing letters imperfectly (e.g., sloppily), with her therapist modeling this behavior. First she wrote imperfectly on blank pieces of paper, then on notes that she later sent to others, and finally on important forms and documents such as financial statements and bank checks. Jill also practiced this exposure between sessions.

At the third and fourth sessions, Jill practiced rearranging items in the therapist's office so that they were "not balanced." For example, she tilted the therapist's picture frames slightly to the right and shifted books on the bookshelves to the right. Jill's homework assignments involved gradually rearranging items in her own home so that they seemed "out of order." This assignment began with items in the living room and eventually involved items in her bedroom. Jill was instructed to remind herself that these items were "out of order," but to also refrain from urges to rearrange them in the "correct" way.

The fifth session involved confrontation with the word *left* in the absence of the word *right*. Jill practiced saying "left" and even writing it on the back of both of her hands. Homework exposure involved further exposure to "left." She also kept a piece of paper with this word in her pocket at all times. Jill's therapist helped Jill learn to accept the feelings of incompleteness and imbalance as normal and not harmful. Jill was able to see that although distressing at first, these feelings dissipated more and more quickly with each successful exposure practice.

Session 6 involved continued exposure to the word *left*, as well as to purposely noticing left–right imbalance and not performing any "balancing" rituals. To provoke this type of discomfort, Jill and her therapist walked though the clinic and purposely pointed out "unevenness" and "imbalance" in the environment (e.g., door handles and light switches on the right side of doors, the fact that more people were sitting on the right side of the waiting room than on the left side, more papers on the left side of the desk than the right side). Jill also purposely brushed against objects such as walls and desks on either her left *or* her right side without "balancing" this out (and making sure that she *never* was able to achieve this type of balance). She completed similar exposures between sessions. In addition, she was instructed to leave her belt buckle slightly off center (facing left) and to tie her left shoe noticeably more tightly than her right shoe.

Sessions 7 through 16 involved repeated exposure to left–right imbalance in various contexts. For example, Jill created this imbalance in her bedroom and encouraged her family to do the same in various parts of the house. Treatment was successful largely because Jill learned that she could manage her temporary feelings of incompleteness, which passed without creating any harmful or negative consequences. Prior to her therapy Jill had always ritualized, which prevented her from learning this lesson on her own.

ADDITIONAL RESOURCES

Radomsky, A. S., & Rachman, S. (2004). Symmetry, ordering and arranging compulsive behaviour. *Behaviour Research and Therapy, 4*, 893–913.

Summerfeldt, L. J. (2004). Understanding and treating incompleteness in obsessive–compulsive disorder. *Journal of Clinical Psychology, 60*, 1155–1168.

Summerfeldt, L. J. (2006). Treating incompleteness, ordering, and arranging concerns. In M. Antony, C. Purdon, & L. J. Summerfeldt (Eds.), *Psychological treatment of OCD: Fundamentals and beyond* (pp. 197–208). Washington, DC: American Psychological Association Press.

Summerfeldt, L. J. (2008). Symmetry, incompleteness, and ordering. In J. Abramowitz, D. McKay, & S. Taylor (Eds.), *Clinical handbook of obsessive–compulsive disorder and related problems* (pp. 44–60). Baltimore, MD: Johns Hopkins University Press.

Part III

Special Considerations in the Use of Exposure Techniques

The third and final section of this book covers special topics in the delivery of exposure therapy. The following chapters present practical advice for facing some of the complex challenges associated with the use of exposure therapy in the treatment of patients with anxiety problems. First, in Chapter 16, we discuss conceptual and practical issues in adapting exposure therapy for patients whose presentation is complex as opposed to straightforward. Next, in Chapter 17, we cover special considerations for using exposure therapy with children. Anxiety problems often have an interpersonal dimension in which significant others are involved in either accommodating symptoms or contributing to increased stress by arguing with the sufferer, both of which may contribute to the maintenance of fear and complicate treatment. Accordingly, in Chapter 18 we discuss the role that significant others play in anxiety problems and present strategies for involving family members in the patient's treatment. Chapter 19 is devoted to discussing the effects of medications—both positive and negative—on exposure therapy, as well as supplying strategies to improve outcomes for patients receiving combined treatment. Chapter 20 then outlines strategies for maintaining improvement and preventing relapse. The book closes with Chapter 21, which highlights the unique ethical and safety concerns associated with this treatment approach.

16

Exposure Therapy with Complex Cases

As anyone who specializes in the treatment of clinical anxiety will testify, comorbidity and complexity are the rule rather than the exception. Some clinicians, however, are hesitant to use exposure with patients who present with complicating diagnoses or other complexities. As a result, exposure may be abandoned based on the belief that alternative treatment approaches are more appropriate. Of course, using exposure therapy with complex cases can be challenging, and it requires additional time and planning (McKay, Abramowitz, & Taylor, 2009). However, this approach is still the most appropriate intervention and can be used within the context of a broader treatment strategy. As such, the current chapter opens with a discussion of some general considerations for using exposure with complex patients. Next, we address how the clinician can deal with specific obstacles that commonly complicate matters, including considerations for treating anxiety in the context of comorbidity.

GENERAL CONSIDERATIONS FOR COMPLEX CASES

Before discussing specific factors that increase the complexity of providing exposure therapy, we review some general principles for managing complicated cases. These themes are intended to help the therapist sort through the myriad of competing concerns and arrive at a workable treatment plan. In addition, refocusing on these and other core principles can help reduce the feeling of being overwhelmed by a challenging case.

Adhere to the Theoretical Foundation and Functional Assessment

When initial exposure sessions are unsuccessful, it may be tempting to consider the patient "resistant to exposure" and look for alternative paradigms to explain and treat his or her problem. But rather than placing the blame with the patient (or his or her symptoms), we encourage therapists to bear in mind that the problem might lie in the exposure plan itself or how it is being implemented. For instance, treatment may not lead to symptom relief if items chosen for exposure do not match to the patient's fears, if exposure is not practiced frequently enough, if the patient does not remain exposed until habituation occurs, or if there is a problem with how response prevention is being implemented. In our own clinical work, and in supervising many therapists, we find that in the majority of instances clinical complexity can be dealt with successfully by "going back to the drawing board." This process entails making sure that the functional assessment is complete, determining that the exposure plan follows from this assessment, and ensuring that exposures are applied in ways that serve to disconfirm the patient's fears.

Consider Richard, a 32-year-old man diagnosed with social phobia and agoraphobia who spent the better part of the last 5 years in his parents' home unable to hold a job or go to school. Curiously, when attempting to create an exposure hierarchy to public situations Richard insisted that he was neither fearful of being evaluated by others, nor of having a panic attack. In fact, he performed at local bars with his band several nights per month without the slightest bit of anxiety. Richard's extreme avoidance behavior led to the suspicion that he was simply trying to manipulate his family. His therapist subsequently shifted away from a cognitive-behavioral approach toward a more psychodynamic one. A functional assessment of this patient's fears, however, revealed that he was fearful of *vomiting* in public. Questioning revealed that the patient was only able to perform with his band outside the home if he avoided eating for 6 hours before leaving. Once the details of the patient's fears were understood via functional assessment, treatment involving exposure to vomit-related triggers (including eating heavy foods) and situations (being in social gatherings where there was alcohol) was extremely successful in helping him return to a normal life.

Assess the Connection between Symptoms

Complicated cases often involve overlapping concerns. Understanding the connections between the patient's symptoms can help the therapist develop an effective treatment plan. For instance, Ginny, a 24-year-old woman with OCD, also had comorbid panic disorder. Although Ginny met criteria for two different anxiety disorders, functional assessment revealed that the symptoms of both her conditions were closely related: Ginny's panic attacks were triggered by the anxious arousal she experienced when having obsessional thoughts and doubts about her faith (e.g., "Do I have *enough* faith in God?"). Her compulsive praying functioned to reduce her obsessions and to prevent panic attacks, which she feared would result in a loss of control. Since her dread of panic attacks prevented her from engaging in ERP for her obsessions, the therapist decided to begin treatment with interoceptive exposures to arousal-related body sensations. Once Ginny learned that feeling anxious was not likely to lead to loss of control, she was able to successfully complete exposures to obsessional stimuli (e.g., books about atheism and the devil), that previously would have been avoided because of the severe panic attacks they provoked.

In other circumstances, a single underlying cause can lead to superficially distinct anxiety problems. For example, high levels of anxiety sensitivity (i.e., fear of one's own anxiety response) can be manifested as *panic disorder* if one fears dying from anxiety symptoms, or as *social phobia* if one fears being negatively evaluated for exhibiting anxiety symptoms. In both instances, treatment targets the underlying fear of the anxiety response; thus a single intervention involving interoceptive exposure (perhaps combined with situational exposure to social situations) could be used to treat both problems. At other times, however, co-occurring conditions are fairly independent. For instance, a patient may suffer from a gambling addiction as well as social phobia. In such cases, there may not be a meaningful connection between symptoms, and two separate treatment approaches might be necessary.

Prioritize Treatment

Regardless of the complexity of a given presenting complaint, the therapist and the patient need to agree on which symptoms to address first. When prioritizing treatment goals therapists should consider the severity of each symptom and its impact on the patient's functioning. Symptoms that put the patient's safety at risk or interfere with therapy need to be addressed first (Linehan, 1993). Suicide attempts, self-harming behavior, and substance abuse would be included in this category. Symptoms that are *not* dangerous but may interfere with implementing exposure include panic attacks (as in the example described above) and agoraphobia (e.g., inability to leave the home). Frequent cancellation of appointments, consistently arriving late for sessions, distrust of the therapist, and persistent avoidance of exposure practices (e.g., stalling by raising less important topics in the session) are also therapy-interfering behaviors. Until these factors are addressed, it is unlikely that exposure-based treatment will be successful.

Once safety and a working relationship have been established, the therapist and the patient should collaborate in determining which symptoms to address next. One approach is to begin with the most pressing concerns. For instance, if a child is afraid to attend school, feels depressed, and is fighting with his parents, treatment might begin by addressing the school phobia in order to avoid developing additional problems with grades and friendships. Alternatively, one might elect to begin by working on a less severe, yet more amenable, symptom. For example, a 48-year-old woman decided to conquer her fear of elevators before working on her phobia of bees since elevators were readily accessible (during winter, when she sought treatment) and less frightening. Success with elevator exposures increased her confidence when it came time to address the more challenging fear of bees during the following spring. When applicable, therapy can be most efficient when targeting symptoms that cause or contribute to other problems, such as panic disorder that has lead to depression. By successfully treating the primary symptoms (panic attacks), the secondary concerns (depression) may resolve as well.

Although there are no hard-and-fast rules regarding which problem to address first, once a plan has been agreed upon it is advisable to stick with it until substantial progress has been made. It is important for the patient to experience a decrease in his or her symptoms and to gain confidence in the therapeutic process before changing focus. Yet exceptions can be made when necessary. For example, one 16-year-old girl began with exposures to feared contaminants, which were her most pressing problem. But this patient also suffered from social anxiety, and the focus of exposure had to be shifted briefly to public speaking when she became extremely anxious about an upcoming presentation she had to give orally in front of her class. Similarly, if a patient experiences a significant loss, such as a death in the family or loss of a job, these issues can be addressed immediately, using techniques other than exposure, at the patient's and the therapist's discretion.

Collaborate with Other Professionals

Patients with complex symptom profiles may require treatment from multiple professionals. Such care can be provided concurrently, such as when a patient receives medication or couple therapy (from a separate therapist) while also participating in exposure treatment, or consecutively, such as treating OCD after manic symptoms have been stabilized. In either circumstance, but especially when another therapist will *continue* to be involved with the patient, it is important for the providers to communicate with one another. Communication allows providers to clearly define their own roles and avoid providing overlapping services or conflicting advice. This allows the exposure therapist to set appropriate expectations regarding what can be addressed through exposure therapy.

COMMON COMPLICATING FACTORS AND OBSTACLES IN THE USE OF EXPOSURE THERAPY

In the above section, we reviewed some general principles to keep in mind when working with challenging patients. Next, we turn to a discussion of specific factors that can complicate the use of exposure and affect the outcome of treatment. We have organized these factors into three categories: (1) characteristics of the treatment itself, (2) patient-related factors, and (3) characteristics of the patient's environment. These are also listed in Table 16.1.

Characteristics Related to Exposure Treatment

Treatment-Related Symptoms

Sometimes a patient's anxiety may become focused on the exposure exercises themselves and impede treatment. We have observed this phenomenon most often among people with OCD as opposed to other anxiety problems. For instance, a 42-year-old man with obsessions that his family would die if he did not repeat certain actions (e.g., turning out a light) in sets of three made good initial progress with exposures. However, toward the end of treatment, he began to have obsessional thoughts that if he did not repeat his exposure practices three times, his treatment would be incomplete and his OCD would worsen. Thus, he was in a bind: he believed that both completing and refraining from exposures would be detrimental. When the

---

TABLE 16.1. Common Obstacles to the Successful Use of Exposure Therapy for Anxious Patients

Characteristics related to exposure treatment

- Treatment-related symptoms
- Extreme anxiety during exposure
- Minimal anxiety during exposure
- Negative outcomes during exposure

Patient-related factors and comorbid conditions

- Readiness for change
- Coexisting medical conditions
- Comorbid psychological symptoms and disorders

Characteristics of the patient's environment

- Environmental stressors
- Relationship stress

---

patient was instructed to do his exposures "incorrectly" (i.e., once or twice, rather than in threes), his treatment-related symptoms abated. Other aspects of treatment can also become entangled in the anxiety symptoms. Another 34-year-old man with OCD had urges to confess his perceived wrongdoings, mostly related to causing cancer by spreading asbestos. Completing daily symptom monitoring forms thus became a ritual since he believed that the therapist would review them and not let him do anything truly dangerous. Therefore, it was necessary to discontinue the use of these forms and limit the amount of information the patient provided the therapist about his behaviors during the week.

Extreme Anxiety during Exposure

Some exposures elicit overwhelming anxiety that may not decrease as expected. If anxiety does not begin to habituate following a reasonable amount of time, it may suggest that the exposure exercise was too difficult for the patient. In such instances a less anxiety-provoking stimulus should be identified, and the patient should confront this alternate target as an "intermediate" exposure before reattempting the initial exercise. Alternatively, if the patient has the time and resolve, the exposure may be continued in a prolonged manner until habituation occurs. We have occasionally conducted exposures in which it takes an hour or more for the patient's anxiety to habituate (e.g., holding a spider).

At other times, anxiety may remain constant because the patient is worrying about something other than the exposure at hand. For instance, an early (and less anxiety-provoking) exposure may remind a patient about more anxiety-provoking exercise planned for later in treatment. When a patient begins worrying about another topic during an exposure, it is helpful to encourage him or her to rate SUDS based only the anxiety related to the current task, emphasizing that later exposures may seem less difficult once early exposures have been successfully completed. In addition, the patient can be assured that the therapist will not *force* the patient to confront highly anxiety-provoking stimuli if the patient prefers not to do so.

Sometimes, anxiety does not habituate simply because the exposure stimulus is highly distressing. For instance, one patient with social anxiety reported that her SUDS remained very high throughout the duration of an exposure to reading out loud in front of a small audience. Under these circumstances, the therapist should point out that (1) although anxiety did not decrease, the patient was able to *manage* the anxiety and complete the exposure exercise; (2) the anxiety did not *escalate*, lead to a loss of control, medical emergency, or death; and (3) performing the same exposure is likely to be easier the next time it is attempted.

Minimal Anxiety during Exposure

At the other extreme, an exposure task might evoke little or no discomfort. On the one hand, this could be an encouraging sign—perhaps the once feared stimulus no longer provokes anxiety because the patient's expectations of threat have been modified. This is most likely to be the case toward the end of treatment, once the patient has gained confidence with using exposure techniques. However, if early exposures evoke little or no anxiety, it is wise to troubleshoot rather than assume that the patient has improved very rapidly. Absence of anxiety during exposure could result if the key anxiety-evoking aspect(s) of the feared situation has not been incorporated into the exposure. For example, some patients with panic attacks require the provocation of very intense body sensations during interoceptive exposure before they show signs of anxiety. The possibility that the exposure is not adequate can be assessed and resolved by directly asking the patient why the exposure did not evoke anxiety or how the situation could be made more anxiety-provoking. The planning of subsequent exposures must then take this information into account.

A second possibility is that the patient has nullified the exposure with a safety behavior. For example, a patient with fears of vomiting took Zofran (an antiemetic medication) prior to exposure to eating at a restaurant where her friend once vomited. Another patient who had OCD and was strictly religious prayed before her exposure session so that God would understand that she didn't mean the sacrilegious thoughts she was about to provoke as part of the ensuing exposure. This absolved her of anxiety, yet prevented her from benefitting from the exposure exercise, the aim of which was to help her manage uncertainty associated with blasphemous thoughts. If the therapist suspects subtle use of avoidance or safety behaviors during exposure, he or she should inquire about this (e.g., "Is there anything you are doing, or anything you are telling yourself, that might make the exposure less distressing?"). The use of safety behaviors may signal the need for further discussion of the rationale for exposure. Some patients underreport anxiety as a means of avoiding or prematurely terminating an exposure exercise. In these cases, the selected exposure task may be too frightening, and a less distressing one should be considered.

Negative Outcomes during Exposure

Although one aims to engineer exposure tasks that involve minimal risk, *minimal risk* is not the same as *no risk*. As a result, exposures sometimes result in negative outcomes. Some examples from our experience include the following:

- A woman who was afraid of embarrassment was laughed at by a stranger when she deliberately spilled a cup of water in a public place.
- A man with fears of contamination from fruit ate a fairly large quantity of fruit for an exposure. That evening he encountered problems with diarrhea which seemed to reinforce his fear of contamination.
- A woman conducting exposure to driving while being distracted with loud music accidentally made a wrong turn into a one-way street.

Such occurrences might initially seem like setbacks since exposure is supposed to *disconfirm* such fears. Recall, however, that anxious patients overestimate both the *probability* and the *severity* of negative outcomes. Thus, if an exposure produces an undesirable outcome, the clinician can salvage the exercise by helping the patient to modify beliefs about the severity or "awfulness" of the outcome, while acknowledging that such negative events are *possible*. Put another way, the therapist can point out that although something negative occurred as a result of exposure, (1) the result was probably not as bad as the patient had anticipated, and (2) the patient was able to manage the situation appropriately. When negative outcomes are hypothetically possible, they should be discussed prior to the exposure to prepare the patient for this possibility and make it easier to troubleshoot afterward.

Here's how each of the exposures described above were resolved:

- The woman with social anxiety felt very uncomfortable at first, but this soon dissipated and she realized that she could handle the temporary distress associated with being laughed at.
- The patient who experienced diarrhea after eating fruit discussed the incident with his wife, who happened to be a dietitian and perceptively pointed out that the diarrhea was probably a normal gastrointestinal response to the sudden change in diet (increase in fiber). After all, the patient had been avoiding eating any fruit for a long time!
- The woman conducting the driving exposure quickly corrected her mistake and, although she was distressed at making the wrong turn, realized that she could recognize such errors and correct them quickly and safely (even while being distracted). She concluded that her driving skills were probably better than she had thought.

Patient-Related Factors and Comorbid Conditions

Readiness for Change

Patient ambivalence about engaging in treatment can certainly impede progress. If one considers the commitment it takes to repeatedly face one's greatest fears, such reluctance is understandable. In addition, some patients view their symptoms as an important part of who they are, such as a 20-year-old woman with OCD scrupulosity symptoms (i.e., religious obsessions) who believed that her underlying motivation to always be pure and nonoffensive was integral to her personality despite the distress caused by her rituals. Other patients may even see their anxiety as beneficial. For instance, some patients with generalized anxiety are reluctant to reduce their worry because they believe it helps them prevent disasters or to achieve at high levels. In these situations, treatment may begin with an examination of the patient's readiness for change (Prochaska, 2000). In addition, motivational interviewing techniques may be an effective adjunct to cognitive-behavioral therapy with ambivalent patients (Westra & Dozois, 2006).

Coexisting Medical Conditions

The interface between anxiety and medical conditions can increase the complexity of assessment and exposure therapy. As mentioned in Chapter 4, some medical conditions such as hyperthyroidism, pheochromocytoma, hypoglycemia, mitral valve prolapse, asthma, allergies, and gastrointestinal problems can trigger panic attacks or mimic anxiety symptoms. If a patient has not been examined by a general practitioner within the past year, such an exam should be an important first step. For some conditions, such as hyperthyroidism, medical treatment is necessary to reduce symptoms. For others, such as asthma, although medical treatment may reduce symptoms, exposure therapy can be very useful for reducing fears and worries associated with the medical problem itself (Rosqvist, 2005).

Additional issues arise when treating anxiety in the context of a known medical condition. Consider a 58-year-old man with panic disorder as well as a history of multiple heart attacks. A complication here is that the recommended response to a heart attack (immediate activation of emergency medical procedures) and to a panic attack (manage the symptoms independently) are diametrically opposed! In such situations it is important to work closely with the patient's physician to determine guidelines regarding what physical sensations are suggestive of a heart attack (and the need for emergency medical attention) versus panic. Additionally, exposure exercises themselves should be approved as medically safe before beginning them (e.g., interoceptive exposure to climbing stairs for someone with heart disease; exposures to bathroom germs for a cancer survivor with a weakened immune system).

A dilemma sometimes encountered by exposure therapists when treating medically ill patients is that physicians may have a conservative bias toward patient behavior (i.e., "better safe than sorry") that is at odds with exposure therapy's emphasis on encouraging patients to face their fears and tolerate uncertainty. To take one rather extreme example, a 19-year-old medically healthy woman with panic disorder and concerns about having a heart attack was told by her physician to avoid intense physical exertion "just to be on the safe side." The therapist was thus in the uncomfortable predicament of recommending interoceptive exposure tasks (e.g., pushups, running in place) that directly contradicted the physician's advice. Collaboration with medical providers, including education about the theory and practice of exposure therapy, is often useful in navigating such situations, as it was in this particular case.

Comorbid Psychological Symptoms and Disorders

As we have discussed earlier in this chapter, exposure therapy can be complicated by the presence of concurrent psychopathology. Other psychological disorders can involve symptoms that appear similar to anxiety or present obstacles to the completion of exposures. Although an exposure therapist does not need to be able to treat all mental health problems, he or she should be able to identify them and determine if they are likely to interfere with treatment. Next, we review some of the more prominent conditions that co-occur with anxiety or that present obstacles to successful exposure.

Multiple Types of Anxiety. Although it is common for patients to have multiple domains of fear and worry (Kessler, 1995), exposure exercises can usually be applied to each. When multiple anxiety complaints are present, treatment planning should include prioritizing treatment goals. Challenges may occur, however, when one set of worries impacts the treatment of others, such as social anxiety interfering with completing other types of exposures that necessitate going into public places (e.g., exposure to public bathrooms). Pervasive worrying may also require the use of cognitive therapy as an adjunct to exposure (Hansen, Vogel, Stiles, & Gotestam, 2007). Although treating one anxiety symptom sometimes leads to improvement in others (Borkovec, Abel, & Newman, 1995), the therapist may need to focus specifically on helping the patient generalize the effects of exposure from one anxiety domain to another.

Depression. Depression and anxiety frequently co-occur (Kessler, 1995), yet problems with anxiety typically precede the onset of depression (Merikangas et al., 2003). For instance, a 35-year-old man presented for treatment for depression following years of struggling interpersonally because of social anxiety. Accordingly, it is usually appropriate to target the anxiety and fear with the expectation that the depressive symptoms will resolve once the fear and anxiety have improved. However, it is important to keep in mind that severe depression can adversely affect the outcome of exposure (Abramowitz, Franklin, Street, Kozak, & Foa, 2000; Ledley et al.,

2005). For example, although the man in the example above was interested in decreasing his anxiety, his depressive symptoms (e.g., extreme hopelessness and lethargy) made it difficult for him to generate the confidence, optimism, or enthusiasm to complete exposures on his own. In such situations it may be necessary to first target the depression, for example, by using cognitive therapy, behavioral activation, and perhaps antidepressant medication.

Substance Abuse and Dependence. Anxiety also occurs frequently among those with substance use disorders (Grant et al., 2004) and sometimes contributes to their onset (Cowley, 1992). In general, the presence of active substance abuse is predictive of poor response to exposure therapy since psychoactive substances impair one's ability to consolidate information learned during exposure (Oei & Loveday, 1997). Moreover, the use of substances before, during, or after exposure may artificially reduce anxiety and interfere with the natural process of habituation. We recommend that therapists carefully screen for substance abuse or dependence when considering the use of exposure therapy (and throughout the course of treatment); and if present, address such difficulties before initiating exposure therapy. For some patients, such as the socially anxious individual who uses alcohol to reduce anxiety in social settings, substance abuse functions as a safety behavior. If such patients can control the use of this substance, it may be worthwhile beginning exposure treatment while trying to gradually fade the substance use along with other safety behaviors as treatment progresses.

Disordered Eating. When food or eating is the object of fear and worry, anxiety symptoms must be differentiated from an eating disorder. For instance, patients with a phobia of certain foods (e.g., due to a fear of choking or vomiting) may restrict their eating, lose weight, and be difficult to distinguish from those with anorexia nervosa. In addition, eating and anxiety disorders can co-occur, as with an adolescent girl with anorexia who also had obsessions that she would absorb calories (and gain weight) by merely *touching or looking at* food. If a patient is underweight, careful consideration should be given to health implications, as well as the potential for cognitive impairment which could prevent learning during exposure. That is, exposure therapy might be delayed until a healthy weight can be maintained. In instances where a specific phobia (e.g., of choking on food) has resulted in significant weight loss that threatens the patient's health, a combined exposure and weight restoration approach may be required.

Personality Disorders. Some personality disorders (PDs) and traits are likely to hinder response to exposure therapy (Hansen et al., 2007). For example, anxious (e.g., obsessive–compulsive) and dramatic (e.g., histrionic) traits might interfere with developing rapport and adhering to instructions for exposure assignments. The interpersonal crises that frequently accompany some personality traits (e.g., borderline PD) have the potential to derail the focus on exposures. That said, if a strong therapeutic alliance can be developed, exposure can be successful despite these traits. Individuals with personality traits in the odd or eccentric cluster (e.g., schizotypal PD) also present a challenge to exposure therapy because of their reduced ability to consolidate the corrective information that is normally obtained during confrontation with feared stimuli. We therefore advise the reader to *consider* using exposure therapy for anxious individuals with comorbid anxious or dramatic personality traits, while heeding the potential problems discussed above. On the other hand, when odd or eccentric personality disorders or traits are present, other sorts of anxiety management strategies may be preferable to exposure.

Psychotic Symptoms and Mania. As with substance abuse and dependence, psychotic and uncontrolled manic symptoms attenuate the effects of exposure because they interfere with normal perception, cognition, and judgment and impede the ability to follow treatment instructions and consolidate corrective information gleaned through exposure exercises. Therefore, services aimed at bringing such conditions under control (e.g., antipsychotic or antimanic medications) should be sought prior to attempting exposure therapy for anxiety.

Developmental Disorders. Given the cognitive impairments frequently associated with developmental disorders, such as mental retardation and pervasive developmental disorders, exposure-based treatments may be more feasible than comparatively abstract cognitive strategies to address anxiety. However, the deficits associated with these disorders can also interfere with the success of exposure. For instance, a propensity to think concretely and perseverate, as well as difficulties seeing another's perspective, can interfere with the habituation of anxiety within exposures in addition to the ability to generalize from in-session exposure exercises to experiences outside the therapeutic setting. Moreover, some fears and worries in individuals are realistic, perhaps the result of actual skill deficits that make daily situations challenging. For instance, interpersonal deficits, weaknesses in cognitive abilities, and executive processing deficits can make social interactions, transitions, and unexpected changes extremely stressful. Finally, stereotyped movements, self-stimulating behavior, and rigid adherence to routines can superficially resemble problems with anxiety (i.e., obsessions and compulsions) and should be differentiated from these symptoms when planning exposures.

When working with such patients, clinicians should emphasize skill building (Cardaciotto & Herbert, 2004; Reaven & Hepburn, 2003). For instance, before addressing anxiety it may be necessary to improve a patient's social or organizational skills. At other times, environmental adaptations that reduce stress related to unrealistic demands, such as providing classroom accommodations, may be more appropriate than asking the patient to change his or her reactions to an overstimulating situation, such as the noise and chaos of a crowded classroom.

Suicidal Ideation and Self-Injurious Behavior. The therapist's first responsibility is to monitor and ensure the patient's safety. Self-destructive methods for managing negative emotions can pose a threat to a patient's well-being. For example, a 22-year-old woman with severe health anxiety stated that the distress she felt when she was preoccupied with having fatal diseases was so overwhelming that she would cut herself and contemplate suicide. Suicidal ideation can also be associated with other factors in a patient's life such as relationship problems. As mentioned above, regardless of the ultimate cause of self-harm, the safety of the patient should be established before exposure treatment is initiated. If anxiety symptoms lead to unsafe behavior and the anxiety cannot be addressed before safety is established, hospitalization should be considered.

It is important to bear in mind that not all violent thoughts indicate increased risk for harm. As discussed in Chapter 10, some obsessions involve recurrent thoughts of harmful behaviors (e.g., killing family members, molesting children). The presence of such symptoms can be unnerving for a therapist. Thus, when attempting to ascertain a patient's level of risk, it is helpful to evaluate the patient's affective response to the harmful ideation. Patients who react to their violent thoughts with horror or fear are most likely experiencing "ego-dystonic" (i.e., mood-*incongruent*) intrusive thoughts that are unlikely to be acted upon. In addition, the occurrence of such thoughts is often independent of the patient's emotional state and may occur while they are feeling happy, sad, or indifferent.

In contrast, patients at risk to harm themselves or others tend to have mood-*congruent* thoughts. In such instances suicidal thoughts occur when the patient is already feeling sad and hopeless. Although these thoughts may be distressing, suicide may be perceived as an escape from one's problems. Likewise, true intentions to harm others are typically accompanied by anger at a person or a desire for retribution. Such thoughts, especially when they occur in people with a history of violence, should be viewed as a serious threat.

Characteristics of the Patient's Environment

Environmental Stressors

Differentiating between an anxiety disorder (exaggerated estimates of threat where little actual risk is present) and stress (a reasonable response to a realistic threat) is a crucial diagnostic decision that has clear treatment implications. To reduce the former, patients must learn that their fears are unfounded. In contrast, treating stress involves minimizing the impact of the stressor. For example, a child who is afraid of golden retrievers has a phobia that can be treated with exposure. In contrast, one who is afraid of a neighbor's dangerous guard dog is responding accurately to a realistic threat and needs to be protected from attack. A more subtle distinction might involve a college student's worries regarding school achievement, which may be a sign of GAD, the result of an overly demanding professor, or an undiagnosed learning disability. When a patient's fears and worries are related to environmental stress, the appropriate intervention is to help reduce or manage that threat. For example, before treating a woman for PTSD stemming from domestic violence, it is necessary to ensure that she is no longer at risk for being attacked.

Relationship Stress

Anxiety symptoms can also be related to stressful relationships, such as that of a 40-year-old man who was concerned that his wife was going to ask him for a divorce. If this anxiety reflects marital discord, then couple therapy would likely be indicated. However, if these worries were intrusive thoughts in the absence of relationship problems, imaginal exposure and cognitive therapy might be more appropriate.

CONCLUSIONS

This chapter covers general and specific factors that can complicate the use of exposure therapy for anxiety and fear. When complexities arise, we encourage the clinician to adhere to the basic principles of a carefully conducted functional assessment and the cognitive-behavioral conceptualization of the maintenance and treatment of anxiety. With these tools at hand, exposure-based treatment can be applied to anxiety symptoms under a wide variety of seemingly complex circumstances. The presence of comorbidity and other complicating factors should not necessarily discourage therapists from providing exposure therapy, except in instances such as unmanaged psychosis, manic symptoms, and substance abuse. We also believe it is important that when complications and comorbidity are present, the clinician limit his or her intervention to the symptoms that fall within his or her areas of competence and collaborate with other specialists as indicated.

ADDITIONAL RESOURCES

Foa, E. B., & Emmelkamp, P. M. G. (Eds.). (1983). *Failures in behavior therapy.* New York: Wiley.

McKay, D., Abramowitz, J. S., & Taylor, S. (Eds.). (2010). *Cognitive-behavioral therapy for refractory cases: Turning failure into success.* Washington, DC: American Psychological Association.

17

Exposure Therapy with Children

Throughout this book our discussion of exposures has focused primarily on working with adults. Yet because most anxiety symptoms occur across the lifespan, we also need to address the application of exposure therapy to children and adolescents. The basic approach to using this technique is largely the same for adults and youth; thus therapists are encouraged to apply the information presented in Parts I and II to their work with younger patients. However, therapists face a number of challenges and opportunities that should be considered when they intervene with anxious children. In this chapter, we review characteristics of treatment, therapeutic techniques, and anxiety symptoms that are particularly salient when working with this population.

The use of exposure therapy with children has been documented as early as the 1920s when the technique was successfully applied to a 2-year-old with fears of white rats (Jones, 1924). Since these initial "classic" experiments, exposures have been incorporated into comprehensive cognitive-behavioral treatments for a variety of childhood anxiety conditions including social phobia (Beidel, Turner, & Morris, 2000), specific phobia (Ollendick et al., 2009), OCD (March & Mulle, 1998), separation anxiety disorder, and GAD (Kendall, 2000). The effectiveness of such treatment packages have been supported by numerous randomized controlled studies and by meta-analytic reviews (James, Soler, & Weatherall, 2009; Watson & Rees, 2008). Although treatment protocols typically include multiple techniques, such as cognitive restructuring and relaxation strategies, exposure is the primary component of treatment (Beidel et al., 2000; Bouchard, Mendlowitz,

Coles, & Franklin, 2004; Davis & Ollendick, 2005; Kazdin & Weisz, 1998; Kendall et al., 2005; Silverman & Kurtines, 1996).

TREATMENT CHARACTERISTICS

A number of considerations are important when using exposure therapy with children and adolescents. While some of these factors may increase the complexity of the case, and even become obstacles to improvement, others can provide additional opportunities for therapeutic change. In the following section we review characteristics of therapists, families, and children that can impact treatment. This information is summarized in Table 17.1.

Therapist Factors

Despite the proven effectiveness of exposure therapy in the treatment of childhood anxiety, many practitioners opt not to use this technique (Freiheit et al., 2004; Storch et al., 2007; Valderhaug, Gotestam, & Larsson, 2004). For some, this choice stems from a belief that exposure does not fit with their particular theoretical orientation or clinical style (Freiheit et al., 2004). Others are reluctant to purposely provoke a child's anxiety, especially when he or she is already suffering from a disproportionate amount of fear and worry. Clinicians often enter the mental health field with the desire to *reduce*, as opposed to *produce*, distress; and as a result, they prefer using techniques such as cognitive restructuring, relaxation training, or non-CBT approaches that do not involve evoking even temporary distress (Freiheit et al., 2004; Valderhaug et al., 2004). Regrettably, however, this decision often deprives anxious children of the treatment that is most likely to relieve their suffering over the long term.

The process of overcoming a hesitancy to use exposure methods is similar to employing exposure therapy itself. Only by conducting exposures with patients, and learning through one's own experience the provoked anxiety they experience is temporary, and that such exercises often lead to long-term improvement, will one become comfortable with using this approach. It may be helpful to begin with cases, such as animal phobias (see Chapter 7), that involve a relatively straightforward application of exposure. As one experiences success and gains confidence, one will find it easier to attempt more specialized applications of exposure exercises such as working with contamination fears (Chapter 12) and UITs (Chapter 10). Consultation with an experienced exposure therapist who can provide supervision and guidance will likely make this process more palatable. In addition, the information in this book may offer direction and structure to a therapist's efforts to broaden his or her use of exposure therapy.

TABLE 17.1. Overview of Considerations for Using Exposure Therapy with Children

Factors	Potential obstacles	Interventions
Therapist	• Reluctance to use Exposures	• Mentoring • Gradual adoption
Family	• Multiple perspectives • Genetic risk factors • Parental overprotection and criticism • Family stress (marital conflict, parental depression)	• Interviewing parent and child • Working with parents on their reactions to child's anxiety • Referring parents to individual or couple therapy
Child	• Concrete cognitive abilities • Dependence on family • Safety • Social acceptability	• Using modeling and stories • Involving parents in treatment • Focusing on behavioral methods • Consulting with parents when planning exposures

Family Factors

It is important to take into account the influence that the family system may have on the development and maintenance of a child's anxiety symptoms (Ginsburg, Siqueland, Masia-Warner, & Heddtke, 2004). Since anxiety has a genetic component, it is not surprising that many anxious children have parents with high levels of anxiety or other psychopathology. Thus, some children inherit an anxious temperament that can be seen from an early age in the form of reactivity to new situations and a heightened tendency to avoid perceived threats. Over time, anxious parental behavior and the parent's accommodation of a child's fears may also contribute to the maintenance or exacerbation of the child's problems with anxiety. Since most young children learn about the world in large part from watching and mimicking their parents, they react to their parents' fears by modeling their anxious behavior. Finally, research suggests that parents of anxious children tend to be overly protective in their efforts to help their children avoid anxiety and distress (Merlo, Lehmkuhl, Geffken, & Storch, 2009; Rapee, Schniering, & Hudson, 2009). Consequently, children can acquire their fears from their parents through both biological (genetic) and environmental (learning) mechanisms.

A note of caution is warranted when exploring or discussing family factors related to childhood anxiety. Just as is the case with precipitating events, it is rarely possible to identify family factors that clearly led to the development of a child's anxiety disorder. In addition, parents may interpret a discussion of these factors as implying that their own anxiety or their poor parenting is to blame for the child's symptoms. Thus, discussion of family factors should focus on parental reactions that may contribute to the *maintenance* of the child's anxiety and can be changed as part of treatment. In addition, these topics should be addressed later in therapy, after a positive therapeutic relationship has been established.

On a broader level, children generally thrive on structure and routine that allows them to explore and develop in a safe and relatively predictable environment. Family and contextual factors that disrupt this foundation can also contribute to anxiety. These factors include marital conflict, financial problems, parental depression, siblings with behavioral problems, and medical problems within the family. Many of these issues can also increase the frequency with which parents criticize their children or are overly controlling, factors that contribute to child anxiety (Ginsburg et al., 2004). These and other family stressors may also contribute to the maintenance of anxiety symptoms or interfere with the family's ability to participate in treatment.

By the time a child comes to the attention of a therapist, all of these family factors, including the parents' decision to seek treatment, have shaped the family's perception of the problem. Thus, therapists need to assess both the child's and the parents' perspectives concerning the presenting complaint, although each party may provide conflicting information, particularly when the child does not wish to participate in treatment. For instance, one father expressed concern that his 12-year-old son was anxious around his peers and spent too much time at home alone, while the child maintained that he was very sociable at school and often got together with his friends over the weekends. In such situations the therapist might endeavor to collect additional information, such as behavioral observations of the child in various contexts, as well as reports from the child's teacher. For instance, if the child appears very anxious in the therapist's office or is not participating in extracurricular activities despite parental urging, he may be minimizing his anxiety.

When child and parent disagree about the presence of an anxiety problem, exposure tasks can be used as an assessment tool to provide additional information. For instance, therapy with the boy mentioned above began by asking the child to complete a few tasks, such as calling a friend to make plans for the weekend, prior to the next appointment. The next week he and his father reported that he had not called a friend and had become visibly upset when his father prompted him to do so. This reaction suggested that the child had minimized his social anxiety. Moreover, the exercise provided a basis for planning further exposures. If the assignment had been accomplished relatively easily, the therapist might have accepted the child's view and decided that treatment for social anxiety was not required as long as the child continued to meet some basic requirements, for example, call a friend once per week.

Given the impact of parental and family functioning on child anxiety, it is important to assess this information during the initial interview. Many factors, such as modeling and criticism, may need to be addressed in treatment (which we discuss later in this chapter). In some instances, however, it is necessary to encourage parents to seek treatment for their own symptoms, such as anxiety or depression, or to refer them for couple therapy.

Child Factors

For the present chapter, the term *child* refers to a wide age span covering preschool children to adolescents. This range includes multiple developmental stages associated with distinct symptom presentations and treatment needs. For example, problems with separation typically occur in younger children while social phobia is more frequent in adolescents (Costello, Mustillo, Erkanli, Keeler, & Angold, 2003). Particularly important is the fact that younger children tend to have more concrete cognitive abilities, less understanding of emotions, less independence from family, and are more present-oriented (Piacentini & Bergman, 2001). However, rather than contraindicating the use of exposures, these cognitive limitations necessitate the use of primarily behavioral interventions since strategies to identify and challenge distorted thoughts will be too developmentally advanced (Bouchard et al., 2004; Piacentini & Bergman, 2001). Thus, rather than uniformly applying adult treatment techniques to youngsters, therapists must tailor their methods for helping children face their fears to the child's developmental level.

Changes to treatment are apparent in the structure of sessions and the process of presenting information. For instance, parental involvement appears to be more important for younger children than for adolescents (Barrett, Dadds, & Rapee, 1996). Thus, treatment with the former will likely involve concurrent parent interventions to teach them how to assist their child with exposures, while work with the latter may more closely resemble adult therapy. Within sessions, the delivery of psychoeducation will also vary depending on the age of the child. When treating young children, therapists will often need to be very concrete, providing ample therapist modeling and use of stories or developmentally appropriate analogies (Piacentini & Bergman, 2001). For instance, when explaining the cognitive-behavioral conceptualization of anxiety and its treatment, therapists might find it helpful to begin with a basic example, such as a fear of dogs, and then apply this model to the child's particular symptoms. In addition, use of visual aids with pictures can also be helpful. Moreover, use of analogies, such as horror movies and roller-coasters being less scary the second time, or adjusting to the temperature in a swimming pool, can help children understand the concept of habituation.

Therapists should also consider the child's developmental level when planning and implementing exposure exercises. It is important to make sure that initial fear hierarchy items are relatively easy, particularly with young children, so that they experience initial success and are willing to continue with treatment. This task can be challenging since some children have difficulty predicting how anxious they might feel in different situations (Bouchard et al., 2004). Getting feedback from parents about how a child responds to a given situation at home can help determine if an item is manageable enough to be a starting point. For instance, one 7-year-old boy stated that he was only afraid of big dogs, although his mother noted that he also avoided a friend's small beagle. Thus, the therapist decided to begin exposures with a small, slow-moving dog even though the child predicted it would be too easy. An overly easy exposure can provide an initial confidence-building experience.

In addition to making sure exposure hierarchy items are objectively safe (although not necessarily 100% risk-free), the exercises need to be appropriate for the child's developmental level. This issue is particularly salient with imaginal exposures in which the child identifies, elaborates, and repeats an upsetting UIT until it no longer elicits anxiety or distress. Such exercises can frequently involve topics (e.g., sex and violence) from which adults wish to shelter their children. Here, the therapist should explain to concerned parents that during exposure, the child may be asked to elaborate on *existing* unwanted thoughts, but will not be exposed to thoughts he or she has not already experienced. We, for instance, have helped children confront the following types of UITs in imaginal exposure: a 14-year-old boy's thoughts of engaging in sex with another boy, an 11-year-old girl's intrusions about being tortured in hell, a 15-year-old girl's thoughts of murdering her mother and committing suicide, and a 12-year-old boy's thoughts of his parents death (he wrote an obituary that described his thoughts of his parents dying in a car accident). Parents are often more open to this approach when they know that imaginal exposure is based on the child's preexisting intrusive thoughts. As we described in previous chapters, imaginal exposure helps individuals experience UITs in a systematic and therapeutic way.

In some situations the therapist may need to provide examples of his or her own violent or sexual thoughts. For instance, if a child is feeling embarrassed or has difficulty elaborating on his or her UITs, the therapist can offer examples that the child can endorse or reject. Providing examples of other thoughts (e.g., the therapist' own) can also normalize the child's experience and reduce feelings of shame. However, since most adults can generate more graphically violent and sexually explicit thoughts than the average child, it is necessary to use appropriate caution. Thoughts that the therapist offers should be consistent with the vocabulary and concepts with which the child is likely to be familiar. When making these judgments it can be helpful to talk with the parent about the child's knowledge of that topic, what types of words he or she would use at home, or what the child has told them in past. Moreover, it is advisable to thoroughly discuss the general content of the thoughts with parents prior to conducting exposures to ensure that the family feels comfortable with the exercises.

ADDITIONAL CONSIDERATIONS AND THERAPEUTIC TOOLS

In this section we describe a number of considerations and supplementary techniques that are helpful when conducting exposure therapy with children and families.

Experience Working with Children

Prior to using exposure therapy with children, therapists should have appropriate knowledge and skills for work with this special population. This includes, but is not limited to, knowledge of child development and psychopathology, as well as training in providing mental health services to children and their families. Clinical anxiety problems are often accompanied by comorbid conditions such as depression and externalizing disorders, family conflict, and impaired academic functioning. Thus, therapists need to have the skills to assess and treat the symptoms and issues generally associated with childhood mental health care. These skills, in addition to an understanding of the fundamentals of exposure presented in Part I, provide the foundation for treating childhood anxiety problems.

Working with Parents

Involving parents in treatment may be especially helpful for younger children (Barrett, Healy-Farrell, & March, 2004). Most experts suggest that therapists incorporate parents to some degree when working with children of all ages (Bouchard et al., 2004). Within this broad recommendation, there are differences in the extent to which parents have been included in treatment, ranging from a minimal number of concurrent sessions (Kendall, 2000) to being a primary conduit of change (Silverman & Kurtines, 1996). The specific roles that parents can play in treatment include helping in assessment, participating in exposures, and providing emotional support.

Helping in Assessment

Because (particularly younger) children tend to be more focused on the present than the past or the future, parents often provide an important perspective on the child's history. However, child reports should never be discounted, as parents may be unaware of certain symptoms, particularly worries that occur in the absence of behavioral manifestations. The role of parents as assessors can continue throughout treatment. For instance, parents can monitor the presence of new symptoms and provide feedback about the child's success conducting exposures. In addition, parents can offer examples of the child's improvement that the child may have overlooked. For example, one 9-year-old girl stated that her worries about making mistakes were "about the same" until her mother pointed out that it had been over a week since she had asked for reassurance about mistakes. A note of caution is warranted, however: as in all aspects of psychological treatment, it is important for the parent–child relationship to remain collaborative. Thus, parents should be focused on "catching" *positive* behavior and avoid becoming overly concerned with "catching" the child doing something wrong or beginning each appointment with a list of problems that occurred between sessions.

Participating in Exposure Practice

Parents can also be encouraged to take an active role in implementing exposure practices outside of the office. Without consistent home practice it is unlikely that reductions in anxiety will transfer to everyday life. Since conducting exposures at home and in the community is hard work, it is often difficult for children to perform regularly on their own. Younger children especially will need parents to schedule times to complete exposures and help them remain in the situation until their anxiety dissipates. This type of structure can be useful for adolescents as well, although a method of communicating should be worked out ahead of time to minimize potential conflicts. There are a number of resources for clinicians that describe various methods for instructing parents on how to assist their child to actively cope with anxiety (Mendlowitz et al., 1999; Silverman & Kurtines, 1996; Whiteside, Brown, & Abramowitz, 2008).

Providing Emotional Support

Parents should be instructed to encourage adaptive anxiety management and provide emotional support in general. By the time children are referred for treatment, their anxiety often has become a primary focus of the family. For instance, some parents have reported spending hours sitting outside their child's bedroom or school because of separation fears. Since parental attention is a powerful motivator, it is important to shift this attention to more positive behaviors. Specifically, therapists can encourage parents to focus on brave behavior, rather than responding with criticism or nurturance to anxious behavior. Providing less attention to an anxious child can be particularly difficult as it means that parents must *tolerate* their child's anxiety without trying to *fix* it. Expecting a child to continue a behavior at home, *after* he or she has confronted a particular situation in the office, can add structure to this process. For example, once a child practices making telephone calls to other children in the office, he should be expected to make such calls himself at home. Parents should be trained to provide warm praise and support when the child attempts to manage his or her anxiety independently and to refrain from giving in to anxiety or criticizing the child for being anxious.

Behavior Management

Completing exposure tasks can be difficult for anyone, let alone small children. This is especially true of strong-willed children or those who do not view their symptoms as problematic. In these situations, or whenever a child is having difficulty completing exposures, behavior management techniques can be helpful. These strategies can be summarized as involving the use of firm expectations and contingent rewards and negative consequences to shape the child's behavior in the direction of doing something that he or she is not inclined to do otherwise.

Most children with anxiety problems desperately want to feel better and are motivated to participate in therapy. Their current distress, combined with a general tendency to be cooperative, frequently is sufficient to propel them to engage in exposure. In such situations, reductions in symptoms as well as praise (from the therapist and parents) for hard work may be all that is necessary to keep therapy moving along smoothly. For other children, however, these rewards may be too intangible or distant to overcome the initial distress associated with exposure exercises. In such cases, therapists may find it useful to implement contingencies in which rewards are delivered on a more frequent (fixed) schedule.

Contingencies can be used both in the office and at home. During the session younger children may respond well to being permitted to select a sticker or an inexpensive prize (e.g., from a "toy chest") after successfully completing (or even attempting to complete) an exposure task. Additionally, the therapist can reserve a fun activity until after the exposure task as been completed. Similar systems can be adapted for home and for older children and adolescents. For instance small, medium, and large prizes can be connected to practicing exposure to more difficult items on the fear hierarchy. Other reward systems such as earning points, marbles in a jar, check marks, money, or coloring in steps on a path can all be adapted to reward progress with exposure therapy. Social rewards, such as having a friend sleep over, can also be highly motivating; thus rewards need not be large or material. When working with adolescents, it is important to involve them in setting their own goals and taking an active role in designing an appropriate reward system. Examples of rewards are listed in Table 17.2.

For children who are generally compliant, but resistant to completing exposures despite a reward system, it may be necessary to implement mild negative consequences for not completing such exercises (see examples at the bottom of Table 17.2). For instance, one young girl with OCD responded well to in-session exposures but had intense anger outbursts when her parents suggested she try them at home. In response, her mother and therapist explained that exposures were like schoolwork that had to be completed before she could play outside or watch TV. In addition, she was told that it was okay to become angry at her OCD but that hitting other people and screaming were not an acceptable expression of her frustration. The child's parents were instructed to calmly place her in a time-out when she became aggressive. Fortunately, through a combination of rewards and negative consequences, this child was able to complete her therapy homework.

Of note, parents (and therapists) should ensure that the exposure tasks to be conducted are at an appropriate level for the child (i.e., likely to be successfully completed) before implementing negative consequences for noncompliance. In addition, it should be made clear to the child that although acting-out behavior will be met with negative consequences (e.g., loss of privileges), efforts to deal effectively with anxiety will be met with enthusiastic parental support among other (perhaps more tangible) rewards.

Anxious children who have problems with uncooperative, oppositional, and defiant behavior in general often have great difficulty complying with exposure therapy. In these situations it may be necessary to implement a full behavioral modification system before beginning exposure treatment. Such an approach includes instruction in parent management techniques including special one-on-one time, effective commands, ignoring, praise, reinforcement, logical consequences, and time-out (Barkley, 1997). As one can see, these skills are very similar to the behavior encouraged of parents above and thus provide a good foundation for later addressing anxiety symptoms.

Play

Children will be most apt to work hard and complete exposure tasks if they find therapy fun—to put it simply, they will want to please a therapist

TABLE 17.2. Examples of Rewards and Consequences for Use with Children

Category	Examples
Natural rewards	• Symptom relief
	• Ability to participate in desired activities
	• Praise from parents
	• Praise from therapist
	• Sense of accomplishment
	• Pride
Additional rewards	• Extra play time
	• Staying up 30 minutes later
	• Having a friend over
	• Going to the zoo
	• Special dessert
	• Choosing dinner
	• Going to a movie
	• Going out for dinner
	• Car privileges
	• Extended curfew
Negative consequences	• Delay enjoyable activities until exposures are completed each day
	• Time-out for aggressive behavior
	• Loss of privileges

whom they like (Bouchard et al., 2004). Play can be a tool for creating this environment with younger children. Specifically, therapists may choose to play a game at the outset of therapy to reduce the child's anxiety about beginning treatment and establish therapy as an enjoyable activity. In addition, as mentioned previously, playing games and other fun activities can be used at the end of each session as a reward for working hard. Play can also be used as a vehicle for conducting exposures. For instance, a board game with the added rule that each player has to state out loud how many spaces he or she moved and whose turn it is next may be an effective way to help a young child with social anxiety begin to talk. "Contaminating" game pieces with "germs" may also be useful for a child with OCD contamination concerns.

Equally as important as the therapist's use of play itself is the adoption of a playful *attitude*. Attempts to interject humor or silliness can make the experience more tolerable for the patient, the parent, and the therapist. In addition, if a child can laugh and enjoy him- or herself it suggests that the exposure he or she is completing is not as dangerous as he or she initially feared. Still, it is important to keep play in perspective and not let it become the focus of treatment or detract from conducting exposures.

ANXIETY SYMPTOMS IN CHILDHOOD

Despite the consistency between anxiety symptoms in childhood and adulthood, there are a number of presentations that are unique to children. In the following section we review the application of exposure exercises to anxiety symptoms that are primarily seen in children and were not covered in Part II.

Separation Anxiety

Separation anxiety is a normal part of development that abates over time for most children. Clinical problems with separation are most common in younger children and frequently are associated with increased external demands for independence, such as beginning preschool or kindergarten. Symptoms include intense fear and resistance to separating from caregivers, typically parents. A prototypical example is that of a 4-year-old boy who screams, cries, and clings to his mother's leg until he is restrained by the teacher when he is dropped off at preschool. It is not unusual for children's anxiety to dissipate fairly rapidly after the parent's departure and then for the child to function well throughout the rest of the day. Other symptoms of separation anxiety include a refusal to be in a room at home alone, go on overnights at friends' houses, or stay with a baby-sitter. In addition, children may make frequent phone calls to parents when separation is unavoidable.

   Exposures exercises can involve having the child practice being apart from his or her parents for increasingly longer periods of time in progressively challenging situations. A sample hierarchy for such a patient is presented in Figure 17.1. Initial exposures can begin in the office with having the parent(s) going out to the waiting room. The intensity of the exposure can be increased by having the therapist leave the room as well or by having the parents leave the building to run errands (depending on the functional assessment of the child's fear). Initially, children will likely require exact information regarding how long the separation will last and where their parents will be. However, later exposures should introduce uncertainty regarding these variables. Similar steps can be taken at home to encourage children to play alone in a room by themselves (perhaps on a different floor,

FIGURE 17.1. Sample separation anxiety hierarchy.

Description of the exposure task	SUDS
Stay in office with therapist	60
Allow parents to leave building while in office with therapist	70
Stay in office alone	75
Play in room alone at home for 5 minutes Increase time in room alone	80
Go to friend's house without parents	95
Sleep overnight at friend's house	100

if applicable), rather than following their parents around the house. Additional exposure exercises will likely include having the child spend time at a friend's house, spend the night there, or stay at home with a baby-sitter.

Exposures will almost certainly need to be augmented with differential attention and possibly behavioral management. For instance, as long as crying and clinging are effective at maintaining parental attention, this reaction is likely to continue. Thus, to encourage a child to separate at preschool, a father might be instructed to speak warmly and affectionately to his daughter while she is walking bravely to the door, but to leave immediately if she begins to cry, beg him to stay, or cling to his leg. It may also be necessary to reward the child for discontinuing anxious behaviors during the separation process. For example, the child could earn a sticker if she separates without clinging even if she is still crying. Subsequently, the child will need to display greater levels of calmness to earn a sticker. Similarly, rather than responding to a child when he is hovering in the same room, the parent can check in on the child and praise him for playing independently in another room.

As with all exposures, it is important to be mindful of developmental expectations. For older children it is appropriate to have them practice staying home without a parent. Since younger children are not expected to be home alone, exposures might focus on being in a room unaccompanied or staying with a nonparent caregiver. A useful set of guidelines for planning separation exposures are as follows: children under age 7 should never be left alone, 8- to 10-year-olds can be left alone for 3 hours, and 11- to 13-year-olds can be on their own for up to 12 hours (Olmstead County Child and Family Services, 2007).

School Refusal

School refusal provides an excellent example of the importance of a thorough behavioral assessment. Children may avoid school for a variety of reasons including anxiety or other negative emotions, attempts to seek attention, or a desire to participate in more enjoyable activities (Kearney, 2006). Sometimes children's refusal is related to a tangible stressor such as a learning disability or bullying. In cases where a child is avoiding school because of fear or worry, it is important to determine the particular cues for the anxiety. For instance, some children may wish to avoid school due to social anxiety regarding asking questions of teachers or interacting with peers at lunch. Other children may not have a problem with school per se but are extremely nervous about separating from their parents. Some children, even model students, may be extremely anxious about their grades, getting in trouble, or have other worries about performance. Finally, some children may not be able to identify any specific fear other than that they will feel scared or sick while they are in school and not be able to get help.

Once the therapist has a functional understanding of the child's fears, he or she can design an exposure-based plan for school reentry. The centerpiece of this plan will include having the child gradually return to school. Figure 17.2 presents an example hierarchy for a 13-year-old boy who had been absent from middle school for a considerable amount of time. Although he could not identify what precipitated his fears, embarrassment around his absence increased his anxiety about returning. If a functional analysis indicates the presence of specific fears that are interfering with school attendance (i.e., social anxiety), exposures to these items may be completed concurrently or after the child has returned to school. In more severe instances, such as when a child has been absent for a considerable amount of time, such exposures may need to be completed before reentry is possible. In many cases, a structured behavioral plan will be necessary to facilitate return to school. Such a plan would likely include earning privi-

FIGURE 17.2. Sample school refusal hierarchy.

Description of the exposure task	SUDS
Get up on time and get ready for school	5
Ride with parents to school and then return home	15
Go into school after hours	20
Meet with tutor at school during the day	60
Meet with tutor and attend math class	80
Meet with tutor, attend math and English classes	90
Go to school all morning Add afternoon hours one by one	97
Ride bus to and from school	100

leges and rewards for meeting attendance goals and removal of enjoyable activities as a consequence for absence.

Selective Mutism

Extreme social anxiety in children can take the form of selective mutism in which children who converse and interact freely in some settings (particularly home) do not speak at all in other settings. Although an approach similar to that outlined in Chapter 9 on social anxiety is appropriate for these children, the initial exercises will likely need to focus on the basics of communication. Oftentimes, to accomplish an initial goal of having the child speak with the therapist, it is necessary to break communication into basic fundamental steps. Such exposures may involve communicating nonverbally, whispering to parents, or making the basic movements or sounds of speech. For instance, one young girl was able to progress from blowing bubbles, to humming and forming words through a kazoo, to eventually providing one-word answers. Another child gradually whispered to her mother louder and louder while moving farther from her ear until she was talking to the therapist directly.

Once the child is able to talk with the therapist, it is important to generalize this accomplishment to other people. If possible, it can be helpful to bring extended family members or peers into the therapist's office. Within the safety of the session, the child can repeat the steps she used to speak with the therapist or play games that require speaking. Additionally, it is typically necessary to have parents and/or teachers organize enjoyable small-group activities outside of the office during which the child can gradually increase her communication with peers. Other potentially useful strategies include using behavioral reinforcement, modeling, and splicing together video segments to create a movie of the child answering questions posed by her teacher or classmates (Viana, Beidel, & Rabian, 2009).

CONCLUSIONS

The current chapter highlights important topics that therapists should consider when conducting exposure therapy with children. Because the basic principles of exposure treatment are the same for children and adults, the topics covered in this chapter should be combined with the detailed information on conducting exposures presented in Part II. The following additional resources can assist therapists who are interested in increasing their knowledge of the treatment of childhood anxiety disorders.

ADDITIONAL RESOURCES

Barkley, R. A. (1997). *Defiant children: A clinician's manual for assessment and parent training, 2nd ed.* New York: Guilford Press.

Chorpita, B. F. (2007). *Modular cognitive-behavioral therapy for childhood anxiety disorders.* New York: Guilford Press.

Kendall, P. C. (2000). *Cognitive-behavioral therapy for anxious children: Therapist manual* (2nd ed.). Ardmore, PA: Workbook Publishing.

March, J. S., & Friesen, K. M. (1998). *OCD in children and adolescents: A cognitive-behavioral treatment manual.* New York: Guilford Press.

18

Involving Significant Others in Treatment

In the previous chapter we discussed the inclusion of parents in exposure therapy for childhood anxiety disorders. We now expand this consideration of anxiety as an interpersonal phenomenon to include the role of partners, spouses, and other family members or close friends. We begin by describing two ways that relationships can impact anxiety disorders. One way is through symptom accommodation—when loved ones inadvertently maintain symptoms by "helping" with avoidance and safety behaviors. The second is when anxiety problems create relationship distress and conflict, which exacerbates anxiety. Since these two directions of influence are likely to act concurrently, we discuss important areas to assess when planning exposure therapy for individuals involved in relationships. Finally, we present strategies for intervening with anxious individuals from this interpersonal perspective.

SYMPTOM ACCOMMODATION

Family members often become intricately involved with their loved one's anxiety symptoms. They may participate in safety behaviors and rituals, facilitate avoidance, assume daily responsibilities, or resolve problems that have resulted from the patient's anxious behavior. Such actions are commonly referred to as *accommodation* (e.g., Calvocoressi et al., 1999; Shafran et al., 1995). The following example illustrates this phenomenon:

Jack, a 60-year-old grandfather, had suffered with OCD for over 30 years. His primary obsessions concerned unacceptable sexual thoughts (e.g., of molestation and incest) which were triggered by the sight of children, including his own grandchildren. As a result, Jack avoided activities such as playing with his grandchildren and watching certain TV shows that might have children or "sexy" actors (e.g., *Dancing with the Stars*). He and his wife, Norma, refrained from discussing their grandchildren, did not put pictures of them up around their home, and could not have these children stay with them. They also only watched the Weather Channel and the Food Network on TV to avoid Jack's obsessions. Although what had become the status quo was extremely upsetting to Norma (who was very proud of her grandchildren), she was willing to go along with Jack's wishes because she cared about him and didn't like to see him become angry or very anxious.

Accommodation can be subtle or extreme, and may even be found within seemingly "happy" couples and families. Norma, for example, boasted that she and Jack never argued about Jack's OCD. In such instances, the nonanxious partner or family members might be so concerned about making sure his or her loved one doesn't become anxious that he or she goes to great lengths to minimize distress. Such accommodation, however, creates a system that may fit with the anxiety symptoms to perpetuate the vicious cycle that maintains the anxiety disorder. We have worked with family members of OCD (contamination obsessions) sufferers who routinely cleaned car keys with bleach, undressed and showered immediately upon entering the house, laundered clothes and made beds for their adult children on a daily basis, retraced the individual's path home to ensure that he did not hit someone with the car, and drove to an adult child's home every morning to prepare his meals.

Accommodation, however, is not limited to OCD. Family members may also complete all household errands to allow someone with agoraphobia to remain at home, or accompany the same person on all outings. They might handle all phone calls for a loved one with social phobia, repeatedly check in by phone to relieve GAD-related worries, or assume all driving responsibilities for a spouse or partner with a driving phobia. In addition to helping a loved one avoid feared activities, family members may also work to protect the person from negative consequences associated with the functional impairment of clinical anxiety. For instance, parents may continue to support an adult child who is not working, intervene with a teacher or employer to excuse absences or incomplete projects, pay exorbitant water bills resulting from excessive showering, buy extra soap or toilet paper to accommodate compulsive cleaning rituals, and provide excuses to friends for not attending social engagements. Table 18.1 shows some common patterns of accommodation across various anxiety disorders.

TABLE 18.1. Examples of Family Accommodation

Anxiety disorder	Accommodation behaviors by others
OCD	• Washing for the patient • Doing extra laundry • Repeating answers until "just right" • Avoiding discussing certain topics
GAD	• Checking in frequently • Providing reassurance
Social phobia	• Answering questions for the patient • Providing excuses for absences • Cancelling social engagements
Panic disorder/agoraphobia	• Going shopping for patient • Accompanying patient on all errands • Providing reassurance of safety
PTSD	• Avoiding certain areas associated with the traumatic event • Checking on the status of an assailant • Accompanying patient on outings
Specific phobias	• Driving for the patient • Going to upper floors of a building to retrieve something for the patient • Checking for dogs, storms, snakes, etc.

To fully appreciate the effects of family accommodation, these actions need to be understood within the conceptual model of anxiety and its maintenance discussed in Chapter 3. Individuals with pathological anxiety cannot correct their exaggerated beliefs about the danger posed by feared situations and stimuli (and thus will remain fearful) if safety behaviors and avoidance continue to occur. Therefore, when family members accommodate a patient's anxiety, their behaviors inadvertently contribute to its persistence. For instance, by accommodating his wife's agoraphobic avoidance, a husband prevents his spouse from learning that she can manage intense anxiety and panic and that her fears of having a medical catastrophe for which help won't be available are unfounded.

In addition to preventing corrective learning there are a number of other consequences of accommodation that may maintain or worsen a family member's problems with anxiety. To begin with, accommodation often decreases an individual's motivation to participate in exposure therapy because he or she might not perceive good reasons to change the status quo—especially if doing so involves something as distressing as facing his or her fears. For instance, the mother of a 34-year-old man with OCD that we worked with paid rent for her son's apartment and made herself available so that when he became anxious about contamination, she could go and clean his bathroom, handle and clean his dirty laundry, and make his bed. Although the patient reported that he regretted the impact of OCD on his life, he struggled to begin contamination exposures partly because he didn't view such exercises as worthwhile. That is, his mother's excessive efforts to care for him had diminished the consequences of having OCD to the point that his obsessions and compulsions seemed tolerable relative to confronting his fears in exposure therapy. Meanwhile, this patient's mother was extremely distressed over her son's OCD—which had now become *her* problem. In fact, his mother was much more interested in him seeking treatment than he was.

In some relationships, accommodation becomes a chief way in which the unaffected partner expresses warmth, caring, and compassion for his or her loved one. For example, one man prided himself on the fact that whenever or wherever his wife with OCD needed reassurance that she had not come into contact with a dead animal (e.g., if she drove past roadkill), he would travel to where she was to calm her down, "assess" the situation, and reassure her that she was not going to contract rabies. This became an important way for the man to show his affection for his wife. Not only does such accommodation maintain pathological fear and anxiety in the ways we have discussed previously, it also begets additional accommodation as the couple's relationship develops around this sort of pathologically "affectionate" behavior.

As the reader can see, efforts by family members to accommodate a loved one's anxiety can take numerous forms that maintain, if not exacerbate, symptoms. In addition, these actions can interfere with an individual's participation in treatment. In fact, family accommodation has been found to be related to worse symptoms and to predict poorer long-terms outcomes of OCD treatment (Calvocoressi et al., 1999; Merlo et al., 2009). Consequently, when conducting exposures, therapists often need to address the roles that family members play in a patient's symptoms.

RELATIONSHIP CONFLICT

Relationship stress and conflict also plays an important role in anxiety problems (Byrne, Carr, & Clark, 2004; McCarthy & Shean, 1996; Monson, Guthire, & Stevens, 2003; Weissman, 1991; Whisman, 1999). For instance, couples in which one partner suffers with anxiety often report problems with interdependency, unassertiveness, and avoidant communication patterns (Marcaurelle, Belanger, Marchand, Katerelos, & Mainguy, 2005; McCarthy & Shean, 1996). In all likelihood, anxiety and relationship distress influence each other, rather than one exclusively leading to the other. For example, a husband's contentious relationship with his wife might contribute to overall anxiety and uncertainty that develops into GAD. Conversely, his excessive checking, reassurance seeking, and overly cautious actions could lead to frequent disagreements and marital conflict. In the next section, we review interaction patterns that therapists should be aware of when conducting exposure therapy.

Effects of Family Functioning on Anxiety

Family or relationship dysfunction, such as poor communication patterns, may contribute to the onset of anxiety problems (Baucom, Stanton, & Epstein, 2003). In fact, relationship dissatisfaction predicts the expression of anxiety and depression among individuals susceptible to these symptoms (South & Krueger, 2008). Aspects of a relationship that increase distress include poor problem-solving skills, hostility, and criticism. For example, avoidance of problem solving is related to more severe panic symptoms (Marcaurelle et al., 2005). Moreover, relationship dysfunction and communication problems can also adversely affect the outcome of exposure therapy for clinical anxiety. For instance, communication patterns characterized by criticism, hostility, and emotional overinvolvement are associated with premature discontinuation and symptom relapse, whereas those characterized by empathy, hopefulness, and assertiveness are associated with improved outcomes with exposure (Chambless & Steketee, 1999; Craske, Burton, & Barlow, 1989; Steketee, 1993).

To illustrate these patterns, consider the example of a middle-age couple that had difficulty handling disagreements. Rather than effectively reaching a compromise, they typically avoided discussing their differing opinions until an issue came to a head and resulted in arguing. Over time the wife began to develop anxiety and worry over everyday decisions, particularly a fear that any decision she made would lead to an angry outburst from her spouse. As her anxiety increased, she began to doubt the quality of her decisions in other areas, such as work. She sought treatment for chronic worry and anxiety. As part of her treatment, exposure exercises were developed in which she was to discuss difficult topics with her husband. However, given the couple's history of poor communication, the therapist had both partners attend the initial sessions in order to improve their communication and problem-solving skills.

Effects of Anxiety on Relationship Satisfaction

Anxiety likely impacts relationships via multiple avenues (Caughlin, Huston, & Houts, 2000). It may reduce relationship satisfaction by contributing to increased arguing, criticism, and complaining by the sufferer and partner. Given the negative impact of anxiety on relationships, it is not surprising that a variety of anxiety disorders have been associated with marital problems (Byrne et al., 2004; Emmelkamp, de Haan, & Hoogduin, 1990; McCarthy & Shean, 1996; Monson et al., 2003; Weissman, 1991; Whisman, 1999).

To illustrate, consider a 48-year-old man with GAD who presented for treatment after his symptoms had significantly strained his marriage. Conflict with his wife arose around his frequent attempts to reduce his anxiety by taking extra safety precautions and requesting that she do so as well. His wife began to resent his suggestions as implying that she did not care enough for him and their children. In addition, she increasingly responded to his checking and reassurance seeking with hostility because his actions interfered with their daily lives. By the time the patient presented for treatment, his wife had given him an ultimatum that he either seek help for his anxiety or they would separate.

Anxiety symptoms also lead to the reduction of relationship satisfaction by decreasing the number of positive interactions and increasing the number of hostile interactions between individuals. For example, social phobia or agoraphobia symptoms may restrict the range of activities a couple participates in, thereby reducing opportunities for enjoyment. Emotional numbing associated with PTSD may interfere with an individual's ability to give or receive affection, leading to resentment or misunderstandings by both partners (Monson et al., 2003). In the absence of other positive interactions, accommodation of a loved one's anxiety symptoms may become a primary mechanism for communicating warmth and nurturance. Yet despite this, individuals with anxiety disorders still often perceive their partner as unsupportive (McCarthy & Shean, 1996).

ASSESSMENT

In conducting exposure-based therapy for anxious individuals affected by family or relationship distress, the clinician must assess how the interpersonal aspects interact with the anxiety disorder, particularly what Rohrbaugh, Shoham, Spungen, and Steinglass (1985) refer to as "symptom–system fit." Specifically, this refers to how the individual, couple, or family unit has structured the environment so as to accommodate anxiety symptoms (i.e., avoidance and safety behaviors). As discussed previously, accommodation often occurs within seemingly "happy" family and romantic relationships (i.e., "good" symptom–system fit). Other couples and families evidence a poor system–symptom fit in which nonanxious partners and family members refuse to accommodate to anxiety or overtly resent how the anxiety disorder has negatively impacted the family or intimate relationship. Such relationships are likely to be characterized by conflict regarding the anxiety problem. Table 18.2 includes a list of suggested questions for assessing symptom–system fit and the specific ways in which partners or family members relate concerning anxiety symptoms. When it is clear that interpersonal issues contribute to the maintenance of the patient's anxiety disorder, we recommend devoting an entire session (with a partner and family member present) to discussing the answers to these questions. The information gleaned from a discussion of the interpersonal aspects of a patient's anxiety problems can enhance how exposure therapy is implemented. Strategies for involving partners and relatives in treatment are presented later in this chapter.

Although a goal of exposure therapy is to help nonanxious individuals cease their accommodation of anxiety symptoms, this decision must be made in an agreeable manner. Negative and sarcastic reactions to anxiety symptoms are common, yet they increase discord in the family or rela-

---

TABLE 18.2. Questions for Assessing Symptom–System Fit within a Couple or a Family

- When did the partner/family first become aware of the patient's anxiety problem?
- How did they become aware of it?
- What effects have anxiety symptoms (fear, avoidance, safety behaviors) had on the relationship/family in terms of daily life? (Solicit the patient's response and the partner/family's response.)
- If there are any patterns that seem to have developed because of the patient's anxiety problems, what are they? (Solicit the patient's response and the partner/family's response.)
- How does/do the partner/family members think their life together might be different if the patient did not have difficulties with anxiety? (Solicit the patient's response and the partner/family's response.)
- Is there anyone else (e.g., children) who is affected in any way by the patient having problems with anxiety? (If so, explore who and how.) (Solicit the patient's response and the partner/family's response.)
- What types of strategies have the couple/family used to try to cope with the patient's anxiety?
- When the patient either is experiencing fear or engaging in a safety behavior (e.g., ritual), does it ever lead to anger or arguments? What happens in these situations? Does the partner/family member ever have a tendency to help the patient escape from the anxiety, avoid situations that cause anxiety, or assist with safety behaviors to lower the anxiety?
- How well has this worked?
- How often do you discuss the anxiety problem and what does your communication tend to be like at those times?

tionship and maintain the anxiety disorder. Nonanxious family members might initially try to resist accommodating, yet end up giving in after the anxious person makes repeated pleas or raises the stakes by making threats. For example, a 25-year-old man with OCD living at home with his parents repeatedly insisted that his mother clean all of the family's dishes in a certain ritualized way. At first, his mother refused to comply with the cleaning rituals, saying that she would not take part in such excessive behaviors. Yet after persistent nagging from her son, she became angry and washed the dishes in the ritualized way under his careful observation. We have observed some anxious patients resort to threatening violence (on themselves or others) in an effort to manipulate others to accommodate symptoms.

INVOLVING SIGNIFICANT OTHERS IN TREATMENT

Given the role that family members might play in the maintenance of anxiety symptoms, we suggest therapists consider including significant others in treatment. The remainder of this chapter discusses various roles that family members can play in exposure therapy. We recommend a brief assessment of any nonanxious partner or family member who might become involved in exposure treatment. Specifically, it is important to note whether this individual experiences any psychopathology of his or her own, and what factors might have contributed to the development of an interpersonal system in which the patient's anxiety disorder flourishes. For instance, a woman whose first husband died of a heart attack was especially sensitive to her current husband's panic attacks and thus willingly did everything she could to keep him from becoming even slightly anxious, thereby contributing to the maintenance of his problem.

Psychoeducation

Family members are frequently interested in learning about their loved one's symptoms and how they should respond when the patient struggles with anxiety (Shafran et al., 1995). Information about the conceptual model of anxiety (presented in Chapter 3) can help normalize the family's experience, begin to alleviate feelings of guilt and frustration, and reduce a partner's or family member's expressions of resentment and criticism. Similarly, learning about how exposure therapy works and the evidence for its effectiveness can increase hopefulness and reduce feelings of helplessness and of being overwhelmed. To illustrate, when a young woman began to understand that her husband's resistance to spending time with her side of the family arouse from his social anxiety, rather than from dislike, she became less critical of him and his behavior. Knowing that he would be participating in an effective treatment further increased her patience with his anxiety.

Partner-Assisted Exposure

Once a significant other understands the principles underlying exposure therapy, he or she can be taught how to assist with exposure exercises by serving as a coach. Some treatment outcome studies have indicated that involving close relatives in this way improves the effectiveness of CBT as well as the patients' interpersonal relationships (Mehta, 1990). However, we have found that partner-assisted exposure is optimally successful when there is little or no relationship or family conflict and when there is minimal symptom accommodation by others. By adopting the role of "coach," the family member or partner learns to offer emotional support to the patient as he or she completes difficult exposures within and outside of the session. The coach is also taught to provide gentle, but firm reminders not to engage in avoidance or safety behaviors. Most importantly, the coach is trained to help the patient implement exposures correctly by making sure sufficient anxiety is provoked, that exposure continues until anxiety has decreased (habituation), and that no safety behaviors are used.

Preparation for Exposure

Significant others should be involved in developing the exposure hierarchy. Perhaps partners and family members are aware of avoidance behaviors and rituals that the patient is either not aware of or that were overlooked during hierarchy development. Next, the therapist teaches the patient and coach how to work together to help the patient confront his or her hierarchy items. The process of confronting an anxiety-provoking stimulus can be broken down into four components, as we describe next.

   Discussing the Exposure Task. Initially, the therapist teaches the patient and coach to clarify the specifics of the exposure task. Both parties are encouraged to discuss how each is feeling about the upcoming practice and to identify potential obstacles. The patient is helped to specify how he or she would like the coach to help out with the exercise. Below we illustrate how a therapist might present this information to a couple. In the example, the patient, Brooks, suffers from a phobia of escalators. His wife, Connie, is serving as his exposure coach.

> THERAPIST: Brooks, when you know ahead of time that you won't be able to avoid using an escalator, you probably start to worry about how awful it will be. Maybe you've even asked Connie to help

you avoid the anxiety or calm you down. When we do exposure, though, I'll want you to try something different—to *confront* the escalator and work together as a team to get through the anxiety—*not to avoid it*. Connie, instead of helping Brooks *avoid* becoming anxious, I want you to help him *confront* the escalator. Your job is to help him get *through* the anxiety, not to make the anxiety go away. Tell me about how this is similar or different from how things usually go.

BROOKS: It's very different. We've never tried that before. I make Connie hold my hand if I absolutely have to get on the escalator.

CONNIE: Yeah, and sometimes it takes a few minutes to calm him down so that he can even step onto it. He'll get very anxious and upset if I don't help him.

THERAPIST: Okay, I understand. So, this new approach will be something different. I'd like the two of you to discuss the exposure before you start. Focus on what's likely to be difficult, and how you'll deal with the situation and anxiety. Brooks, I don't want Connie to try to calm you down when you do the exposure. Remember that your job is to face the anxiety.

Confronting the Feared Situation. The second component involves actually confronting the exposure hierarchy item. The patient is encouraged to express his or her feelings to the coach, and the coach is encouraged to listen carefully. If the patient becomes anxious, the coach should acknowledge this and reinforce the patient's hard work with lots of praise (e.g., "You're doing such a great job, I'm really proud of you!"). The coach should continue to compliment the patient on handling the situation throughout the exercise and avoid making negative statements. The coach must also resist the temptation to distract the patient or provide reassurance that everything will be okay. Table 18.3 provides a list of things for an exposure coach to tell (and avoid telling) the patient during exposures. Brooks's therapist gave the following instructions to Brooks and Connie:

"Once you're actually on the escalator, Brooks, your goal is to remain focused on the situation. Go with the anxiety. Accept that it's there, rather than trying to control or avoid it. Don't turn to Connie for help either; you are learning to break that pattern. Also, do not try to overanalyze whether anything bad is going to happen to you. This will just feed your anxiety and make it seem worse.

"Connie, I'd like you to be there with Brooks when he starts the exposure. However, just being nearby might make Brooks feel more at ease, which is similar to a safety behavior. The eventual goal is to have

TABLE 18.3. Statements for Exposure Coaches to Use (or Avoid) during Exposure Exercises

When the patient reports anxiety:
- "I know this is hard, but you're doing a great job."
- "Think of how good you'll feel when you're through."
- "Remember the anxiety is temporary."

When the patient requests reassurance or safety behaviors:
- "I can't give you that guarantee—I just don't know for sure."
- "How can I help you without doing safety behaviors for you?"
- "If I did that for you, it would only be making your problem worse. How else can I help you?"
- "It sounds like you are asking for reassurance, but the therapist said it's not helpful for me to give you assurance."

When the patient wants to end an exposure prematurely:
- "I know it is difficult. Let's talk with the therapist about the problems you're having getting through this."
- "If you stop now, you'll only make the fear stronger."
- "You have made it so far, let's not let anxiety win now."

Comments for coaches to avoid:
- "I know everything is going to be fine, don't worry."
- "I've done this before; your fears are irrational."
- "Believe me, the therapist wouldn't make you do this if it was dangerous."
- "You'd better do what the therapist says or I'll. ..."

Brooks ride escalators on his own. So, at first, it's okay for Connie to be there to provide support—but it will be important for her to phase this out so Brooks can learn to manage anxiety in these situations.

"If Brooks says he is getting anxious in anticipation of getting on the escalator, your job, Connie, is to encourage him to keep going in spite of the anxiety. Sympathize with how hard it is, but don't dwell on it, and don't let him off the hook!

"Finally, Connie, if Brooks becomes upset, or if he blames you or criticizes your attempts to be helpful, remind him that this is very hard work. But whatever you do, don't argue with Brooks during an exposure. This will make things worse. Instead, suggest that you discuss the problem when it won't interfere with an exposure, and ask Brooks what you could do at the moment to help him cope with the anxiety."

Dealing with Overwhelming Anxiety. If the patient becomes overwhelmed with extreme anxiety, he or she should express these feelings to the coach, who should acknowledge that the task is difficult but also note that eventually the anxious feelings will lessen. If the patient absolutely cannot continue with the exposure, a brief time-out can be taken. During a time-out, the partner provides support in ways the patient would like (but *not* using reassurance or safety behaviors). The two parties should also discuss what went wrong and how they will approach the exposure when it resumes. Although the coach should remind the patient of the importance of resuming the exposure, the decision to stop or continue is ultimately up to the patient. A partner should never encourage stopping exposures but at the same time must not force the patient to continue.

Evaluation. The fourth component involves the patient and coach evaluating how the exposure went. How did the patient feel about how the exposure went? How did the patient feel about the coach's help? The coach should also let the patient know how he or she felt about the exposure and, when appropriate, provide copious praise for a job well done.

Who Is a Good Exposure Coach?

Unfortunately, not all family members or partners will be good exposure coaches. To be a good coach one needs to be patient, considerate, nonjudgmental, supportive, and optimistic about treatment. In addition, the coach and patient should have a stable relationship. If a considerable amount of conflict exists within a couple, for example, it may not be a good idea to enlist the patient's partner or spouse as a coach. For instance, if a patient and her husband argue and criticize each other over daily issues, such as paying bills, they are likely to continue this pattern over a stressful exercise, such as exposure, in which the partner also assumes a position of authority. In addition, if the partner has extreme difficulty tolerating the other's anxiety, he or she may not be prepared to assume the role of coach. In these situations other family interventions discussed below may be necessary before, or instead of, training a significant other to be an exposure coach.

Eliminating Accommodation

When symptom accommodation is a noteworthy part of the clinical picture, the therapist may need to involve significant others in interventions outside of formal exposure exercises. In such interventions, the therapist begins by describing accommodation and its deleterious effects, as in the sample dialogue below for a patient with panic disorder and agoraphobia (Margaret):

THERAPIST: When a loved one has a serious problem, the whole family has to figure out ways to adapt to the problem that allows them to keep functioning. For example, if one family member develops a medical illness, that person often will be relieved of some of his or her chores or responsibilities, and the family might try to be emotionally supportive to let him or her know that they care. This makes lots of sense and is very reasonable, but if you are not careful, it can have some unintended, negative effects. Let's say that in order to recover from a medical problem you need to get lots of physical exercise. If your family does all of your chores for you, then you might not get the exercise that you need, and this could slow your recovery.

The same thing can happen when someone has panic attacks and agoraphobia. That is, a family member, spouse, or partner can get involved, and even with the best of intentions, still do things that don't help the person get over the anxiety problems. This might happen in a couple of ways. First, family members may take over certain roles to help the person avoid becoming anxious— for example, by always travelling outside the home with the person. Likewise, over time, the family might learn to stay away from certain situations or objects that trigger anxiety and panic. For example, a couple might avoid having sex because of the anxious person's discomfort with the feeling of sexual arousal. Can you think of ways your family divides roles to help Margaret avoid becoming anxious or things that you as a family avoid or just don't do to prevent her anxiety?

FAMILY MEMBER: Yes. We go out of our way to avoid shopping at certain stores and eating in certain restaurants where Margaret has had panic attacks. Also we can't take trips to certain areas if they don't have good cell phone reception in case Margaret needs to call doctor. We don't like what has become of our lives, but we do it for Margaret's sake.

THERAPIST: We often help loved ones avoid these situations because we don't want to see them become anxious or upset. At other times, the person with panic attacks is so distressed that he or she demands or insists that the family help him or her avoid anxiety. So whether it is out of concern or to avoid arguments, one way that families get involved is by helping the person avoid anxiety-producing situations. But as we know, in order to get over panic and agoraphobia, people have to confront the situations that create anxiety. So, our goal today will be to think through the different ways in which your family accommodates Margaret's anxiety and panic symptoms.

As treatment progresses, the therapist also helps the patient and significant others develop healthier patterns of relating outside the context of the anxiety problem, another important part of changing detrimental interaction patterns. Below is an example of a discussion of this topic with a patient with PTSD (Lauren) following a sexual assault:

> THERAPIST: One of the things we want to be careful about is that many families come to express their care and concern around problems like PTSD. So, as her mother and father, you might express your caring and love for Lauren by doing things that keep her from experiencing anxiety. Of course, we don't want to disrupt your sense of togetherness, closeness, or ability to relate as a family. However, we do want to make sure that your family's closeness is not just based on Lauren's anxiety. So I want you to think about things you would like to do together with Lauren, ways to enjoy her company and feel close to her, that you haven't done recently or as much as you would like. What are some things you would like to do as a family that you have had to stop because of Lauren's PTSD? I want you to get back to enjoying each other and feeling close to each other in ways that are not related to the PTSD.
>
> PATIENT'S FATHER: We have stopped going out at night as a family because Lauren has become afraid of being attacked at night. But we would love to be able to enjoy this again.
>
> THERAPIST: That's a great example.

Next, the family (or couple) chooses an activity that has become hampered by anxiety-related avoidance or safety behaviors and the therapist facilitates a problem-solving discussion about how they can try to handle this situation differently in order to promote the idea of exposure. In other words, without creating specific exposure hierarchies, they work on building exposure and response prevention into their everyday life. For example, in the case of Margaret described earlier, her relatives might resume vacations, shopping at the avoided stores, and eating at restaurants that had been off-limits. They might also agree to stop accompanying Margaret everywhere she goes. In the case of Lauren with PTSD, her family might agree to have nighttime outings, perhaps gradually spending more and more time outside at night (of course, refraining from venturing into unsafe areas of town).

As with partner-assisted exposures, in these specific family or couple interventions, the goal is to work toward a life in which the family or couple confronts the things the patient has been avoiding, and stays in the situation rather than using safety behaviors to lower the anxiety.

CONCLUSIONS

Anxiety disorders often affect, and are affected by, interpersonal relationships. Significant others can influence anxiety symptoms and treatment by accommodation, as well as through conflict. Consequently, clinicians are encouraged to consider including family members in exposure-based treatments when appropriate. In the absence of significant symptom accommodation or conflict, the training of a family member as an exposure coach and source of support can facilitate a patient's recovery. When accommodation plays a significant role in the persistence of anxiety symptoms, the clinician can work with the patient and family members to identify how this is a problem and to develop specific interventions with the aim of lessening this maladaptive pattern of behavior.

ADDITIONAL RESOURCE

Baucom, D. H., Stanton, S., & Epstein, N. B. (2003). Anxiety disorders. In D. K. Snyder & M. A. Whisman (Eds.), *Treating difficult couples: Helping clients with coexisting mental and relationship disorders* (pp. 57–87). New York: Guilford Press.

19

Combining Exposure Therapy with Medication

As we noted in Chapter 2, firm evidence indicates that exposure-based therapy is an effective treatment for pathological anxiety and fear. It is not, however, the most commonly used intervention for these problem. By a large margin, more patients receive pharmacotherapy for their anxiety symptoms than exposure (or any psychological intervention, for that matter; Stein et al., 2004). Medications such as selective serotonin reuptake inhibitors (SSRIs), tricyclic antidepressants (TCAs), monoamine oxidase inhibitors (MAOIs), and benzodiazepines (BZs) are effective anxiety disorder treatments in their own right that often produce short-term benefits comparable to those produced by exposure therapy (Fedoroff & Taylor, 2001; Gould, Buckminster, et al., 1997; Gould, Otto, et al., 1997; Mitte, 2005). Owing to the popularity of pharmacotherapy, most individuals presenting for psychological treatment are likely to already be taking one or more medications. Accordingly, clinicians need to understand the manner in which medications can influence the process and outcome of exposure therapy.

The observation that exposure and pharmacotherapy are both effective treatments raises the question as to whether it is advantageous to combine them. It is possible that exposure therapy and pharmacotherapy affect anxiety in different ways and thus patients could receive the major advantages of both treatments (e.g., Hegel, Ravaris, & Ahles, 1994). Similarly, medication could dampen patients' anxiety symptoms, thereby improving their ability to tolerate the distress provoked by exposure practices. However, there are also reasons to doubt that such an additive effect exists. For instance, antianxiety medication might diminish physiological arousal to the point that fear cannot be activated during exposure. As we have discussed in previous chapters, some medications (e.g., BZs) are used by individuals to prevent panic and anxiety, which may interfere with the disconfirmation of inaccurate beliefs during exposure or lead the patient to attribute any improvement to their medication instead of to exposure (Powers, Smits, Whitley, Bystritsky, & Telch, 2008). In this chapter, we review research on the effects of combining pharmacotherapy with exposure therapy for different anxiety disorders. Then we highlight clinical issues that arise in the context of combined treatment.

DOES MEDICATION ENHANCE THE EFFECTS OF EXPOSURE THERAPY?

Panic Disorder and Agoraphobia

Several large-scale studies investigating the effects of combining various psychotropic medications (TCAs, SSRIs, and BZs) with exposure-based CBT have been conducted with panic patients (e.g., Barlow, Gorman, Shear, & Woods, 2000; de Beurs, van Balkom, Lange, Koele, & van Dyck, 1995; Sharp et al., 1996; van Apeldoorn et al., 2008). The results from these studies provide some evidence that immediately following treatment, the combination of exposure-based CBT and antidepressants is superior to CBT alone. However, this finding has not been consistently replicated, and variations in the way exposure was conducted (e.g., use of interoceptive vs. situational exposure) across studies make it difficult to ascertain the extent to which antidepressants augment the psychological treatment. Moreover, long-term results suggest no advantage of combined treatment over monotherapy with CBT. These studies also show that adding antidepressants lead to higher drop-out rates than exposure therapy alone. With regard to BZs, research suggests few advantages of combination treatment and clear disadvantages over exposure therapy alone after drug taper. When BZs are prescribed for use "as needed" (PRN; i.e., when anxiety or panic occurs), they may impede the acute and long-term effects of exposure therapy. However, through avoiding PRN dosing and initiating a slow taper that occurs during the administration of exposure, the problematic effects of BZs may be minimized.

Obsessive–Compulsive Disorder

As with panic disorder, a number of carefully controlled studies have investigated whether the combination of exposure-based therapy (i.e., exposure and response prevention; ERP) and medication are more effective than ERP alone in the treatment of OCD (e.g., Cottraux et al., 1990; Foa et al., 2005; for a review, see Franklin, 2005). The findings of these studies can be summarized in the following way: Generally, there seems to be little advantage to augmenting ERP with pharmacotherapy in the treatment of OCD. The longer term effects of combined treatment are largely unknown, although 6-month follow-up analyses conducted by Cottraux et al. (1990) suggest that ERP alone is equivalent to combined treatment. Importantly, there is no evidence to suggest that pharmacotherapy *interferes* with the effects of exposure; rather, medication appears largely superfluous for patients with OCD who are undergoing treatment with ERP. Longer term studies are necessary to examine whether ongoing pharmacotherapy or its discontinuation interferes with the durability of ERP. Initial evidence suggests that patients who begin ERP while taking an antidepressant respond as well as patients who are medication-free (Franklin, Abramowitz, Bux, Zoellner, & Feeny, 2002).

Social Phobia

Despite a handful of controlled studies, it is difficult to draw reliable conclusions about the effects of combining pharmacotherapy with exposure therapy in the treatment of social phobia. One large and well-designed trial clearly indicated no advantage of adding fluoxetine (an SSRI) to exposure-based CBT (Davidson et al., 2004). Other studies have highlighted a trend for pharmacotherapy to produce more rapid reductions in social phobic symptoms, although exposure therapy appears to "catch up" with pharmacotherapy by the end of acute treatment and may produce more long-lasting effects (Blomhoff et al., 2001; Haug et al., 2003; Heimberg et al., 1998; Liebowitz et al., 1999).

Posttraumatic Stress Disorder

Surprisingly little research exists on the effectiveness of combination treatment for patients with PTSD. At the time of this writing, no published clinical trials have compared exposure-based CBT to combined treatment in the acute treatment of PTSD. One study found that exposure therapy improved outcomes for patients who had previously failed to benefit from pharmacotherapy (Otto et al., 2003). A second reported that the SSRI sertraline did not improve outcomes for patients who failed to benefit from exposure therapy (Simon et al., 2008).

Specific Phobia

Little research is available on the effects of combined treatments, or pharmacotherapy more generally, in the treatment of specific phobias. A small number of older studies have examined the effects of combined treatment with the BZ diazepam (Whitehead, Robinson, Blackwell, & Stutz, 1978) and imipramine (Zitrin, Klein, & Woerner, 1978; Zitrin, Klein, Woerner, & Ross, 1983). In each case, the authors concluded that concurrent pharmacotherapy did improve treatment response beyond that obtained with exposure alone.

Generalized Anxiety Disorder

Only one published clinical trial has examined the effects of combined treatment for GAD. Power, Simpson, Swanson, and Wallace (1990) compared the effectiveness of CBT, the BZ, and their combination in the treatment of GAD. A pill placebo condition was also included. CBT (either alone or in combination with diazepam) was associated with significantly better outcomes than diazepam and pill placebo, which did not differ from each other.

Childhood Anxiety

A limitation of the anxiety treatment literature is the paucity of studies on combined treatments for children and adolescents. The Pediatric OCD Treatment Study (2004) is an important exception to this trend. In this two-site study, children and adolescents with OCD were randomly assigned to receive ERP, the SSRI sertraline, their combination, or pill placebo for 12 weeks. ERP consisted of 14 one-hour sessions over 12 weeks. At posttreatment, all three active treatments were superior to pill placebo. Combined treatment was more effective than either ERP alone or sertraline alone, which did not differ from each other. Interestingly, there were site differences in outcomes. At the University of Pennsylvania site, which housed expertise in ERP, this treatment (ERP alone) was as effective as combined treatment, while at Duke University, which specializes in pharmacotherapy, combined treatment (ERP + sertraline) was more effective than ERP alone. The authors concluded that children and adolescents with OCD should receive either combined treatment or ERP alone.

Aside from this study, only one other large, randomized controlled trial for childhood anxiety disorders has been published. Walkup et al. (2008) reported findings from a comparison of exposure-based CBT, sertraline, their combination, and pill placebo in 488 children (ages 7 to 17 years) diagnosed with separation anxiety disorder, GAD, or social phobia. CBT was administered in 14 hour-long sessions. The findings indicated a clear advantage of combined treatment over exposure therapy alone, and the study authors concluded that sertraline and exposure-based CBT are both effective treatments for childhood anxiety, yet their combination offers the best chance for a positive outcome.

Summary of Research on Combined Treatments

Carefully conducted controlled studies provide little convincing evidence that using pharmacotherapy facilitates exposure therapy for adults with anxiety problems. A number of studies have reported evidence for a short-term advantage of combined treatment for patients with panic disorder. However, high dropout rates and increased risk of relapse following medication discontinuation caution against recommending combination treatment as a matter of course. Taking into account research on the short- and long-term effects of combined treatment, as well as its greater expense and increased risk of medication side effects and attrition, there is little reason to recommend this treatment over exposure-based CBT alone as a first-line treatment for any anxiety disorder.

Additional research is needed on the effects of combined treatment for childhood anxiety. Presently, it is not clear whether concurrent pharmacotherapy for patients with these disorders is helpful, unnecessary, or harmful. Given that most anxious patients presenting for exposure therapy are already taking medications, more research is needed on treatment outcomes for such individuals and how to optimally sequence multiple therapeutic modalities. Fortunately, the available evidence suggests that in most cases ongoing pharmacotherapy regimens do not interfere with a patient's ability to benefit from exposure.

Results of clinical trials of combined treatments do not support the idea that the therapeutic effects of pharmacotherapy and exposure will synergistically combine to produce a superior treatment. Rather, it appears that exposure therapy and traditional psychotropic medications for anxiety disorders work through different mechanisms that are not complementary, and may be contradictory in some instances. However, researchers have recently discovered an exciting exception to this trend that may constitute a breakthrough in combination therapy. Below, we discuss emerging research on the beneficial effects of augmenting exposure therapy with medications known as "cognitive enhancers."

PHARMACOLOGICAL ENHANCEMENT OF EXPOSURE THERAPY: THE FUTURE OF COMBINED TREATMENT?

Perhaps two primary approaches to the pharmacotherapy of anxiety disorders during the last half-century have been BZs (e.g., alprazolam, clonazepam), which dampen the physiological arousal that accompanies anxiety, and antidepressants (SSRIs or MAOIs), which are believed to reduce anxiety symptoms via their effects on neurotransmitter (i.e., serotonin) activity. Although often effective as monotherapies (Stein, Hollander, & Rothbaum, 2010), as reviewed above, neither of these approaches consistently improve the effectiveness of exposure therapy.

A radically different approach to combined treatment involves augmenting exposure therapy with medication that has no antianxiety effect per se, but that may enhance learning and facilitate fear extinction during exposure. D-cycloserine (DCS), an FDA-approved drug for tuberculosis for over 20 years, has been shown in animal studies to enhance the neural learning process underlying fear extinction (e.g., Ledgerwood, Richardson, & Cranny, 2003). Researchers have begun studying the clinical benefits of combining DCS with exposure therapy with quite promising results. The use of DCS to augment exposure therapy is fundamentally different from combination treatment with BZs or SSRIs or MAOIs because the sole purpose of DCS is to enhance the effects of exposure, rather than produce a general state of sedation or correct a presumed biological dysfunction as with other pharmacological strategies. We next review the research that has been conducted to date on the use of DCS for this purpose.

In the first study of DCS with humans, Ressler et al. (2004) randomly assigned 27 adults with acrophobia (fear of heights) to receive two sessions of virtual reality exposure combined with either pill placebo, 50mg of DCS, or 500mg of DCS. The DCS or placebo was ingested 2 to 4 hours prior to each exposure session. Patients in each group had equivalent levels of fear during the first exposure session. However, during the second exposure session, 1 week later, and at 3-month follow-up, patients who had received either dose of DCS were less afraid during the exposures than were placebo patients. The beneficial effects of DCS extended beyond the virtual world, as patients receiving DCS reported fewer real-world acrophobic symptoms than those receiving placebo at each assessment.

Numerous studies have independently replicated these findings. For example, Wilhelm et al. (2008) compared the effectiveness of DCS to pill placebo in augmenting ERP for 23 patients with OCD. Patients took a tablet of either DCS (100 mg) or placebo 1 hour prior to each of 10 exposure therapy sessions. The longer duration of treatment in this study, unlike the two-session intervention used by Ressler et al. (2004), more closely approximates the real length of treatment in actual clinical practice. Those patients receiving DCS improved more quickly by midtreatment and had markedly fewer obsessions and compulsions at posttreatment and a 1-month follow-up assessment than patients receiving placebo. They also had significantly fewer symptoms of depression.

Additional clinical trials have examined the effects of combining DCS with exposure in the treatment of social phobia, panic disorder, OCD, and specific phobias (see Norberg, Krystal, & Tolin, 2008, for a review), and in all but one study (Storch et al., 2007), adding DCS (relative to placebo) to exposure led to moderately large benefits at both posttreatment and follow-up (Norberg et al., 2008). The effects of DCS appear to vary according to the dose (lower is better) and timing of DCS administration (shortly before exposure is better), and its benefits appear most pronounced early in therapy. Thus, perhaps the effects of DCS are time-limited, with the greatest benefits obtained during initial exposure sessions and the effects diminishing gradually over time and repeated administrations of DCS.

A variety of other medications are being studied that may, like DCS, help to facilitate fear extinction in exposure therapy. Augmenting exposure therapy for claustrophobia with yohimbine, a selective competitive alpha2-adrenergic receptor antagonist, has been shown to substantially improve outcomes in comparison with placebo augmentation (Powers, Smits, Otto, Sanders, & Emmelkamp. 2009). Similarly, administration of the glucocorticoid cortisone prior to exposure tasks produced significantly improved outcomes for patients with social phobia and spider phobia (Soravia et al., 2006). Future cutting-edge research on combining exposure therapy with DCS and other "cognitive enhancers" holds significant promise for improving the lives of individuals suffering from anxiety disorders.

Despite the appeal of using medications like DCS to augment exposure therapy, there are formidable barriers that may hinder the widespread adoption of this approach by prescribers. First, prescribing medication exclusively for the purpose of enhancing the effects of a psychological treatment (i.e., exposure), rather than for the purpose of changing presumed neurobiological dysfunctions (e.g., serotonin dysregulation), constitutes a major paradigm shift for psychiatrists and other physicians who might view anxiety disorders as "brain diseases" caused by abnormally functioning neurotransmitter systems. Second, physicians prescribing DCS would be assuming the role of a "secondary treatment provider," helping the exposure therapist implement his or her treatment more effectively, rather than serving as the primary (or sole) treatment provider. This, too, represents a paradigm shift from the current thinking in many medical centers that psychological treatments are secondary to drug treatment (Abramowitz & Piacetini, 2006). Assuming that additional research findings continue to support the use of DCS and related medications to augment exposure, there may be increasing pressure on exposure therapists to work with prescribers in the treatment of their anxious patients, and on prescribers to reconsider their assumptions about the goals and process of pharmacotherapy.

CLINICAL ISSUES ASSOCIATED
WITH COMBINED TREATMENTS

Given that most patients presenting for psychological treatment of anxiety are already using one or more psychotropic medications, exposure therapists need to be ready to address certain key issues regarding combined treatment. Next, we discuss how to convey a treatment rationale for seemingly contradictory approaches (medicine and exposure), how to manage the possible context effects of medication use, and how to best collaborate with those prescribing the patient's psychotropic medicines.

Conveying an Integrated Treatment Rationale

In contrast to the basis for exposure therapy (as presented in Chapter 3 and discussed across the chapters in Part II), the basis for most pharmacotherapy for anxiety is a biological model that emphasizes the role of neurotransmitter dysregulation in the development of anxiety disorders (e.g., Krystal, Deutsch, & Charney, 1996; Pigott, 1996). This "chemical imbalance" model may be disseminated by prescribing physicians, as well as the pharmaceutical industry through the popular media. Thus, patients are typically familiar with the theory that their symptoms are caused by a "chemical imbalance in the brain" that may be "corrected" with medication.

Although the basis for exposure and for medication may each have some validity, they often appear incongruous to patients whose treatment providers have not attempted to integrate them. That is, a chemical imbalance explanation might seem incompatible with the notion that anxiety symptoms are associated with modifiable cognitive and behavioral factors. As a result, poor compliance with either medication or exposure therapy may occur if the patient perceives either treatment may be superfluous (Deacon & Lickel, 2009).

To avoid this potential pitfall, exposure therapists (and ideally, prescribers) should convey an integrated treatment rationale that acknowledges the role of biology but emphasizes the need to target the psychological processes that maintain pathological anxiety. Biological factors (e.g., genetics, neurotransmitter dysregulation) may be described as one of many variables that contribute to the development of an anxiety problem. These factors may increase an individual's vulnerability to anxiety in general, and as such they are legitimate targets for intervention via pharmacotherapy. However, the content and persistence of the patient's exaggerated threat-related beliefs are best viewed as the product of psychological processes that may be modified by exposure therapy. From this perspective, pharmacotherapy may facilitate recovery by producing symptom relief, while the task of directly modifying problematic cognitive and behavioral responses is targeted with exposure (as well as other CBT techniques).

Although we find that this integrated model is understood by most anxiety patients, some express skepticism regarding how psychological treatment will benefit them if their symptoms are caused by biochemical factors. In such instances, it may be helpful to inform patients that exposure-based CBT is often as effective as combination treatment and that it produces observable changes in brain functioning comparable to what is produced by medication (e.g., Baxter et al., 1992). The latter may be especially useful in correcting the pervasive but incorrect assumption that symptoms attributed to faulty brain chemistry can only be improved with pharmacotherapy.

This integrated model is most applicable when combined treatment includes pharmacotherapy with SSRIs that do not produce an immediate anxiety-reducing effect. The circumstances are markedly different when patients present for exposure therapy while using BZs on a PRN schedule as discussed earlier in this chapter. In such cases, it may be difficult to integrate the competing rationales for exposure and BZ treatment. In fact, it may be unwise to do so in light of research findings that combined treatment with BZs interferes with the effects of exposure (e.g., Marks et al., 1993). The recommended course of action with such patients is to incorporate the use of BZ into the exposure-based model in which BZ use functions as a safety behavior. The possibility of gradually discontinuing the BZ during exposure therapy (as directed by the prescribing physician) can also be discussed. If the patient is amenable to this approach, he or she may still derive substantial benefit from exposure provided that BZ taper occurs slowly and is completed before the termination of exposure therapy (Spiegel & Bruce, 1997). If the patient is unwilling to consider altering his or her BZ use at some point during exposure therapy, it may be best not to initiate treatment as this essentially constitutes the refusal to give up a safety behavior.

Managing Context Effects

Exposure therapy facilitates safety learning by demonstrating to patients that the stimuli they fear are not threatening *in any context* (Bouton, 2002). Thus, the effects of exposure are partially dependent on the context in which this learning occurs. A patient with a spider phobia who spends an exposure session holding a spider, for example, does so in a specific context which may include (among other things) the office where the session took place, the presence of the therapist, the physical characteristics of the spider, and so on. Therapists should not assume that learning in one context will fully generalize to different contexts.

The use of pharmacotherapy during exposure introduces a number of potential contexts and conditions that may attenuate the effects of exposure when a change in context occurs. One such context is the internal state created by the pharmacological effects of the medication. For example, internal cues associated with the context of imipramine include dry mouth, sweating, and increased heart rate (Mavissakalian, Perel, & Guo, 2002). A large randomized controlled trial of combined treatment for panic disorder with imipramine (Barlow et al., 2000) provides powerful evidence of an internal context effect. Following imipramine discontinuation, patients in combined treatment (who had previously responded quite well) experienced a marked increase in their panic symptoms. This did not occur for patients in combined treatment who discontinued placebo medication. The most likely explanation for these findings is that learning that occurred in the internal context created by imipramine did not generalize to the new context in which the pharmacological effects of the medication were absent. Practically speaking, the context effect of internal drug state increases the risk of relapse after patients discontinue their medication. The negative effects of this context shift may be managed by discontinuing medication during ongoing exposure therapy, which provides patients with the opportunity to actively acquire safety learning in this new internal context.

An additional pharmacotherapy-induced context effect occurs when medications diminish the physiological symptoms of anxious arousal. In this context, the safety learning produced by exposure may be conditional on the experience of no more than moderate arousal (e.g., "I am unlikely to have a heart attack *provided that my heart doesn't beat too rapidly*"). For patients who fear physiological arousal itself (i.e., who are anxiety-sensitive), the context of diminished anxiety may interfere with safety learning by preventing exposure to sufficiently intense body sensations.

Medications are especially likely to interfere with learning in psychotherapy when they are used as safety aids. This phenomenon is observed when patients take BZ medication PRN to avert or cope with perceived threat. When used in this manner, these medications may acquire in the minds of their users the power to prevent the very catastrophes that exposure seeks to disconfirm. To illustrate, take the example of a 35-year-old woman with panic disorder who described an intense fear of suffocation during her panic attacks. When asked why she continued to fear this consequence despite its failure to occur in hundreds of previous attacks, she responded that only by taking alprazolam (a BZ) during each attack had she managed to prevent suffocation.

This case exemplifies two problematic cognitive effects of using medications as safety aids. First, patients are effectively prevented from acquiring information that might disconfirm their inaccurate threat-related beliefs. Second, these beliefs may actually be strengthened on the basis of the notion that the nonoccurrence of catastrophe constitutes a "near-miss" that was achieved only through the power of the medication. Beyond the deleterious effects on cognition, the use of medications in this manner may interfere with improvement during psychotherapy by strengthening escape behavior (i.e., taking a pill to short-circuit increasing anxiety), effectively preventing patients from learning that high anxiety in the presence of fear cues will eventually dissipate without the use of safety behaviors. Discouraging the use of medications as safety aids may require the exposure therapist to educate prescribers who instruct patients to use their pills in this manner.

Collaborating with Prescribers

It is often helpful for therapists to work directly with prescribers to facilitate the integration of psychotherapy and pharmacotherapy. The failure of prescribers and psychological treatment providers to collaborate sometimes results in the delivery of two seemingly incompatible treatment modalities, leaving the patient caught in the middle and left to decide how to navigate these competing approaches. Ideally, the prescribing physician and the exposure therapist present an integrated treatment rationale that leaves room for the role of both exposure and pharmacotherapy. However, as discussed earlier, this ideal may not reflect the clinical reality in which psychotherapists and physicians often present a one-sided psychological or biological rationale. A related problem involves a situation in which well-meaning prescribers instruct patients to use their medications in ways that directly contradict the process of exposure therapy; for example, patients are sometimes instructed to carry BZs on their person and ingest a pill when they become anxious. It is especially important that exposure therapists consult with prescribers in these circumstances in order to coordinate the treatment rationale and plan.

The informed consent process in combined treatment should include discussion of the possibility of relapse upon medication discontinuation. Patients who plan on taking medication for the foreseeable future are often willing to accept this risk. However, individuals who wish to discontinue their medication in the near future may express concern about their prognosis. For such individuals, it may be useful to taper off medications during ongoing psychotherapy so that fear extinction during exposure generalizes to the new internal context of being medication-free. Because withdrawal symptoms and other adverse effects may occur during drug discontinuation, this process should always occur under the supervision of an adequately trained prescriber.

Luckily, many prescribers are interested in learning about evidence-based psychological treatments and are willing to consider prescribing medications in a circumspect manner or not at all in cases for which effective nonpharmacological treatment options are available. Proactive clinicians may have the opportunity to educate prescribers, particularly those with little mental health training, about how to optimally integrate pharmaco-therapy and psychotherapy. Therapists who foster collaborative relation-ships with prescribers may avoid the aforementioned problems associated with combined treatment and facilitate consistently better outcomes for their patients.

CONCLUSIONS

Most patients who participate in exposure therapy also take medication for their anxiety symptoms. Unfortunately, relatively little is known about how concurrent pharmacotherapy affects the outcome of exposure for most anxi-ety disorders. The research literature suggests that combined treatment does not necessarily augment the effects of exposure-based therapy. When longer term outcomes are considered, exposure may actually be more effective than combined treatment in some circumstances (e.g., after medication discon-tinuation). Existing research does not support the assumption that exposure therapy and traditional pharmacotherapies like SSRIs and BZs synergisti-cally combine to produce uniquely robust therapeutic effects. Instead, these treatment modalities likely exert their effects through noncomplementary mechanisms. The emerging literature on the use of DCS to facilitate fear extinction during exposure is promising, yet additional research is necessary before this approach is ready for widespread use.

ADDITIONAL RESOURCE

Otto, M. W., McHugh, R. K., & Kantak, K. M. (2010). Combined pharmacother-apy and cognitive-behavioral therapy for anxiety disorders: Medication effects, glucocorticoids, and attenuated treatment outcome. *Clinical Psychology: Sci-ence and Practice, 17,* 91–103.

20

Maintaining Improvement after Treatment

Exposure therapy is, by design, a brief treatment in which patients are encouraged to develop the skills necessary to conduct the therapy independently. Exposure therapists assume an active, expert role early in treatment as they educate patients about the nature of anxiety, the cognitive-behavioral conceptual model, and the rationale and procedures for exposure. Once exposure sessions begin, the therapist's role gradually transitions from "teacher" to "coach" and "cheerleader." This process entails gradually transferring the primary responsibility for conducting the "work" of therapy to the patient. Once the patient has demonstrated the ability to successfully conduct exposures to the most feared hierarchy items in various contexts, the therapist's main task is to teach the patient to become his or her own therapist. For patients who understand the theory and practice of exposure therapy and use this knowledge to overcome their fears, continued participation in treatment may seem unnecessary, which marks the ideal end to exposure therapy. In this chapter, we discuss clinical strategies for encouraging long-term recovery from pathological anxiety and preventing relapse following treatment.

WHEN IS TREATMENT COMPLETE?

A first step in promoting continued recovery is ensuring that the patient has indeed *completed* treatment. But how is this determined? When is further treatment for an anxiety problem unnecessary? In this section, we review markers of improvement that are important indicators of success in exposure therapy and promote the long-term maintenance of treatment gains.

Completion of All Hierarchy Items

Exposure therapy is not considered complete until the patient has successfully faced the highest item on the exposure hierarchy. This typically requires confrontation with the most feared stimuli or situations, and perhaps "overlearning" by confronting them directly and in ways that might not routinely occur in everyday life (Antony & Swinson, 2000)—for example, handling a snake or spider, sitting on a bathroom floor, spending an hour in a small closet, making a pact with the devil, *wishing* bad luck on a relative, purposely embarrassing oneself, and the like. Facing one's worst fear without the use of safety behaviors is a powerful and courageous act that is considered a key index of recovery in exposure therapy.

Although confronting the most feared hierarchy item is necessary for full improvement, it may not be sufficient. Depending on the specific anxiety problem and the patient's goals, it may be important to conduct the exposure repeatedly and in a variety of contexts in order to fully correct maladaptive threat beliefs. For example, one patient with social phobia whose most feared situation was striking up conversations with strangers at parties needed to complete this task on numerous occasions, and with different conversational partners, before she believed that social catastrophes were unlikely to occur in such a situation. Another patient with a dog phobia had to interact with several dogs of different breeds until she came to believe that dogs in general, as opposed to the specific dogs used for the exposure tasks, were unlikely to attack her.

The Patient No Longer Meets Diagnostic Criteria for the Anxiety Disorder

By definition, patients who no longer meet DSM criteria for the anxiety disorder(s) being treated have experienced a significant decrease in their anxiety symptoms and an improved ability to function. The absence of an anxiety disorder diagnosis provides a simple and categorical measure of improvement that is often favored by scientists who conduct clinical trials. However, failure to meet the threshold for a DSM diagnosis does not necessarily indicate the absence of significant anxiety symptoms. Moreover, improvement in anxiety symptoms may occur without modification of maladaptive threat beliefs and avoidance. To illustrate, patients who stop experiencing panic attacks through frequent use of benzodiazepine medications may still view panic as harmful and take efforts to avoid situations that might trigger a panic attack. For these reasons, the patient's diagnostic status is insufficient as a sole index of recovery in exposure therapy.

Maladaptive Beliefs Have Been Corrected

As we discussed in Chapter 3, anxious patients hold a number of characteristic maladaptive beliefs that underlie their fears. Exposure therapy is a learning process designed to correct these maladaptive beliefs by instilling in patients a sense of unconditional learned safety. When successful, exposure teaches patients that the dreaded outcomes associated with feared stimuli are unlikely to occur, and for certain feared consequences (e.g., blushing) are manageable even if they were to occur. Patients should come to believe that the experience of anxiety itself is harmless, unavoidable, and tolerable. They should also be convinced that safety behaviors are, in most cases, unnecessary to prevent feared outcomes from occurring. Lastly, patients should evidence a willingness to accept some degree of uncertainty about the possible occurrence of feared outcomes in situations where disaster is unlikely.

How can exposure therapists determine whether their patients' maladaptive beliefs have been sufficiently corrected? One strategy is to formally assess them throughout the course of therapy using validated self-report questionnaires such as the Anxiety Sensitivity Index (Reiss, Peterson, Gursky, & McNally, 1986), the Obsessive Beliefs Questionnaire (Obsessive–Compulsive Cognitions Working Group. 2001), or the Appraisal of Social Concerns Scale (Telch et al., 2004). Therapists can administer relevant measures to their patients at pretreatment and again during therapy, either on an ongoing (e.g., session-by-session) basis or toward the end of treatment. Scores in the normal range provide objective evidence that the patient's maladaptive beliefs have been sufficiently corrected. The *Practitioner's Guide to Empirically Based Measures of Anxiety* (Antony, Orsillo, & Roemer, 2001) is a useful reference that provides copies of dozens of questionnaires for various anxiety problems and lists normative data for both nonclinical and anxiety samples for each measure (when available).

Informal assessment of maladaptive beliefs occurs on an ongoing basis during therapy sessions, particularly during and immediately following exposure practices. The desired pattern is for patient ratings of the probability and/or the cost of feared consequences to decrease throughout treatment. One index of improvement is reduction in threat estimates within exposure practices, such that predictions of harm decrease to low levels by the end of the exercises. A second index is a reduction in threat estimates across sessions, such that similar exposure tasks are rated as progressively less dangerous over consecutive therapy sessions. By the time the patient has completed all exposure tasks, the estimated probability and/or cost of previously feared catastrophes should be low and proportionate to the actual degree of risk. If the patient continues to exhibit exaggerated threat beliefs at the end of treatment, a functional analysis should be conducted to determine the nature of such beliefs and the kinds of exposure tasks that might serve to promote unconditional learned safety.

Safety Behaviors Have Been Eliminated

The patient's use of safety behaviors provides an objective indicator of improvement in exposure therapy. Ongoing use of one or more safety behaviors likely indicates the presence of lingering maladaptive threat beliefs that have not been adequately addressed in treatment. Likewise, continuing insistence on having access to safety aids (e.g., carrying benzodiazepine medication in one's purse) should be considered problematic. The use of self-monitoring may assist therapists and patients in determining the extent of safety behavior use during therapy. In addition, a number of validated questionnaires have been developed to assess the degree of safety behavior use for patients with different anxiety disorders, such as the Texas Safety Maneuver Scale (Kamphuis & Telch, 1998) for panic disorder and the Liebowitz Social Anxiety Scale (Liebowitz, 1987) for social phobia. As before, the *Practitioner's Guide to Empirically Based Measures of Anxiety* (Antony et al., 2001) is a useful reference for identifying such measures.

Patients who have become truly convinced through exposure therapy that previously feared stimuli are not dangerous should not exhibit safety behaviors (Why go out of the way to prevent a disaster that is unlikely to occur?). Clinical experience suggests that patients who have the best outcomes in exposure are those whose maladaptive threat beliefs have been corrected so completely that they are willing, even eager, to face previously avoided stimuli in order to prove to themselves that they have nothing to fear. These patients seem to have a "Bring it on!" attitude toward exposure tasks. Properly conducted exposure therapy aims to elicit such an attitude. This, along with the absence of safety behaviors, is a good indication that exposure therapy is nearing completion and that the patient will likely maintain his or her gains following termination.

Functioning and Quality of Life Have Improved

Although the immediate goal of exposure therapy is the correction of the maladaptive cognitive and behavioral processes that maintain pathological anxiety, the outcomes of this treatment extend far beyond these symptom-based changes. One of the most harmful effects of clinical anxiety is restricted participation in daily activities such as driving, flying, using the bathroom, practicing one's religion, and dating. Inability to participate in such activities often exerts a profoundly negative effect on patients' quality of life, psychological well-being, and even physical health. Exposure therapy fosters substantial improvement in patients' quality of life by removing the formidable barrier posed by pathological anxiety.

By encouraging participation in valued but previously avoided situations and activities through exposure tasks, exposure therapy directly promotes an improved quality of life. Patients who have completed their exposure hierarchy should demonstrate both reduced distress in feared situations and increased participation in valued but previously avoided activities. Someone who previously suffered from agoraphobia should be able to watch a movie in a crowded theater (even sitting in the middle of the row). An individual who presented with social anxiety should be able to talk to an authority figure or ask someone out for a date. A patient with needle phobia should be able to undergo a medically necessary surgical procedure. Evidence that patients are actively participating in activities that improve the quality of their lives indicates that an important goal of exposure therapy has been reached. Together with the above criteria, markedly improved quality of life may be considered a sign that further treatment is unnecessary. Of course, there is more to quality of life than the absence of clinically significant distress and functional impairment. Overcoming an anxiety problem doesn't necessarily equate with happiness and fulfillment. Therapists who wish to extend treatment beyond the realm of anxiety reduction into direct enhancement of quality of life per se may benefit from the use of positive psychology and cognitive therapy techniques, as well as values-based strategies from acceptance and commitment therapy (e.g., Eifert & Forsyth, 2005).

MAINTAINING GAINS AND PREVENTING RELAPSE

As our literature review in Chapter 2 makes clear, exposure therapy is neither universally nor completely effective for reducing anxiety. Even in the best-case scenario, individuals undergoing exposure are likely to remain with at least some degree of residual symptoms. But even so, the patient has gained invaluable skills for managing times when fear and anxiety strike. As treatment draws to a close, there are a number of steps therapists can take to promote the longer term maintenance of gains and prevent relapse. We describe these next.

Spread Out Therapy Sessions toward the End of Treatment

We recommend fading the frequency of therapist-supervised exposure sessions as treatment progresses toward its later stages. For example, formerly weekly sessions may be scheduled biweekly, and then monthly, and then "as needed." The type of therapist support may also transition from face-to-face visits to telephone "check-ins." The practice of gradually slowing the pace of therapy is consistent with research on the short- and long-term effects of massed versus spaced learning on memory retention (e.g., Bjork & Bjork, 1990; Schmidt & Bjork, 1992). Specifically, longer and more varied intervals between practice trials enhance long-term retention of learning because they provide increased opportunities to use what has been learned in varied contexts (Bjork & Bjork, 1990; Schmidt & Bjork, 1992). The implications of this research for exposure therapy are very clear: spacing out the treatment sessions toward the end of therapy increases the opportunities the patient has to consolidate what was learned during in-session exposures. This fosters the long-term maintenance of treatment gains because it protects against the return of fear (Rachman, 1979; Rowe & Craske, 1998).

Plan for Ongoing Self-Directed Treatment

Given that exposure therapy is a method for acquiring skills for managing anxious thinking and behavior, it naturally follows that those skills need to be maintained over time. Ost (1989) drew a useful analogy to learning to drive a car for discussing this issue with patients. After obtaining a driver's license, one is not yet a highly skilled driver. It is necessary to continue driving, in different road conditions and environments, to learn to effectively handle these situations and refine one's skills. If one rarely drives after obtaining the driver's license, driving skills may deteriorate to the point that they become worse than they were when the license was obtained. Thus, if one were unexpectedly asked to drive after a long period of not driving, his or her driving skills might have declined to the point that he or she is not able to drive very well. This analogy is easy for patients to understand and makes it clear that they need to continue to practice exposure even after formal therapy has been completed.

A written maintenance plan may be used to specify strategies for continued self-directed treatment. The plan should include specific exposure tasks to be conducted, as well as the frequency with which the practices should occur. Patients should continue using homework monitoring forms as needed. Ongoing self-directed treatment encompasses both planned exposures and "lifestyle exposures" in which individuals are encouraged to face feared situations that naturally arise in the course of everyday life. In addition, safety behaviors should be monitored and eliminated during both planned and lifestyle exposures. Patients are encouraged to contact the therapist if they encounter difficulties in the course of self-directed treatment.

An example of a written maintenance plan for a patient with panic disorder and agoraphobia was described by Deacon (2007b). The patient, a 38-year-old woman, participated in a 2-day, intensive exposure treatment that targeted her fear of arousal-related body sensations as well as her tendency to faint while experiencing panic symptoms. Following treatment, the therapist and the patient collaboratively developed a written four-part relapse prevention plan (see Figure 20.1). The first section prescribed conducting frequent, planned interoceptive and situational exposures such as hyperventilation and aerobic exercise. The second involved eliminating avoidance in her normal routine by conducting exposures when the chance arose in everyday life. Third, the patient was urged to identify and eliminate all safety and avoidance behaviors related to her panic and vasovagal symptoms. Fourth, she was encouraged to use applied tension to prevent fainting in situations in which she felt the clear onset of a vasovagal reaction. A telephone contact 1 month after the final session was arranged, and the patient was encouraged to contact the therapist on an as-needed basis with any questions or concerns.

Anticipate Potential Triggers for Symptom Exacerbation

Awareness of "high-risk" situations and stimuli that are likely to trigger anxiety symptoms may help prevent the patient from slipping back into dysfunctional thinking and behaving patterns when such stimuli are encountered. A number of circumstances may trigger an exacerbation of anxiety symptoms

FIGURE 20.1. A written maintenance plan for a patient with panic disorder and agoraphobia who occasionally fainted during panic attacks.

1. **Conduct frequent, planned exposure practices (not part of normal routine).**

Interoceptive exposures:	Spin in swivel chair, shake head from side to side, hold breath, engage in vigorous exercise, make self hot (e.g., sit in sauna, wear hot clothing)
Situational exposures:	Eat at crowded restaurants, ride crowded elevators, attend kids' sporting events, attend church, shop at crowded stores/malls

2. **Eliminate avoidance in normal routine (conduct exposures when opportunity arises).**

3. **Eliminate harmful safety behaviors.**

   Leaving work when anxious, elevating legs, monitoring breathing, carrying and eating protein bars, carrying cell phone when walking, relying on safe person in public places, distracting self from anxiety symptoms, using diaphragmatic breathing to reduce anxiety symptoms

4. **Use applied tension to prevent fainting (as needed).**

following exposure therapy (Antony & Swinson, 2000). One candidate is the experience of stressful life events. A major illness, loss of job, breakup of a relationship, or death of a loved one may lead to emotional distress, catastrophic thinking, aversive body sensations, and an increase in anxiety symptoms. Unexpected encounters with new and difficult situations not tackled during exposure practices may also provoke anxiety. For example, a patient who was successfully treated for social phobia experienced an unexpected bout of high anxiety when attending a wedding reception and dancing with the bride on an otherwise empty dance floor in front of hundreds of onlookers. Experiencing a trauma in the context of one's previously feared situation may also trigger a return of fear. For example, a man who completed a successful trial of exposure for his fear of injections experienced a return of fear 1 year later when he fainted and hit his head during a routine blood draw. In each of these circumstances, patients should be encouraged to actively engage in self-directed exposure to once again acquire learned safety. A small number of "booster sessions" of therapist-supervised exposure might also be considered.

Discontinuing anxiety medication can also trigger an increase in anxiety symptoms. Indeed, panic symptoms tend to worsen after patients who participate in combined treatment discontinue their antidepressant (Barlow et al., 2000) or benzodiazepine (Marks et al., 1993) medication. In some cases, the potential for relapse can be mitigated by following a program designed to integrate medication taper with exposure exercises (e.g., Otto, Jones, Craske, & Barlow, 1996). Patients who attribute their improvement during exposure therapy to medication are at particular risk of relapse when the medication is discontinued (Basoglu, Marks, Kilic, Brewin, & Swinson, 1994). Thus, therapists should be alert for the possible misattribution of safety to pharmacotherapy among patients taking medication along with exposure. This problem is especially likely when medication and exposure are initiated simultaneously. To mitigate this problem, the patient's efforts at behavioral change in exposure therapy should be highlighted by the therapist, and patients may be encouraged to produce a written description of what they did to produce treatment gains and what they learned during exposure therapy (Taylor, 2000).

Educate the Patient about the Difference between Lapse and Relapse

Patients should be aware that at some point following treatment, anxiety symptoms are likely to reemerge. We have observed that a temporary return of fear can occur even for individuals who respond extremely well to exposure therapy. Thus, therapists should help patients set realistic expectations for experiencing anxiety after treatment. For example, it is useful to remind the patient that anxiety symptoms are universal and unavoidable, yet harmless. The transient experience of anxiety symptoms is therefore to be expected, and it is important for patients not to misinterpret such symptoms as though their anxiety disorder has returned.

Patients should understand the critical distinction between a *lapse* (also called a "setback") and a *relapse*. A lapse consists of the occurrence of anxiety symptoms, such as panic attacks, avoidance, fear, or unexpected difficulty managing a situation one has previously managed adequately. In contrast, a relapse denotes a complete return of symptoms such that the patient is back to where he or she started from prior to exposure therapy. Whether or not a lapse evolves into a relapse depends on how the patient chooses to react to his or her return of symptoms. In other words, longer term success is defined not in terms of being symptom-free but rather by being able to successfully manage the reemergence of symptoms if and when they occur. Naturally, the preferred response is to conduct exposures, challenge maladaptive beliefs, and practice therapy skills to stop the renewed anxiety in its tracks. Indeed, a lapse may be thought of as an opportunity to practice exposure (and other CBT skills) in order to once again prove to oneself that formerly held beliefs about anxiety and feared stimuli are inaccurate. It is critical to emphasize that the same therapy skills that led to improvement during exposure therapy may be used to manage lapses following the completion of treatment.

Have a Plan for How to Respond to a Lapse

Exposure therapists should prepare their patients with an action plan for managing setbacks when they occur. Ost (1989) reported guidelines for responding to a setback as part of a comprehensive maintenance program that has shown promising results in numerous studies (McKay, 1997; McKay, Todaro, Neziroglu, & Yaryura-Tobias, 1996; Ost, 1989). A simplified presentation of these steps, adapted from Taylor (2000), is as follows:

1. *Remember that a lapse is not the same thing as a relapse.* It is simply a temporary failure to manage a situation. Occasional lapses are to be expected and are not problematic if they are dealt with properly.
2. *Analyze the situation.* Try to understand what might have caused the lapse. Was the patient engaging in catastrophic thinking? Were safety behaviors used? Was there something distinct about the situation in comparison to other situations in which the patient had conducted exposures?
3. *Practice skills learned in treatment.* Return to the situation and conduct a planned exposure. Remain in the situation until anxiety has

habituated. Test the accuracy of predictions about harm in the situation.

4. *Restrict the lapse.* The patient can think of a lapse as a small fire—which *could* turn into an inferno if it is allowed to spread before it is extinguished. To avoid allowing a return of fear in one situation to spread to other contexts, the patient must plan and conduct exposures and eliminate safety behaviors in any situations in which anxiety symptoms have returned.

5. *If self-directed efforts do not work, contact the therapist as soon as possible.* Arrange for a therapy session to review the situation. The clinician may recommend conducting a number of therapist-assisted exposure sessions.

SUMMARY AND CONCLUSIONS

Exposure therapy is designed to promote long-term recovery by modifying the maladaptive psychological processes that maintain pathological anxiety. Patients should continue conducting exposures and practicing therapy skills well after the end of formal therapy sessions. Even patients who have experienced a complete recovery during exposure may experience a return of fear after treatment has been completed. The probability of temporary anxiety symptoms escalating into a full-blown relapse may be reduced by fostering reasonable expectations for the maintenance of gains and equipping patients with specific strategies for how to respond to an exacerbation of anxiety symptoms. In summary, exposure therapy is most effective in the long term when clinicians actively prepare their patients for life after treatment.

21

A Risk–Benefit Analysis
of Exposure Therapy

Exposure-based CBT is the most scientifically supported psychological treatment for anxiety. As we reviewed in Chapter 2, dozens of randomized controlled trials have demonstrated the *efficacy* of this treatment for different anxiety disorders and the *effectiveness* of this approach when applied in community settings with real-world patients (Stewart & Chambless, 2009). On average, exposure-based therapy leads to as much short-term benefit as the most potent antianxiety and antidepressant medications and is associated with better long-term maintenance of treatment gains. Relative to medications, exposure therapy is also more cost-effective (Heuzenroeder, Donnelly, & Haby, 2004), more acceptable and preferable to patients and their caregivers (Brown, Deacon, Abramowitz, & Whiteside, 2007; Deacon & Abramowitz, 2005), and results in less patient attrition (Hofmann et al., 1998; Huppert, Franklin, Foa, & Davidson, 2003). Taken together, these observations make a strong case for exposure-based CBT as the treatment of choice for anxiety disorders. Indeed, this treatment may have more scientific support than any other psychotherapy of any kind, for any problem.

Yet despite its documented effectiveness, exposure therapy techniques are rarely used by practicing clinicians. To illustrate, Foy et al. (1996) reported that exposure therapy was used to treat fewer than 20% of 4,000 veterans with PTSD in the Veteran's Affairs health care system, and that it was the primary method of treatment in only 1% of cases. More broadly, the majority of patients with any anxiety disorder do not receive evidence-based psychotherapy (Stein et al., 2004); indeed, psychodynamic therapy is received as often as CBT (Goisman, Warshaw, & Keller, 1999). Even clinicians who report using "CBT" with their patients rely primarily on relaxation techniques and seldom use procedures such as interoceptive exposure (Freiheit et al., 2004).

How can we explain the low utilization of exposure by mental health professionals? Without question, one reason is that many therapists have not received sufficient training in the theory and practice of exposure therapy. We believe, however, that many therapists also hold negative beliefs about exposure that keep them from using this set of techniques (Olatunji et al., 2009). For example, we have encountered therapists who think that exposure will *harm* their patients or that subjecting anxious individuals to their feared stimuli is tantamount to torture. As a result of such beliefs, even therapists who are aware of exposure's scientific support may reject it in favor of treatments they deem to be less aversive and more "humane." The all-too-common result of this misplaced compassion is the wasted time and effort, the financial expense, and the continued emotional suffering associated with receiving inadequate treatment.

In this chapter, we begin by considering common negative beliefs about exposure therapy. Next, we discuss an approach for minimizing risks to patient safety when implementing exposure. Last, we review strategies for maintaining ethical boundaries during exposure. By challenging popular misconceptions about exposure-based treatments, we hope this chapter will help persuade clinicians that an objective and evidence-based risk–benefit analysis strongly argues for the use of this treatment with most anxiety patients. Readers interested in a more detailed consideration of these issues are referred to Olatunji et al. (2009).

BELIEFS ABOUT EXPOSURE THERAPY

Exposure therapy has a public relations problem with many in the field of psychotherapy, even among some practitioners who specialize in the treatment of anxiety (Prochaska & Norcross, 1999; Richard & Gloster, 2007). Condemnation of exposure may stem from the fact that this treatment evokes distress (albeit temporarily), rather than soothes it, as one might intuitively expect a treatment for anxiety to do. More specific and widespread negative beliefs about exposure therapy described by Feeny, Hembree, and Zoellner (2003) and Prochaska and Norcross (1999) include the following:

- The ends do not justify its means.
- Exposure is rigid and insensitive to the individual needs of the patient.
- Exposure does not work for complex cases.

- Exposure is only effective in "ivory tower" research settings, and its effects do not generalize to "real-world" clinical settings.
- Exposure involves impersonal techniques that are done "to," rather than "with," anxious individuals.
- Exposure exacerbates anxiety symptoms and causes high rates of attrition.
- Patients are better off suffering from their anxiety disorder than undergoing such an aversive treatment.

Becker, Zayfert, and Anderson (2004) demonstrated that such beliefs are common, particularly among clinicians specializing in the treatment of patients with PTSD. Hopefully, reading through the chapters of this book, one will recognize that these beliefs turn out to be either exaggerations or simply incorrect. What follows next is a more direct critical analysis of the most prevalent of these beliefs:

- *Patients will drop out of therapy.* Critics of exposure therapy often assume that such a presumably aversive treatment must result in unacceptably high dropout rates in therapy. Hembree et al. (2003) tested this assumption by reviewing studies of prolonged exposure for PTSD, which is often considered the most difficult-to-tolerate application of exposure therapy. As we describe in Chapter 13, this empirically supported form of exposure involves helping the patient "relive" his or her trauma by deliberately recounting the details of the traumatic event (e.g., a sexual assault). Outcomes from 25 clinical trials yielded no significant differences in drop-out rates between prolonged exposure (20.6%), exposure combined with cognitive therapy or anxiety management (26.0%), and eye movement desensitization and reprocessing (18.9%). Hembree and Cahill (2007) noted that dropout rates for prolonged exposure for PTSD are comparable to those observed in exposure therapy with other anxiety disorders, and are lower than dropout rates associated with psychotropic medications.

- *Exposure will worsen a patient's symptoms.* Another undesirable outcome commonly attributed to exposure therapy is its perceived potential to worsen anxiety symptoms. This concern is often voiced by therapists who believe that, for example, patients with PTSD will be unable to tolerate the process of reliving traumatic memories via imaginal exposure. Foa, Zoellner, Feeny, Hembree, and Alvarez-Conrad (2002) directly investigated this issue by examining symptom exacerbation during the course of prolonged exposure. Although the majority of PTSD patients did not experience worsening of their symptoms, a temporary exacerbation following the start of imaginal exposure did occur in a minority of individuals. Importantly, patients whose symptoms initially worsened were not at increased risk of either dropping out of therapy or failing to improve. Thus, symptom exacerbation during exposure was both uncommon and of little prognostic value. The results of Foa et al. (2002) support the practice of informing patients that exposure is likely to provoke temporary initial distress, but that experiencing this type of fear will eventually prove beneficial following repeated practice. These findings are also consistent with the notion that, despite some therapists' beliefs to the contrary, most patients are resilient and able to tolerate the distress associated with facing their fears.

• *Patients won't like exposure therapy.* Some therapists assume that their patients will dislike exposure therapy, and will instead prefer to undergo treatment that does not entail the distress associated with having to directly face their fears. This negative perception of exposure appears to pervade public sentiment as well. A study by Richard and Gloster (2007) presented undergraduates and outpatients in a university-based psychotherapy clinic with a series of vignettes describing the application of exposure techniques for different anxiety problems. Some techniques (e.g., interoceptive exposure for panic attacks, exposure and response prevention for OCD, imaginal exposure for PTSD) were perceived as unlikely to be helpful, unacceptable, and even unethical. Others, such as virtual reality exposure therapy for fears of flying and gradual *in vivo* exposure for social phobia, were viewed as more acceptable, helpful, and more ethical.

Despite the reservations of some practitioners, exposure therapy appears to be held in generally high esteem by patients. Compared to pharmacotherapy, anxiety patients perceive exposure-based CBT as more credible, acceptable, and likely to be effective in the long term (Deacon & Abramowitz, 2005; Norton, Allen, & Hilton, 1983). The same can be said of parents of clinically anxious children (Brown et al., 2007). Moreover, exposure therapy is rated as at least as acceptable, ethical, and effective as cognitive therapy and relationship-oriented psychotherapy by undergraduate students and agoraphobic patients (Norton et al., 1983). Among patients completing exposure-based CBT for panic disorder, situational and interoceptive exposure are perceived as highly useful despite lower ratings for likeability (Cox, Fergus, & Swinson, 1994). These findings suggest that therapist reservations about exposure therapy are not shared by most patients who receive this treatment. Why do therapists seem to overestimate the extent to which their patients will dislike exposure therapy? Richard and Gloster (2007) suggest that anxious patients might be less intimidated by the prospect of experiencing heightened anxiety during exposures because such symptoms are simply temporary exacerbations of familiar and long-standing emotional responses.

• *Therapists might get sued if they use exposure techniques.* Clinicians who believe exposure to be inhumane, intolerably aversive, or potentially dangerous may also worry about the legal risks associated with the use of these techniques. They might think it is unwise to leave the office to conduct exposures or have concern about the types of exposure tasks patients are asked to complete. Such reservations are typically based on a misunderstanding of exposure, its efficacy, tolerability, and the manner in which it is ethically and competently conducted. It might also be useful to consider that exposure merely provokes anxiety, which is no different than what patients are already experiencing, and part of the body's natural defense mechanism (i.e., the *fight-or-flight* response). In other words, anxiety is not inherently dangerous to the vast majority of people (and those who might be harmed from provoking physiological arousal are not candidates for exposure) and is therefore generally safe. As such, it poses little legal risk for practicing clinicians.

Richard and Gloster (2007) searched the legal record for court cases involving exposure therapy. Their exhaustive search criteria did not reveal a single instance of litigation related to this treatment. Similarly, none of the 84 members of the Anxiety Disorders Association of America surveyed by Richard and Gloster reported knowledge of any legal action or ethics complaints regarding exposure. This survey approach, however, cannot rule out the possibility that relevant complaints have been filed, but dismissed or settled out of court. Yet the available evidence suggests that exposure therapy is acceptably safe and tolerable, and that it carries little risk of actively harming patients or their therapists.

STRATEGIES FOR MINIMIZING RISK

Ethical principles dictate that psychologists and therapists avoid harming their patients. The admonition against harming patients appears twice in the American Psychological Association's (2002) ethics code, both as a general principle (Principle A: Beneficence and Nonmaleficence; psychologists "take care to do no harm" and "safeguard the welfare and rights" of their patients) and as an ethical standard in human relations (section 3.04; "Psychologists take reasonable steps to avoid harming their patients/clients" and "minimize harm where it is foreseeable and unavoidable"). Does exposure submit patients to an unacceptably high risk of being harmed?

We have previously described research suggesting that exposure does not lead to negative outcomes such as excessive drop-out rates or symptom exacerbation. However, exposure therapy does have the potential to place patients at greater risk of harm in other ways than many traditional forms of verbal psychotherapy. For example, exposure can involve the remote but real potential for physical harm when patients handle snakes, receive injections, or touch "contaminated" objects such as garbage cans. Although these exercises involve acceptably low levels of risk when conducted properly, exposure therapists must carefully consider the patient's safety when designing and implementing exposure practices.

Negotiating Informed Consent

Consistent with the ethical imperative to obtain informed consent in psychotherapy (e.g., American Psychological Association, 2002), exposure therapists must obtain patient consent as soon as possible in treatment. Exposure may be somewhat unique among psychological treatment techniques in that its very nature necessitates constant and inherent vigilance to the process of informed consent. Therapists must explain each new exposure practice to the patient, and the patient must agree to proceed before a given task is begun. Informed consent is thus an ongoing process and patients may, and often do, negotiate or even revoke their consent during treatment sessions. Informed consent for a particular exposure task may be discussed several times each session; for example, consent for a situational exposure involving conversing with others in a shopping mall may be negotiated both in the office while planning the exposure and subsequently in the mall prior to initiating conversations. To increase the likelihood of patient adherence to anxiety-provoking procedures, exposure therapists often place great emphasis on conveying a clear rationale for exposure and a detailed explanation of its requirements. Interestingly, because of the unique demands it places on patients and therapists, exposure therapy is likely an exemplar among psychotherapies for satisfying the ethical principle of informed consent.

Determining Acceptable Risk during Exposure Tasks

The probability of patients being harmed in exposure therapy can be reduced by understanding how to determine when a given exposure task entails an unacceptably high level of risk. In certain cases, tasks might be clearly contraindicated, such as intensive hyperventilation for a patient with severe asthma, walking through a dangerous area of town after dark for an assault survivor, and touching bathroom floors for a patient whose immune system is compromised. In the absence of clear-cut risks of harm, we suggest asking the following question to evaluate whether the risk associated with an exposure is acceptable: *Do at least some people ordinarily confront the situation/stimulus in the course of everyday life without adverse consequences?* The heart-healthy patient with panic disorder who fears cardiac arrest may express concern about the safety of briskly walking up and down a stairway for 30 minutes. However, a trip to the local gym reveals many individuals who engage in this level of vigorous exercise without incident. Someone who has been violently mugged might rebuff the suggestion that she return to using public transportation, yet thousands of other city-dwellers use such conveniences on a regular basis.

Regarding contamination-related OCD, many people suffer no ill effects from the routine touching of door handles and trash cans without washing their hands. Some people even occasionally skip showers, refrain from hand washing after using restrooms, and eat finger foods after petting the dog. Outdoor enthusiasts routinely have close encounters with snakes and spiders without incident, and most everyone has at some point been stuck outside in a thunderstorm without being struck by lightning. An exposure task may be considered to involve acceptable risk if the patient is not at significantly higher risk of experiencing harm than other individuals who engage in the same activity in the course of everyday life largely without incident.

Time Management during Therapy Sessions

Patients whose high anxiety fails to habituate within the allotted session time during exposure therapy may experience demoralization and express doubts about their ability to benefit from the treatment. To prevent such an occurrence, therapists should schedule longer sessions (e.g., 90–120 minutes) to account for individual variation in time to habituation. A recent patient whose anxiety took more than 3 hours to habituate while holding a spider illustrates that even 2-hour sessions may not allow sufficient time for all individuals to show habituation. Framing exposures as "behavioral experiments" designed to test specific anxious predictions may help patients view exposure tasks as useful, even if their anxiety does not habituate. In this context, the failure of habituation to occur may be viewed as a valuable learning experience, such as: "Anxiety is manageable even if it lasts a long time."

Managing Potentially Negative Outcomes

There is no absolute guarantee in exposure therapy, as with life in general, that unanticipated or unwanted outcomes will not occur. Dogs sometimes bite. Repeated spinning in a swivel chair may elicit vomiting. People may forget their lines during a speech. If an exposure task could conceivably result in an undesirable but reasonably harmless outcome, the therapist should consider framing it as a test of both the probability and the cost of the outcome. In this manner, the unintended occurrence of freezing up during a conversation, being negatively evaluated by strangers, or experiencing a panic attack can provide corrective information regarding the actual badness (or lack thereof) of the outcome. Of course, an exposure task should never be conducted if the therapist determines that it involves an unacceptably high probability of resulting in an objectively negative outcome (e.g., serious illness, assault, loss of a valued relationship).

Therapists cannot possibly anticipate all conceivable low-probability outcomes in any given situation. It is possible that exposure therapy could result in a claustrophobic patient being stuck in a cramped elevator for days, a driving phobic suffering a fatal car accident, or a flying phobic boarding a plane that subsequently crashes. As in real life, there is no absolute guarantee of safety in any exposure task. However, the remote possibility of catastrophe should no more preclude a driving exposure than it should prevent the therapist from driving to work.

Therapist Competency

In addition to the strategies described above, risks can be effectively minimized during exposure therapy by ensuring that exposure therapists are adequately trained (or supervised) and deliver this treatment in a competent manner. Although exposure therapy may seem deceptively straightforward to administer, research indicates that optimal delivery of this treatment requires careful consideration of contexts and other factors that can influence the effectiveness of exposure-based treatment (Powers et al., 2007). For example, the mere availability of safety aids during exposure can be highly detrimental to treatment outcome, even if the safety aids are not used (Powers et al., 2004). Therapists interested in using exposure techniques should be adequately trained or supervised by a competent exposure therapist. Castro and Marx (2007) noted that part of protecting client welfare means ensuring that the therapist is both intellectually and emotionally ready to provide adequate and appropriate treatment for each client: "Exposure therapy is not only difficult for the client, it is challenging and strenuous for the therapist. In fact it is not uncommon for the strong emotional responses of the client during exposure therapy to evoke secondary distress in the therapist" (pp. 164–165). This observation indicates that, in addition to skill in implementing exposure methods, competency to conduct exposure therapy requires that therapists have the ability to tolerate the often intense emotional responses of their patients.

Therapist Self-Care

Exposure therapy may pose a risk to the therapist in the form of psychological distress. Such distress is especially likely when conducting imaginal exposure for PTSD, during which the therapist may listen to painfully detailed accounts of truly horrifying trauma narratives. Successfully navigating this demanding work requires exposure therapists to strike a balance between empathy for their patients' pain and maintaining professional distance that allows for therapeutic, professional responses (Foa & Rothbaum, 1998). This balance is difficult to maintain in some instances, and we have each felt a lump in our throat or fought back tears after hearing our patients recount particularly terrible experiences. However, even the most compassionate therapist must remember that it is his or her job to assist the patient in recovery from clinical anxiety, and losing emotional control is incompatible with this goal. Indeed, patients may draw strength from the therapist's outward expressions of confidence in their ability to tolerate the distress associated with particularly difficult exposures. An important part of one's development as an exposure therapist involves learning to cope with and accept the emotional distress patients exhibit during particularly challenging exposures. From time to time, unburdening oneself by talking to colleagues, or seeking distraction in the form of other professional or personal activities, is necessary to cope with the unique demands of exposure therapy.

MAINTAINING ETHICAL BOUNDARIES

As described above, some therapists believe that exposure is unethical based on concerns about its aversiveness and presumed capacity to harm patients. However, negative beliefs about the ethics of exposure may also reflect therapists' concerns about this treatment's potential to create problematic boundary violations and dual relationships. For clinicians whose preferred brand of psychotherapy emphasizes therapist neutrality, passivity, and non-directiveness, exposure may involve an uncomfortably high level of active engagement with the patient. The idea that such engagement might occur in the context of distinctly unconventional therapeutic activities, such as spinning in a swivel chair or touching objects in public restrooms, likely contributes an additional measure of discomfort. In addition, the practice of leaving the office to conduct exposures may be troubling for therapists who fear that doing so will fundamentally alter the professional nature of the therapeutic relationship. Below we review these issues in the context of ethical principles regarding boundaries and discuss strategies for conducting exposure therapy in an optimally ethical manner.

A *boundary crossing* in psychotherapy refers to a deviation from the typical practice of traditional, strict forms of therapy (Zur, 2005). Therapists have traditionally been encouraged to maintain strict boundaries in order to create a therapeutic context that is in the patient's best interest. Examples of boundaries include time, place, touch, self-disclosure, gifts, and money (Barnett, Lazarus, Vasquez, Moorehead-Slaughter, & Johnson, 2007). Among these, the practice of violating the "only in the office" boundary is particularly relevant to exposure therapy. Traditionally, psychotherapy has been conducted without the need to leave the office. Exposure therapy, however, sometimes requires that therapists leave the office with their patients to conduct exposures to feared stimuli that cannot easily be brought into in the office. As a result, exposure therapy for many patients involves at least occasional boundary crossings.

Boundary crossings in the form of out-of-the-office exposures carry the possibility of eroding the strict boundaries inherent in traditional notions of the therapist–patient relationship. Indeed, the conduct of exposure therapy outside the office walls may increase the probability of less formal interactions, some of which may not be strictly therapeutic. Interactions with patients outside the office have traditionally been considered unadvisable as they are seen as laying the groundwork for dual relationships, including sexual relationships with patients (Barnett et al., 2007). From this viewpoint, exposure field trips may be viewed as a step down a "slippery slope" that may lead to increasingly inappropriate behaviors and ultimately exploitative sexual encounters or other dual relationships. To discourage clinicians from traveling down this slippery slope, the "only in the office" rule has been proposed to ensure that clinicians provide treatment that is in the best interests of their patients (Smith & Fitzpatrick, 1995).

Within the context of traditional forms of psychotherapy, the "only in the office" boundary is a logical prescription. However, rigid adherence to this traditional notion of boundaries would severely restrict therapists' ability to practice exposure therapy in an effective manner with many patients. Accordingly, temporarily crossing boundaries for therapeutic purposes is not necessarily unethical or harmful (Lazarus, 1998). Indeed, the failure to do so may be considered unethical, or at the very least suboptimal, in the exposure-based treatment of some patients with anxiety disorders. Thus, boundary *crossings* do not necessarily lead to boundary *violations*; neither do boundary crossings necessarily place the clinician on a "slippery slope" (e.g., Zur, 2001, 2007).

Crossing some boundaries may be clinically appropriate and even necessary when conducting exposure therapy. Exposure is optimally effective when it is conducted in a therapist-assisted manner (Abramowitz, 1996) and when it occurs in a variety of contexts (Powers et al., 2007). For some patients, exposure outside the office is necessary to ensure that safety learning is not conditional on the presence of specific contexts (e.g., "Heart palpitations aren't dangerous *as long as I experience them in the hospital where emergency medical attention is available*"). When clinically indicated, exposure therapists may cross additional boundaries associated with traditional therapies by extending the length of sessions beyond 1 hour, traveling to the patient's home, or involving strangers in the therapy (e.g., as audience members for a public speaking exposure). Such boundary crossings are not by themselves unethical, nor do they inevitably lead to an increasing series of inappropriate interactions with the patient that ultimately results in an exploitative sexual relationship.

The fact that boundary crossings are not necessarily unethical does not mean that they are always ethical. Likewise, the observation that boundary crossings do not necessarily continue down a slippery slope toward sexual exploitation does not mean that this never occurs. Boundary crossings should only occur when the therapist deems them necessary to assist the patient. If all therapeutic tasks can effectively be conducted inside the office, there is no need to conduct exposures elsewhere. Pope and Keith-Spiegel (2008) outlined a number of steps for practitioners to consider when contemplating a boundary crossing. The most relevant of these is for therapists to imagine the best possible outcome and the worst possible outcome from crossing the boundary and from *not* crossing the boundary. This cost–benefit analysis may be used to determine the overall therapeutic value of engaging in a given boundary crossing during exposure therapy.

CONCLUSIONS

An informed risk–benefit analysis suggests that exposure therapy is generally safe and effective, and should be considered a first-line treatment for anxiety disorders. However, relatively few therapists provide this treatment, and most individuals with anxiety disorders do not receive exposure-based treatment. In this chapter, we review a number of negative therapist beliefs about exposure that serve to impede efforts to make this treatment more widely available to patients. We also discuss strategies for minimizing the unique risks and ethical challenges associated with exposure therapy. We conclude that therapist beliefs about the intolerable and inhumane nature of exposure therapy, as well as its presumed capacity to harm patients and foster unethical therapist–patient interactions, are not supported by the scientific evidence or the clinical experience of adequately trained exposure therapists. In fact, we believe that given its well-established effectiveness, there may be ethical (and perhaps even legal) consequences for failing to consider exposure therapy in favor of less effective or unsubstantiated treatments. This is not to say that this treatment is risk-free; indeed, exposure may place patients at greater risk of temporary emotional discomfort than do other forms of psychological treatment. However, by being aware of this possibility and taking steps to manage it, exposure therapists can significantly decrease the risk of harm to their patients.

The unacceptably large disconnect between the empirically established effectiveness of exposure therapy, on the one hand, and the infrequency with which it used by treatment providers, on the other, is of great concern to us. It is exasperating to encounter patient after patient in our clinical practice who has been suffering for years with distressing anxiety symptoms and, despite having seen numerous mental health practitioners, has never received exposure therapy, or in many cases even been informed of its existence. It is our hope that the information provided in this chapter (and indeed, this book) will help to correct common therapist reservations about exposure and promote its use by fostering a more objective analysis of its risks and benefits.

References

Abramowitz, J. S. (1996). Variants of exposures and response prevention in the treatment of obsessive–compulsive disorder: A meta-analysis. *Behavior Therapy, 27,* 583–600.

Abramowitz, J. S. (1997). Effectiveness of psychological and pharmacological treatments for obsessive–compulsive disorder: A quantitative review of the controlled treatment literature. *Journal of Consulting and Clinical Psychology, 65,* 44–52.

Abramowitz, J. S. (2006). *Understanding and treating obsessive–compulsive disorder: A cognitive-behavioral approach.* Mahwah, NJ: Erlbaum.

Abramowitz, J. S., & Braddock, A. E. (2008). *Psychological treatment of health anxiety and hypochondriasis: A biopsychosocial approach.* Cambridge, MA: Hogrefe & Huber.

Abramowitz, J. S., & Deacon, B. J. (2005). Obsessive–compulsive disorder: Essential phenomenology and overlap with anxiety disorders. In J. S. Abramowitz & A. C. Houts (Eds.), *Concepts and controversies in obsessive–compulsive disorder* (pp. 119–135). New York: Springer.

Abramowitz, J. S., Foa, E. B., & Franklin, M. E. (2003). Exposure and ritual prevention for obsessive–compulsive disorder: Effects of intensive versus twice-weekly sessions. *Journal of Consulting and Clinical Psychology, 71,* 394–398.

Abramowitz, J. S., Franklin, M. E., Schwartz, S. A., & Furr, J. M. (2003). Symptom presentation and outcome of cognitive-behavioral therapy for obsessive–compulsive disorder. *Journal of Consulting and Clinical Psychology, 71,* 1049–1057.

Abramowitz, J. S., Franklin, M. E., Street, G. P., Kozak, M. J., & Foa, E. B. (2000). Effects of comorbid depression on response to treatment for obsessive–compulsive disorder. *Behavior Therapy, 31*(3), 517–528.

Abramowitz, J. S., Huppert, J. D., Cohen, A. B., Tolin, D. F., & Cahill, S. P. (2002). Religious obsessions and compulsions in a non-clinical sample: The Penn Inventory of Scrupulosity (PIOS). *Behaviour Research and Therapy, 40,* 825–838.

Abramowitz, J. S., & Moore, E. L. (2007). An experimental analysis of hypochondriasis. *Behaviour Research and Therapy, 45*, 413–424.

Abramowitz, J. S., & Piacentini, J. (2006). Clinical psychologists in departments of psychiatry: Current issues and a look to the future. *Clinical Psychology: Science and Practice, 13*, 282–286.

Abramowitz, J. S., Whiteside, S. P., & Deacon, B. J. (2005). The effectiveness of treatment for pediatric obsessive–compulsive disorder: A meta-analysis. *Behavior Therapy, 36*, 55–63.

American Psychiatric Association. (2000). *Diagnostic and statistical manual of mental disorders* (4th ed., text rev.). Washington, DC: Author.

American Psychological Association. (2002). *Ethical principles of psychologists and code of conduct.* Available at *www.apa.org/ethics*.

Antony, M. M., Brown, T. A., & Barlow, D. H. (1997). Heterogeneity among specific phobia types in *DSM-IV*. *Behaviour Research and Therapy, 35*, 1089–1100.

Antony, M. M., Orsillo, S. M., & Roemer, L. (Eds.). (2001). *Practitioner's guide to empirically based measures of anxiety.* New York: Kluwer.

Antony, M. M., & Swinson, R. P. (2000). *The shyness and social anxiety workbook: Proven techniques for overcoming your fears.* Oakland, CA: New Harbinger.

Antony, M. M., & Watling, M. A. (2006). *Overcoming medical phobias: How to conquer fear of blood, needles, doctors, and dentists.* Oakland, CA: New Harbinger Publications.

Arntz, A., Rauner, M., & van den Hout, M. (1995). If I feel anxious, there must be danger: *Ex-consequentia* reasoning in inferring danger in anxiety disorders. *Behaviour Research and Therapy, 33*, 917–925.

Baer, L. (1994). Factor analysis of symptom subtypes of obsessive compulsive disorder and their relation to personality and tic disorders. *Journal of Clinical Psychiatry, 55*, 18–23.

Bakker, A., van Balkom, A. J. L. M., Spinhoven, P., Blaauw, B. M. J. W., & van Dyck, R. (1998). Follow-up on the treatment of panic disorder with or without agoraphobia. *Journal of Nervous and Mental Disease, 186*, 414–419.

Bandura, A. (1988). Self-efficacy conception of anxiety. *Anxiety Research, 1*, 77–98.

Barkley, R. A. (1997). *Defiant children: A clinician's manual for assessment and parent training* (2nd ed.). New York: Guilford Press.

Barlow, D. H. (2002). *Anxiety and its disorders: The nature and treatment of anxiety and panic* (2nd ed.). New York: Guilford Press.

Barlow, D. H., & Craske, M. G. (2007). *Mastery of your anxiety and panic* (4th ed.). New York: Oxford University Press.

Barlow, D. H., Craske, M. G., Cerny, J. A., & Klosko, J. S. (1989). Behavioral treatment of panic disorder. *Behavior Therapy, 20*, 261–282.

Barlow, D. H., Gorman, J. M., Shear, M. K., & Woods, S. W. (2000). Cognitive-behavioral therapy, imipramine, or their combination for panic disorder: A randomized controlled trial. *Journal of the American Medical Association, 283*, 2529–2536.

Barnett, J. E., Lazarus, A. A., Vasquez, M., Moorehead-Slaughter, O., & Johnson, W. B. (2007). Boundary issues and multiple relationships: Fantasy and reality. *Professional Psychology: Research and Practice, 38*, 401–410.

Barrett, P. M., Dadds, M. R., & Rapee, R. M. (1996). Family treatment of childhood anxiety: A controlled trial. *Journal of Consulting and Clinical Psychology, 64*(2), 333–342.

Barrett, P. M., Healy-Farrell, L., & March, J. S. (2004). Cognitive-behavioral family treatment of childhood obsessive–compulsive disorder: A controlled trial. *Journal of the American Academy of Child and Adolescent Psychiatry, 43*(1), 46–62.

Basoglu, M., Marks, I. M., Kilic, C., Brewin, C. R., & Swinson, R. P. (1994). Alprazolam and exposure for panic disorder with agoraphobia: Attribution of improvement to medication predicts subsequent relapse. *British Journal of Psychiatry, 164*(5), 652–659.

Baucom, D. H., Stanton, S., & Epstein, N. B. (2003). Anxiety disorders. In D. K. Snyder & M. A. Whisman (Eds.), *Treating difficult couples: Helping clients with coexisting mental and relationship disorders* (pp. 57–87). New York: Guilford Press.

Baxter, L. R., Schwartz, J. M., Bergman, K., Szuba, M., Guze, B., Mazziotta, J., et al. (1992). Caudate glucose metabolic rate changes with both drug and behavior therapy for obsessive–compulsive disorder. *Archives of General Psychiatry, 49,* 681–689.

Beck, A. T., Emery, G., & Greenberg, R. L. (1985). *Anxiety disorders and phobias.* New York: Basic Books.

Beck, A. T., Sokol, L., Clark, D. A., Berchick, R., & Wright, F. (1992). A crossover study of focused cognitive therapy for panic disorder. *American Journal of Psychiatry, 149,* 778–783.

Becker, C., Zayfert, C., & Anderson, E. (2004). A survey of psychologists' attitudes toward utilization of exposure therapy for PTSD. *Behaviour Research and Therapy, 42,* 277–292.

Beidel, D. C., Turner, S. M., & Morris, T. L. (2000). Behavioral treatment of childhood social phobia. *Journal of Consulting and Clinical Psychology, 68*(6), 1072–1080.

Berman, N. C., Abramowitz, J. S., Pardue, C., & Wheaton, M. G. (2010). The relationship between religion and thought-action fusion: Use of an in vivo paradigm. *Behaviour Research and Therapy, 48,* 670–674.

Beutler, L. E. (2004). The empirically supported treatments movement: A scientist-practitioner's response. *Clinical Psychology: Science and Practice, 11,* 225–229.

Biondi, M., & Picardi, A. (2003). Increased probability of remaining in remission from panic disorder with agoraphobia after drug treatment in patients who received concurrent cognitive-behavioural therapy: A follow-up study. *Psychotherapy and Psychosomatics, 72,* 34–42.

Bjork, R. A., & Bjork, E. L. (1990). A new theory of disuse and an old theory of stimulus fluctuation. In A. Healy & R. Shiffrin (Eds.), *From learning processes to cognitive processes: Essays in honor of William K. Estes* (Vol. 2, pp. 35–67). Hillsdale, NJ: Erlbaum.

Blake, D. D., Weathers, F. W., Nagy, L. M., Kaloupek, D. G., Gusman, F. D., Charney, D. S., et al. (1995). The development of a clinician-administered PTSD scale. *Journal of Traumatic Stress, 8,* 75–90.

Blomhoff, S., Haug, T. T., Hellstrom, K., Holme, I., Humble, M., & Wold, J. E.

(2001). Randomised controlled general practice trial of sertraline, exposure therapy and combined treatment in generalized social phobia. *British Journal of Psychiatry, 179*, 23–30.

Borkovec, T. D., Abel, J. L., & Newman, H. (1995). Effects of psychotherapy on comorbid conditions in generalized anxiety disorder. *Journal of Consulting and Clinical Psychology, 63*(3), 479–483.

Borkovec, T. D., & Costello, E. (1993). Efficacy of applied relaxation and cognitive behavioral therapy in the treatment of generalized anxiety disorder. *Journal of Consulting and Clinical Psychology, 61*, 611–619.

Borkovec, T. D., & Roemer, L. (1995). Perceived functions of worry among generalized anxiety disorder subjects: Distraction from more emotional topics? *Journal of Behavior Therapy and Experimental Psychiatry, 26*, 25–30.

Borkovec, T. D., & Whisman, M. A. (1996). Psychosocial treatment for generalized anxiety disorder. In M. Mavissakalian & Prien (Eds.), *Long-term treatment of anxiety disorders* (pp. 171–199). Washington, DC: American Psychiatric Association.

Bouchard, S., Mendlowitz, S. L., Coles, M. E., & Franklin, M. (2004). Considerations in the use of exposure with children. *Cognitive and Behavioral Practice, 11*(1), 56–65.

Bouton, M. E. (2002). Context, ambiguity, and unlearning: Sources of relapse after behavioral extinction. *Biological Psychiatry, 52*, 976–986.

Brown, A., Deacon, B. J., Abramowitz, J. S., & Whiteside, S. P. (2007). Parents' perceptions of pharmacological and cognitive-behavioral treatments for childhood anxiety disorders. *Behaviour Research and Therapy, 45*, 819–828.

Brown, D. (1996). *Flying without fear*. Oakland, CA: New Harbinger.

Burns, D. (1980). *Feeling good: The new mood therapy*. New York: Morrow.

Byrne, M., Carr, A., & Clark, M. (2004). The efficacy of couples-based interventions for panic disorder with agoraphobia. *Journal of Family Therapy, 26*, 105–125.

Calhoun, K. S., & Resick, P. (1993). Posttraumatic stress disorder. In D. H. Barlow (Ed.), *Clinical handbook of psychological disorders: A step-by-step treatment manual* (2nd ed., pp. 48–98). New York: Guilford Press.

Calvocoressi, L., Mazure, C. M., Kasl, S. V., Skolnick, J., Fisk, D., Vegso, S. J., et al. (1999). Family accommodation of obsessive–compulsive symptoms: Instrument development and assessment of family behavior. *Journal of Nervous and Mental Disease, 187*, 636–642.

Cardaciotto, L., & Herbert, J. D. (2004). Cognitive behavior therapy for social anxiety disorder in the context of Asperger's syndrome: A single-subject report. *Cognitive and Behavioral Practice, 11*(1), 75–81.

Cartwright-Hatton, S., Roberts, C., Chitsabesan, P., Fothergill, C., & Harrington, R. (2004). Systematic review of the efficacy of cognitive behaviour therapies for childhood and adolescent anxiety disorder. *British Journal of Clinical Psychology, 43*, 421–436.

Castro, F., & Marx, B. P. (2007). Exposure therapy with adult survivors of childhood sexual assault. In D. C. S. Richard & D. Lauterbach (Eds.), *Comprehensive handbook of the exposure therapies* (pp. 153–167). New York: Academic Press.

Caughlin, J. P., Huston, T. L., & Houts, R. M. (2000). How does personality matter in marriage?: An examination of trait anxiety, interpersonal negativity, and marital satisfaction. *Journal of Personality and Social Psychology*, 78(2), 326–336.

Chambless, D. L. (1990). Spacing of sessions in the treatment of agoraphobia and simple phobia. *Behavior Therapy*, 21, 217–229.

Chambless, D. L., Baker, M. J., Baucom, D. H., Beutler, L. E., Calhoun, K. S., Crits-Cristoph, P., et al. (1998). Update on empirically validated therapies, II. *The Clinical Psychologist*, 51, 3–16.

Chambless, D. L., & Gillis, M. M. (1993). Cognitive therapy of anxiety disorders. *Journal of Consulting and Clinical Psychology*, 61, 248–260.

Chambless, D. L., & Ollendick, T. H. (2001). Empirically supported psychological interventions: Controversies and evidence. *Annual Review of Psychology*, 52, 685–716.

Chambless, D. L., & Steketee, G. (1999). Expressed emotion and behavior therapy outcome: A prospective study with obsessive–compulsive and agoraphobic outpatients. *Journal of Consulting and Clinical Psychology*, 67(5), 658–665.

Ciarrocchi, J. W. (1995). *The doubting disease: Help for scrupulosity and religious compulsions*. Mahwah, NJ: Paulist Press.

Clark, D. M. (1986). A cognitive approach to panic. *Behaviour Research and Therapy*, 24, 461–470.

Clark, D. M. (1999). Anxiety disorders: Why they persist and how to treat them. *Behavior Research and Therapy*, 37, S5–S27.

Clark, D. M., Salkovskis, P. M., Hackmann, A., Middleton, H., Anastasiades, P., & Gelder, M. (1994). A comparison of cognitive therapy, applied relaxation and impiramine in the treatment of panic disorder. *British Journal of Psychiatry*, 164, 759–769.

Clark, D. M., & Wells, A. (1995). A cognitive model of social phobia. In R. G. Heimberg, M. R. Liebowitz, D. A. Hope, & F. R. Schneier (Eds.), *Social phobia: Diagnosis, assessment, and treatment* (pp. 69–94). New York: Guilford Press.

Clum, G. A., Clum, G. A., & Surls, R. (1993). A meta-analysis of treatments for panic disorder. *Journal of Consulting and Clinical Psychology*, 61, 317–326.

Cohen, J. (1977). *Statistical power analysis for the behavioral sciences* (rev. ed.). New York: Academic Press.

Costello, E. J., Mustillo, S., Erkanli, A., Keeler, G., & Angold, A. (2003). Prevalence and development of psychiatric disorders in childhood and adolescence. [see comment]. *Archives of General Psychiatry*, 60(8), 837–844.

Cottraux , J., Mollard, E., Bouvard, M., Marks, I., Sluys, M., Nury, A. M., et al. (1990). Controlled study of fluvoxamine and exposure in obsessive–compulsive disorder. *International Clinical Psychopharmacology*, 5, 17–30.

Cowley, D. S. (1992). Alcohol abuse, substance abuse, and panic disorder. *American Journal of Medicine*, 92(1A), 41S–48S.

Cox, B. J., Fergus, K. D., & Swinson, R. P. (1994). Patient satisfaction with behavioral treatments for panic disorder with agoraphobia. *Journal of Anxiety Disorders*, 8, 193–206.

Craske, M. G., Burton, T., & Barlow, D. H. (1989). Relationships among measures of communication, marital satisfaction and exposure during couples treatment of agoraphobia. *Behaviour Research and Therapy, 27*(2), 131–140.

Curtis, G. C., Magee, W. J., Eaton, W. W., Wittchen, H. U., & Kessler, R. C. (1998). Specific fears and phobias: Epidemiology and classification. *British Journal of Psychiatry, 173*, 212–217.

Davey, G., Tallis, F., & Capuzzo, N. (1996). Beliefs about the consequences of worrying. *Cognitive Therapy and Research, 20*, 499–520.

Davidson, J. R., Foa, E. B., Huppert, J. D., Keefe, F. J., Franklin, M. E., Compton, J. S., et al. (2004). Fluoxetine, comprehensive cognitive behavioral therapy, and placebo in generalized social phobia. *Archives of General Psychiatry, 61*, 1005–1013.

Davidson, P. R., & Parker, K. C. H. (2001). Eye movement desensitization and reprocessing (EMDR): A meta-analylsis. *Journal of Consulting and Clinical Psychology, 69*, 305–316.

Davis, T. E., III, & Ollendick, T. H. (2005). Empirically supported treatments for specific phobia in children: Do efficacious treatments address the components of a phobic response? *Clinical Psychology: Science and Practice, 12*(2), 144–160.

Dawes, R. (1986). Representative thinking in clinical judgement. *Clinical Psychology Review, 6*, 425–441.

Deacon, B. J. (2007a). The effect of pharmacotherapy on the effectiveness of exposure therapy. In D. C. S. Richard & D. Lauterbach (Eds.), *Comprehensive handbook of the exposure therapies* (pp. 311–333). New York: Academic Press.

Deacon, B. J. (2007b). Two-day, intensive cognitive-behavioral therapy for panic disorder: A case study. *Behavior Modification, 31*, 595–615.

Deacon, B. J., & Abramowitz, J. S. (2005). Patients' perceptions of pharmacological and cognitive-behavioral treatments for anxiety disorders. *Behavior Therapy, 36*, 139–145.

Deacon, B. J., & Abramowitz, J. S. (2006a). A pilot study of two-day cognitive-behavioral treatment for panic disorder. *Behaviour Research and Therapy, 44*, 807–817.

Deacon, B. J., & Abramowitz, J. S. (2006b). Anxiety sensitivity and its dimensions across the anxiety disorders. *Journal of Anxiety Disorders, 20*, 837–857.

Deacon, B. J., & Abramowitz, J. S. (2006c). Fear of needles and vasovagal reactions among phlebotomy patients. *Journal of Anxiety Disorders, 20*, 946–960.

Deacon, B. J., & Abramowitz, J. S. (2008). Is hypochondriasis related to OCD, panic disorder, or both?: An empirical evaluation. *Journal of Cognitive Psychotherapy, 22*, 115–127.

Deacon, B. J., & Lickel, J. J. (2009). On the brain disease model of mental disorders. *The Behavior Therapist, 32*, 113–118.

de Beurs, E., van balkom, A. J. L. M., Lange, A., Koele, P., & van Dyck, R. (1995). Treatment of panic disorder with agoraphobia: Comparison of fluvoxamine, placebo, and psychological panic management combined with exposure and of exposure in vivo alone. *American Journal of Psychiatry, 152*, 683–691.

Dimopoulos, V., Robinson, J., & Fountas, K. (2008). The pearls and pitfalls of skull trephination as described in the Hippocratic treatise "On head wounds." *Journal of the History of the Neurosciences, 17*, 131–140.

Di Nardo, P. A., Guzy, L. T., & Bak, R. M. (1988). Anxiety response patterns and etiological factors in dog-fearful and non-fearful subjects. *Behaviour Research and Therapy, 21*, 245–252.

Doogan, S., & Thomas, G. (1992). Origins of fear of dogs in adults and children: The role of conditioning processes and prior familiarity with dogs. *Behaviour Research and Therapy, 30*, 387–394.

Dugas, M. J., Buhr, K., & Ladouceur, R. (2004). The role of intolerance of uncertainty in etiology and maintenance. In R. G. Heimberg, C. L. Turk, & D. S. Mennin (Eds.), *Generalized anxiety disorder: Advances in research and practice* (pp. 143–163). New York: Guilford Press.

Ehlers, A., & Clark, D. M. (2000). A cognitive model of posttraumatic stress disorder. *Behaviour Research and Therapy, 38*, 319–345.

Eifert, G. H., & Forsyth, J. P. (2005). *Acceptance and commitment therapy for anxiety disorders: A practitioner's treatment guide to using mindfulness, acceptance, and values-based behavior change strategies.* Oakland, CA: New Harbinger Publications.

Emmelkamp, P. M., de Haan, E., & Hoogduin, C. A. (1990). Marital adjustment and obsessive–compulsive disorder. *British Journal of Psychiatry, 156*, 55–60.

Emmelkamp, P. M. G., & Kraanen, J. (1977). Therapist-controlled exposure *in vivo* versus self-controlled exposure *in vivo*: A comparison with obsessive–compulsive patients. *Behaviour Research and Therapy, 15*, 491–195.

Fedoroff, I. C., & Taylor, S. (2001). Psychological and pharmacological treatments of social phobia: A meta analysis. *Journal of Clinical Psychopharmacology, 21*, 311–324.

Feeney, N., Hembree, E., & Zoellner, L. (2003). Myths regarding exposure therapy for PTSD. *Cognitive and Behavioral Practice, 10*, 85–90.

Feske, U., & Chambless, D. L. (1995). Cognitive behavioral versus exposure only treatment for social phobia: A meta-analysis. *Behavior Therapy, 26*, 695–720.

Foa, E. B., Franklin, M. E., & Moser, J. (2002). Context in the clinic: How well do cognitive-behavioral therapies and medications work in combination? *Biological Psychiatry, 10*, 987–997.

Foa, E. B., Hembree, E., & Rothbaum, B. O. (2007). *Prolonged exposure therapy for PTSD: Emotional processing of traumatic experiences.* New York: Oxford University Press.

Foa, E. B., & Kozak, M. J. (1986). Emotional processing of fear: Exposure to corrective information. *Psychological Bulletin, 99*, 20–35.

Foa, E. B., & Kozak, M. J. (1995). DSM-IV field trial: Obsessive–compulsive disorder. *American Journal of Psychiatry, 152*, 90–96.

Foa, E. B., Liebowitz, M. R., Kozak, M. J., Davies, S., Campeas, R., Franklin, M. E., et al. (2005). Randomized, placebo-controlled trial of exposure and ritual prevention, clomipramine, and their combination in the treatment of obsessive–compulsive disorder. *American Journal of Psychiatry, 162*, 151–161.

Foa, E. B., & Riggs, S. S. (1993). Posttraumatic stress disorder in rape victims. In J. Oldham, M. B. Riba, & A. Tasman (Eds.), *Americam Psychiatric Press review of psychiatry* (Vol. 12, pp. 273–303). Washington, DC: American Psychiatric Press.

Foa, E. B., & Rothbaum, B. O. (1998). Treating the trauma of rape: Cognitive behavioral therapy for PTSD. New York: Guilford Press.

Foa, E. B., Steketee, G., & Milby, J. B. (1980). Differential effects of exposure and response prevention in obsessive–compulsive washers. *Journal of Consulting and Clinical Psychology, 48,* 71–79.

Foa, E. B., Steketee, G. S., & Rothbaum, B. O. (1989). Cognitive-behavioral conceptualizations of post-traumatic stress disorder. *Behavior Therapy, 20,* 155–176.

Foa, E. B., Zoellner, L. A., Feeny, N. C., Hembree, E. A., & Alvarez-Conrad, J. (2002). Does imaginal exposure exacerbate PTSD symptoms? *Journal of Consulting and Clinical Psychology, 70,* 1022–1028.

Foy, D. W., Kagan, B., McDermott, C., Leskin, G., Sipprelle, R. C., & Paz, G. (1996). Practical parameters in the use of flooding for treating chronic PTSD. *Clinical Psychology and Psychotherapy, 3,* 169–175.

Frank, J. D. (1989). Therapeutic components shared by all psychotherapies. In J. H. Harvey & M. M. Parks (Eds.), *Psychotherapy research and behavior change, Master lecture series, Vol. 1.* (pp. 9–37). Washington, DC: American Psychological Association.

Franklin, M. E. (2005). Combining serotonin medication with cognitive-behavior therapy: Is it necessary for all OCD patients? In J. S. Abramowitz & A. C. Houts (Eds.), *Concepts and controversies in obsessive–compulsive disorder* (pp. 377–390). New York: Springer.

Franklin, M. E., Abramowitz, J. S., Bux, D. A., Zoellner, L. A., & Feeny, N. C. (2002). Cognitive-behavior therapy with and without medication in the treatment of obsessive–compulsive disorder. *Professional Psychology: Research and Practice, 33,* 162–168.

Freeston, M. H., Rheaume, J., Letarte, H., Dugas, M. J., & Ladouceur, R. (1994). Why do people worry? *Personality and Individual Differences, 17,* 791–802.

Freiheit, S. R., Vye, C., Swan, R., & Cady, M. (2004). Cognitive-behavioral therapy for anxiety: Is dissemination working? *The Behavior Therapist, 27,* 25–32.

Freud, S. (1949/1989). *An outline of psychoanalysis.* New York: Norton.

Friedman, L. M., Furberg, C. D., & DeMets, D. L. (1998). *Fundamentals of clinical trials.* New York: Springer.

Frueh, B., Turner, S., & Beidel, D. (1995). Exposure therapy for combat-related PTSD: A critical review. *Clinical Psychology Review, 15,* 799–817.

Furer, P., Walker, J. R., & Stein, M. B. (2007). *Treating health anxiety and the fear of death.* New York: Springer.

Ginsburg, G. S., Siqueland, L., Masia-Warner, C., & Heddtke, K. A. (2004). Anxiety disorders in children: Family matters. *Cogntive and Behavioral Practice, 11,* 28–43.

Goisman, R. M., Warshaw, M. G., & Keller, M. B.(1999). Psychosocial treatment prescriptions for generalized anxiety disorder, panic disorder, and social phobia, 1991–1996. *American Journal of Psychiatry, 156,* 1819–1821.

Goldfried, M. R. (1971). Systematic desensitization as training in self-control. *Journal of Consulting and Clinical Psychology, 37,* 228–234.

Gould, R. A., Buckminster, S., Pollack, M. H., Otto, M. W., & Yap, L. (1997). Cognitive-behavioral and pharmacological treatment for social phobia: A meta-analysis. *Clinical Psychology: Science and Practice, 4,* 291–306.

Gould, R. A., Otto, M. W., & Pollack, M. H. (1995). A meta-analysis of treatment outcome for panic disorder. *Clinical Psychology Review, 8,* 819–844.

Gould, R. A., Otto, M. W., Pollack, M. H., & Yap, L. (1997). Cognitive behavioral and pharmacological treatment of generalized anxiety disorder: A preliminary meta-analysis. *Behavior Therapy, 28,* 285–305.

Grant, B. F., Stinson, F. S., Dawson, D. A., Chou, S. P., Dufour, M. C., Compton, W., et al. (2004). Prevalence and co-occurrence of substance use disorders and independent mood and anxiety disorders: Results from the National Epidemiologic Survey on Alcohol and Related Conditions. *Archives of General Psychiatry, 61,* 807–816.

Grant, J. E., & Potenza, M. N. (2004). Impulse control disorders: Clinical characteristics and pharmacological management. *Annals of Clinical Psychiatry, 16,* 27–34.

Grayson, J. B., Foa, E. B., & Steketee, G. (1982). Habituation during exposure treatment: Distraction vs. attention-focusing. *Behaviour Research and Therapy, 20,* 323–328.

Hansen, B., Vogel, P. A., Stiles, T. C., & Gotestam, K. G. (2007). Influence of comorbid generalized anxiety disorder, panic disorder and personality disorders on the outcome of cognitive behavioural treatment of obsessive–compulsive disorder. *Cognitive Behaviour Therapy, 36,* 145–155.

Harvey, A., Watkins, E., Mansell, W., & Shafran, R. (2004). *Cognitive behavioural processes across the psychological disorders: A transdiagnostic approach to research and treatment.* New York: Oxford University Press.

Haug, T. T., Blomhoff, S., Hellstrom, K., Holme, I., Humble, M., Madsbu, H. P., et al. (2003). Exposure therapy and sertraline in social phobia: One-year follow-up of a randomised controlled trial. *British Journal of Psychiatry, 182,* 12–18.

Hegel, M. T., Ravaris, C. L., & Ahles, T. A. (1994). Combined cognitive-behavioral and time-limited alprazolam treatment of panic disorder. *Behavior Therapy, 25,* 183–195.

Heimberg, R. G., Dodge, C. S., Hope, D. A., Kennedy, C. R., Zollo, L. J., & Becker, R. E. (1990). Cognitive behavioral group treatment for social phobia: Comparison with a credible placebo control. *Cognitive Therapy and Research, 14,* 1–23.

Heimberg, R. G., Liebowitz, M. R., Hope, D. A., Schneier, F. R., Holt, C. S., Welkowitz, L. A., et al. (1998). Cognitive behavioral group therapy vs. phenelzine therapy for social phobia: 12-week outcome. *Archives of General Psychiatry, 55,* 1133–1141.

Hellstrom, K., Fellenius, J., & Ost, L.-G. (1996). One versus five sessions of applied tension in the treatment of blood phobia. *Behaviour Research and Therapy, 34,* 101–112.

Hembree, E. A., & Cahill, S. P. (2007). Obstacles to successful implementation of exposure therapy. In D. C. S. Richard & D. Lauterbach (Eds.), *Comprehensive handbook of the exposure therapies* (pp. 389–408). New York: Academic Press.

Hembree, E. A., Foa, E. B., Dorfan, N. M., Street, G. P., Kowalski, J., & Tu, X. (2003). Do patients dropout prematurely from exposure therapy for PTSD? *Journal of Traumatic Stress, 16,* 552–562.

Heuzenroeder, L., Donnelly, M., & Haby, M. (2004). Cost effectiveness of psychological and pharmacological interventions for general anxiety disorder and panic disorder. *Australian and New Zealand Journal of Psychiatry, 38,* 602–612.

Hicks, T. V., Leitenberg, H., Barlow, D. H., Gorman, J. M., Shear, M. K., & Woods, S. W. (2005). Physical, mental, and social catastrophic cognitions as prognostic factors in cognitive-behavioral and pharmacological treatments for panic disorder. *Journal of Consulting and Clinical Psychology, 73,* 506–514.

Hodgson, R., Rachman, S., & Marks, I. (1972). The treatment of chronic obsessive-compulsive neurosis: Follow-up and further findings. *Behaviour Research and Therapy, 10,* 181–189.

Hofmann, S. G., Barlow, D. H., Papp, L. A., Detweiler, M., Ray, S., Shear, M. K., et al. (1998). Pretreatment attrition in a comparative treatment outcome study on panic disorder. *American Journal of Psychiatry, 155,* 43–47.

Hofmann, S. G., & Otto, M. W. (2008). *Cognitive behavioral therapy for social anxiety disorder.* New York: Routledge.

Hogan, R. A. (1968). The implosive technique. *Behaviour Research and Therapy, 6,* 423—431.

Hohagen, F., Winkelmann, G., Rasche-Rauchle, H., Hand, I., Konig, A., Munchau, N., et al. (1998). Combination of behaviour therapy with fluvoxamine in comparison with behaviour therapy and placebo: Results of a multicentre study. *British Journal of Psychiatry, 173*(Suppl. 35), 71–78.

Houts, A. C. (2005). Behavioral and functional animal models of OCD. In J. S. Abramowitz & A. C. Houts (Eds.), *Concepts and controversies in obsessive-compulsive disorder* (pp. 73–86). New York: Springer.

Huppert, J. D., Franklin, M. E., Foa, E. B., & Davidson, J. R. T. (2003). Study refusal and exclusion from a randomized treatment study of generalized social phobia. *Journal of Anxiety Disorders, 17,* 683–693.

In-Albon, T., & Schneider, S. (2007). Psychotherapy of childhood anxiety disorders: A meta-analysis. *Psychotherapy and Psychosomatics, 76,* 15–24.

Jacobson, E. (1938). *Progressive relaxation.* Chicago: University of Chicago Press.

Jacobson, J. W., Mulick, J. A., & Schwartz, A. A. (1996). A history of facilitated communication: Science, Pseudoscience, and Antiscience Science Working Group on Facilitated Communication. *American Psychologist, 50,* 750–765.

James, A., Soler, A., & Weatherall, R. (2009). Cognitive behavioural therapy for anxiety disorders in children and adolescents. *Cochrane Database of Systematic Reviews, 4,* CD004690.

Johnstone, K. A., & Page, A. C. (2004). Attention to phobic stimuli during exposure: The effect of distraction on anxiety reduction, self-efficacy and perceived control. *Behaviour Research and Therapy, 42,* 249–275.

Jones, H., & Adleman, U. (1959). *Moral theology.* Westminster, MD: Newman Press.

Jones, M. C. (1924). A laboratory study of fear: The case of Peter. *Pedagogical Seminary, 31,* 308–315.

Kamphuis, J. H., & Telch, M. J. (1998). Assessment of strategies to manage or avoid perceived threats among panic disorder patients: The Texas Safety Maneuver Scale (TSMS). *Clinical Psychology and Psychotherapy, 5,* 177–186.

Katon, W. J., & Walker, E. A. (1998). Medically unexplained symptoms in primary care. *Journal of Clinical Psychiatry, 59,* 15–21.

Kazdin, A. E., & Weisz, J. R. (1998). Identifying and developing empirically supported child and adolescent treatments. *Journal of Consulting and Clinical Psychology, 66*(1), 19–36.

Kearney, C. A. (2006). Confirmatory factor analysis of the School Refusal Assessment Scale—Revised: Child and Parent Versions. *Journal of Psychopathology and Behavioral Assessment, 28*(3), 139–144.

Kendall, P. C. (2000). *Cognitive-behavioral therapy for anxious children: Therapist manual* (2nd ed.). Ardmore, PA: Workbook Publishing.

Kendall, P. C., Robin, J. A., Hedtke, K. A., Suveg, C., Flannery-Schroeder, E., & Gosch, E. (2005). Considering CBT with anxious youth?: Think exposures. *Cognitive and Behavioral Practice, 12*(1), 136–150.

Kessler, R. C. (1995). Epidemiology of psychiatric comorbidity. In M. T. Tsuang, M. Tohen, & G. E. Zahner (Eds.), *Textbook in psychiatric epidemiology* (pp. 179–198). New York: Wiley.

Krasner, L. (1971). Behavior therapy. In P. H. Mussen & M. R. Rosenzweig (Eds.), *Annual Review of Psychology: Vol. 22* (pp. 483–532). Palo Alto, CA: Annual Reviews, Inc.

Krasner, L., & Houts, A. C. (1984). A study of the "value" systems of behavioral scientists. *American Psychologist, 49*, 840–850.

Krystal, J. H., Deutsch, D. N., & Charney, D. S. (1996). The biological basis of panic disorder. *Journal of Clinical Psychiatry, 57*(Suppl. 6), 23–31.

Lander, J. A., Weltman, B. J., & So, S. S. (2006). EMLA and amethocaine for reduction of children's pain associated with needle insertion. *Cochrane Database of Systematic Reviews, 19*, CD004236.

Lazarus, A. A. (1994). How certain boundaries and ethics diminish therapeutic effectiveness. *Ethics and Behavior, 4*, 255–261.

Lazarus, A. A. (1998). How do you like these boundaries? *The Clinical Psychologist, 51*, 22–25.

Ledgerwood, L., Richardson, R., & Cranney, J. (2003). Effects of D-cycloserine on extinction of conditioned freezing. *Behavioral Neuroscience, 117*, 341–349.

Ledley, D. R., Huppert, J. D., Foa, E. B., Davidson, J. R. T., Keefe, F. J., & Potts, N. L. (2005). Impact of depressive symptoms on the treatment of generalized social anxiety disorder. *Depression and Anxiety, 22*, 161–167.

Leon, A. C., Portera, L., & Weissman, M. M. (1995). The social costs of anxiety disorders. *British Journal of Psychiatry, 166*(Suppl. 27), 19–22.

Levant, R. (2004). The empirically validated treatments movement: A practitioner's perspective. *Clinical Psychology: Science and Practice, 11*, 219–224.

Liebowitz, M. R. (1987). Social phobia. *Modern Problems in Pharmacopsychiatry, 22*, 141–173.

Liebowitz, M. R., Heimberg, R. G., Schneier, F. R., Hope, D. A., Davies, S., Holt, C. S., et al. (1999). Cognitive-behavioral group therapy versus phenelzine in social phobia: Long-term outcome. *Depression and Anxiety, 10*, 89–98.

Lilienfeld, S. (1996). EMDR treatment: Less than meets the eye. *The Skeptical Inquirer, 20*, 25–31.

Linehan, M. M. (1993). *Skills training manual for treating borderline personality disorder.* New York: Guilford Press.

Marcaurelle, R., Belanger, C., Marchand, A., Katerelos, T. E., & Mainguy, N. (2005). Marital predictors of symptom severity in panic disorder with agoraphobia. *Journal of Anxiety Disorders, 19*(2), 211–232.

March, J. S., & Mulle, K. M. (1998). *OCD in children and adolescents: A cognitive-behavioral treatment manual.* New York: Guilford Press.

Marks, I. (1988). Blood-injury phobia: A review. *American Journal of Psychiatry, 145,* 1207–1213.

Marks, I. M. (1973). New approaches to the treatment of obsessive–compulsive disorders. *Journal of Nervous and Mental Disease, 156,* 420–426.

Marks, I. M., Gray, S., Cohen, D., Hill, R., Mawson, D., Ramm, E., et al. (1983). Imipramine and brief therapist-aided exposure in agoraphobics having self-exposure homework. *Archives of General Psychiatry, 40,* 153–162.

Marks, I. M., Swinson, R. P., Basoglu, M., Noshirvani, H., O'Sullivan, G., Lelliott, P. T., et al. (1993). Alprazolam and exposure alone and combined in panic disorder with agoraphobia: A controlled study. *British Journal of Psychiatry, 162,* 776–787.

Matchett, G., & Davey, G. C. L. (1991). A test of a disease-avoidance model of animal phobia. *Behaviour Research and Therapy, 29,* 91–94.

Mavissakalian, M., Perel, J., & Guo, S. (2002). Specific side effects of long-term imipramine management of panic disorder. *Journal of Clinical Psychopharmacology, 22,* 155–261.

McCabe, R. E., Antony, M. M., Summerfeldt, L. J., Liss, A., & Swinson, R. P. (2003). Preliminary examination of the relationship between anxiety disorders in adults and self-reported history of teasing or bullying experiences. *Cognitive Behavior Therapy, 32,* 187–193.

McCarthy, L., & Shean, G. (1996). Agoraphobia and interpersonal relationships. *Journal of Anxiety Disorders, 10*(6), 477–487.

McGlynn, F., Smitherman, T., & Gothard, K. (2002). Comment on the status of systematic desensitization. *Behavior Modification, 28,* 194–205.

McKay, D. (1997). A maintenance program for obsessive–compulsive disorder using exposure with response prevention: 2-year follow-up. *Behaviour Research and Therapy, 35,* 367–369.

McKay, D., Abramowitz, J. S., & Taylor, S. (Eds.). (2009). *Cognitive-behavioral therapy for refractory cases: Turning failure into success.* Washington, DC: American Psychological Association Press.

McKay, D., Todaro, J. F., Neziroglu, F., & Yaryura-Tobias, J. A. (1996). Evaluation of a naturalistic maintenance program in the treatment of obsessive–compulsive disorder: A preliminary investigation. *Journal of Anxiety Disorders, 10,* 211–217.

McLean, P. D., Whittal, M. L., Thordarson, D. S., Taylor, S., Söchting, I., Koch, W. J., et al. (2001). Cognitive versus behavior therapy in the group treatment of obsessive–compulsive disorder. *Journal of Consulting and Clinical Psychology, 69,* 205–214.

McNally, R. J., & Steketee, G. (1985). The etiology and maintenance of severe animal phobias. *Behaviour Research and Therapy, 23,* 431–435.

Meehl, P. E., (1996). *Clinical versus statistical prediction: A theoretical analysis and a review of the evidence.* Lanham, MD: Aronson. (Originally published 1954)

Mehta, M. (1990). A comparative study of family-based and patient-based behavioural management in obsessive–compulsive disorder. *British Journal of Psychiatry*, *157*, 133–135.

Meit, S. S., Yasek, V., Shannon, K., Hickman, D., & Williams, D. (2004). Techniques for reducing anesthetic injection pain: An interdisciplinary survey of knowledge and application. *Journal of the American Dental Association*, *135*, 1243–12530.

Mendlowitz, S. L., Manassis, K., Bradley, S., Scapillato, D., Miezitis, S., & Shaw, B. F. (1999). Cognitive-behavioral group treatments in childhood anxiety disorders: The role of parental involvement. *Journal of the American Academy of Child and Adolescent Psychiatry*, *38*(10), 1223–1229.

Merikangas, K. R., Zhang, H., Avenevoli, S., Acharyya, S., Neuenschwander, M., & Angst, J. (2003). Longitudinal trajectories of depression and anxiety in a prospective community study: The Zurich cohort study. *Archives of General Psychiatry*, *60*, 993–1000.

Merlo, L. J., Lehmkuhl, H., Geffken, G. R., & Storch, E. A. (2009). Decreased family accommodation associated with improved therapy outcome in pediatric obsessive–compulsive disorder. *Journal of Consulting and Clinical Psychology*, *77*, 355–360.

Meyer, V. (1966). Modifications of expectations in case of obsessional rituals. *Behaviour Research and Therapy*, *4*, 273–280.

Michelson, L., Mavissakalian, M., & Marchione, K. (1985). Cognitive-behavioral treatments of agoraphobia: Clinical, behavioral, and psychophysiological outcome. *Journal of Consulting and Clinical Psychology*, *53*, 913–925.

Miller, W. R., & Rollnick, S. (2002). *Motivational interviewing: Preparing people for change*. New York: Guilford Press.

Mineka, S., & Zinbarg, R. (2006). A contemporary learning theory perspective on the etiology of anxiety disorders: It's not what you thought it was. *American Psychologist*, *61*, 10–26.

Mitte, K. (2005). Meta-analysis of cognitive-behavioral treatments for generalized anxiety disorder: A comparison with pharmacotherapy. *Psychological Bulletin*, *131*, 785–795.

Monson, C. M., Guthire, K. A., & Stevens, S. (2003). Cognitive-behavioral couple's treatment for posttraumatic stress disorder. *The Behavior Therapist*, *26*, 393–402.

Morton, V., & Torgerson, D. J. (2003). Effect of regression to the mean on decision making in health care. *British Medical Journal*, *326*, 1083–1084.

Newman, M. G., Hofmann, S. G., Werner, T., Roth, W. T., & Taylor, C. B. (1994). Does behavioral treatment of social phobia lead to cognitive changes? *Behavior Therapy*, *25*, 503–517.

Norberg, M. M., Krystal, J. H., & Tolin, D. F. (2008). A meta-analysis of D-cycloserine and the facilitation of fear extinction and exposure therapy. *Biological Psychiatry*, *63*, 1118–1126.

Norton, G. R., Allen, G. E., & Hilton, J. (1983). The social validity of treatments for agoraphobia. *Behaviour Research and Therapy*, *21*, 393–399.

Obsessive–Compulsive Cognitions Working Group. (2001). Development and initial validation of the Obsessive Beliefs Questionnaire and the Interpretation of Intrusions Inventory. *Behaviour Research and Therapy*, *39*, 987–1006.

Obsessive–Compulsive Cognitions Working Group. (2005). Psychometric validation of the Obsessive Belief Questionnaire and Interpretation of Intrusions Inventory: Part 2, factor analyses and testing of a brief version. *Behaviour Research and Therapy, 43*, 1527–1543.

Oei, T. P. S., & Loveday, W. A. L. (1997). Management of co-morbid anxiety and alcohol disorders: Parallel treatment of disorders. *Drug and Alcohol Review, 16*, 261–274.

Olatunji, B. O., Deacon, B. J., & Abramowitz, J. S. (2009). Is hypochondriasis an anxiety disorder? *British Medical Journal, 194*, 481–482.

Olatunji, B. O., & McKay, D. (Eds.). (2009). *Disgust and its disorders: Theory, assessment, and treatment implications.* Washington, DC: American Psychological Association.

Olatunji, B. O., Smits, J. A., Connolly, K., Willems, J., & Lohr, J. M. (2007). Examination of the decline in fear and disgust during exposure to threat-relevant stimuli in blood–injection–injury phobia. *Journal of Anxiety Disorders, 21*, 445–455.

Ollendick, T., & King, N. (1998). Empirically supported treatments for children with phobic and anxiety disorders: Current status. *Journal of Clinical Child and Adolescent Psychology, 27*, 156–167.

Ollendick, T. H., & King, N. J. (1998). Empirically supported treatments for children with phobic and anxiety disorders: Current status. *Journal of Clinical Child Psychology, 27*, 156–167.

Ollendick, T. H., King, N. J., & Muris, P. (2002). Fears and phobias in children: Phenomenology, epidemiology, and aetiology. *Child and Adolescent Mental Health, 7*, 98–106.

Ollendick, T. H., Öst, L. G., Reuterskiöld, L., Cederlund, R., Davis, T. E., III, Jarrett, M. A., et al. (2009). One-session treatment of specific phobias in youth: A randomized clinical trial in the United States and Sweden. *Journal of Consulting and Clinical Psychology, 77*, 504–516.

Olmsread County Child and Family Services. (2007). *Home alone: How old is old enough? A guideline for supervision of children.* Rochester, MN: Author. (*www. co.olmsted.mn.us/departments/docs/CS/brochurehomealone.pdf*)

Ost, L.-G. (1989). A maintenance program for behavioral treatment of anxiety disorders. *Behaviour Research and Therapy, 27*, 123–130.

Ost, L.-G. (1991). Acquisition of blood and injection phobia and anxiety response patterns in clinical patients. *Behaviour Research and Therapy, 29*, 323–332.

Ost, L.-G. (1992). Blood and injection phobia: Background and cognitive, physiological, and behavioral variables. *Journal of Abnormal Psychology, 101*, 68–74.

Otto, M. W., Hinton, D., Korbly, N. B., Chea, A., Phalnarith, B., Gershuny, B. S., et al. (2003). Treatment of pharmacotherapy-refractory posttraumatic stress disorder among Cambodian refugees: A pilot study of combination treatment with cognitive-behavior therapy vs. sertraline alone. *Behaviour Research and Therapy, 41*, 1271–1276.

Otto, M. W., Jones, J. C., Craske, M. G., & Barlow, D. H. (1996). *Stopping anxiety medication: Panic control therapy for benzodiazepine discontinuation.* San Antonio, TX: Psychological Corporation.

Page, A. C. (1994). Blood-injury phobia. *Clinical Psychology Review, 1994,* 443–461.

Page, A. C. (2003). The role of disgust in faintness elicited by blood and injection stimuli. *Journal of Anxiety Disorders, 17,* 45–58.

Paul, G. L. (1966). *Insight vs. desensitization in psychotherapy.* Stanford, CA: Stanford University Press.

Pediatric OCD Treatment Study (POTS) Team. (2004). Cognitive-behavior therapy, sertraline, and their combination for children and adolescents with obsessive-compulsive disorder: The Pediatric OCD Treatment Study (POTS) randomized controlled trial. *Journal of the American Medical Association, 292,* 1969–1976.

Perls, F. S. (1969). *Gestalt therapy verbatim.* Lafayette, CA: Real People Press.

Piacentini, J., & Bergman, R. L. (2001). Developmental issues in cognitive therapy for childhood anxiety disorders. *Journal of Cognitive Psychotherapy, 15*(3), 165–182.

Pigott, T. A. (1996). OCD: Where the serotonin selectivity story begins. *Journal of Clinical Psychiatry, 57*(Suppl. 6), 11–20.

Pope, K. S., & Keith-Spiegel, P. (2008). A practical approach to boundaries in psychotherapy: Making decisions, bypassing blunders, and mending fences. *Journal of Clinical Psychology: In Session, 64,* 1–15.

Poulton, R., & Menzies, R. G. (2002). Non-associative fear acquisition: A review of the evidence from retrospective and longitudinal research. *Behaviour Research and Therapy, 40,* 127–149.

Poulton, R., Thomson, W. M., Davies, S., Kruger, E., Brown, R. H., & Silva, P. A. (1997). Good teeth, bad teeth and fear of the dentist. *Behaviour Research and Therapy, 35,* 327–334.

Power, K. G., Simpson, R. J., Swanson, V., & Wallace, L. A. (1990). Controlled comparison of pharmacological and psychological treatment of generalized anxiety disorder in primary care. *British Journal of General Practice, 40,* 288–294.

Powers, M. B., Smits, J. A., Otto, M. W., Sanders, C., & Emmelkamp, P. M. (2009). Facilitation of fear extinction in phobic participants with a novel cognitive enhancer: A randomized placebo controlled trial of yohimbine augmentation. *Journal of Anxiety Disorders, 23,* 350–356.

Powers, M. B., Smits, J. A. J., Leyro, T. M., & Otto, M. W. (2007). Translational research perspectives on maximizing the effectiveness of exposure therapy. In D. C. S. Richard & D. L. Lauterbach (Eds.), *Handbook of the exposure therapies* (pp. 109–126). New York: Elsevier.

Powers, M. B., Smits, J. A. J., & Telch, M. J. (2004). Disentangling the effects of safety-behavior utilization and safety-behavior availability during exposure-based treatment: A placebo-controlled trial. *Journal of Consulting and Clinical Psychology, 72,* 448–454.

Powers, M. B., Smits, J. A. J., Whitley, D., Bystritsky, A., & Telch, M. J. (2008). The effect of attributional processes concerning medication taking on return of fear. *Journal of Consulting and Clinical Psychology, 76,* 478–490.

Prochaska, J. O. (2000). Change at differing stages. In C. R. Snyder & R. E. Ingram (Eds.), *Handbook of psychological change: Psychotherapy processes and practices for the 21st century* (pp. 109–127). Hoboken, NJ: Wiley.

Prochaska, J. O., & Norcross, J. (1999). *Systems of psychotherapy: A transtheoretical analysis* (4th ed.). Pacific Grove, CA: Brooks/Cole.

Rabavilas, A., Boulougouris, J., & Stefanis, C. (1976). Duration of flooding sessions in the treatment of obsessive–compulsive patients. *Behaviour Research and Therapy, 14,* 349–355.

Rachman, S. (1978). *Fear and courage.* San Francisco: Freeman.

Rachman, S. (1979). The return of fear. *Behaviour Research and Therapy, 17,* 164–165.

Rachman, S. (1994). Pollution of the mind. *Behaviour Research and Therapy, 32,* 311–314.

Rachman, S. (1997). A cognitive theory of obsessions. *Behaviour Research and Therapy, 35,* 793–802.

Rachman, S. (1998). A cognitive theory of obsessions: elaborations. *Behaviour Research and Therapy, 36,* 385–401.

Rachman, S. (2002). A cognitive theory of compulsive checking. *Behaviour Research and Therapy, 40,* 624–639.

Rachman, S., & Bichard, S. (1988). The overprediction of fear. *Clinical Psychology Review, 8,* 303–312.

Rachman, S., & de Silva, P. (1978). Abnormal and normal obsessions. *Behaviour Research and Therapy, 16,* 233–248.

Rachman, S., Marks, I., & Hodgson, R. (1971). The treatment of chronic obsessive–compulsive neurosis. *Behaviour Research and Therapy, 9,* 237–247.

Rachman, S., Marks, I., & Hodgson, R. (1973). The treatment of obsessive–compulsive neurotics by modelling and flooding in vivo. *Behaviour Research and Therapy, 11,* 463–471.

Rachman, S., Radomsky, A., & Shafran, R. (2008). Safety behaviors: A reconsideration. *Behaviour Research and Therapy, 46,* 163–173.

Rachman, S., & Shafran, R. (1998). Cognitive and behavioral features of obsessive–compulsive disorder. In R. P. Swinson, M. M. Antony, S. Rachman, & M. A. Richter (Eds.), *Obsessive–compulsive disorder: Theory, research, and treatment* (pp. 51–78). New York: Guilford Press.

Radomsky, A. S., & Rachman, S. (2004). Symmetry, ordering and arranging compulsive behaviour. *Behaviour Research and Therapy, 4,* 893–913.

Rapee, R. M., & Heimberg, R. G. (1997). A cognitive behavioral model of anxiety in social phobia. *Behaviour Research and Therapy, 35,* 741–756.

Rapee, R. M., Schniering, C. A., & Hudson, J. L. (2009). Anxiety disorders during childhood and adolescence: Origins and treatment. *Annual Review of Clinical Psychology, 5,* 311–341.

Reaven, J., & Hepburn, S. (2003). Cognitive-behavioral treatment of obsessive–compulsive disorder in a child with Asperger syndrome: A case report. *Autism, 7*(2), 145–164.

Reiss, S., Peterson, R. A., Gursky, D. M., & McNally, R. J. (1986). Anxiety sensitivity, anxiety frequency, and the prediction of fearfulness. *Behaviour Research and Therapy, 24,* 1–8.

Ressler, K. J., Rothbaum, B. O., Tannenbaum, L. Anderson, P., Graap, K., Zimand, E., et al. (2004). Cognitive enhancers as adjuncts to psychotherapy: Use of

D-cycloserine in phobic individuals to facilitate extinction of fear. *Archives of General Psychiatry*, *61*, 1136–1144.

Richard, D. C. S., & Gloster, A. T. (2007). Exposure therapy has a public relations problem: A dearth of litigation amid a wealth of concern. In D. C. S. Richard & D. Lauterbach (Eds.), *Comprehensive handbook of the exposure therapies* (pp. 409–425). New York: Academic Press.

Rohrbaugh, M., Shoham, V., Spungen, C., & Steinglass, P. (1985). Family systems therapy in practice: A systemic couples therapy for problem drinking. In B. M. Bongar & L. E. Beutler (Eds.), *Comprehensive textbook of psychotherapy: Theory and practice* (pp. 228–253). New York: Oxford University Press.

Rosqvist, J. (2005). *Exposure treatments for anxiety disorders*. New York: Taylor & Francis.

Rothbaum, B., Foa, E., Riggs, D., Murdock, T., & Walsh, W. (1992) A prospective examination of post-traumatic stress disorder in rape victims. *Journal of Traumatic Stress*, *5*, 455–475.

Rowe, M., & Craske, M. (1998). Effects of an expanding spaced vs. massed exposure schedule on fear reduction and return of fear. *Behaviour Research and Therapy*, *36*, 701–717.

Salkovskis, P. M. (1991). The importance of behavior in the maintenance of anxiety and panic: A cognitive account. *Behavioural Psychotherapy*, *19*, 6–19.

Salkovskis, P. M. (1996). Cognitive-behavioral approaches to the understanding of obsessional problems. In R. Rapee (Ed.), *Current controversies in the anxiety disorders* (pp. 103–133). New York: Guilford Press.

Salkovskis, P. M., Clark, D. M., Hackman, A., Wells, A., & Gelder, M. G. (1999). An experimental investigation of the role of safety behaviours in the maintenance of panic disorder with agoraphobia. *Behaviour Research and Therapy*, *37*, 559–574.

Salkovskis, P. M., & Harrison, J. (1984). Abnormal and normal obsessions: A replication. *Behaviour Research and Therapy*, *22*, 549–552.

Salter, A. (1949) *Conditioned reflex therapy*. New York: Capricorn Books.

Sartory, G., Rachman, S., & Grey, S. J. (1982). Return of fear: The role of rehearsal. *Behaviour Research and Therapy*, *20*, 123–133.

Schmidt, N. B., Lerew, D. R., & Trakowski, J. H. (1997). Body vigilance in panic disorder: Evaluating attention to bodily perturbations. *Journal of Consulting and Clinical Psychology*, *65*, 214–220.

Schmidt, R. A., & Bjork, R. A. (1992). New conceptualizations of practice: Common principles in three paradigms suggest new concepts for training. *Psychological Science*, *3*, 207–217.

Shafran, R., Ralph, J., & Tallis, F. (1995). Obsessive–compulsive symptoms and the family. *Bulletin of the Menninger Clinic*, *59*(4), 472–479.

Shafran, R., Thordarson, D., & Rachman, S. (1996). Thought-action fusion in obsessive–compulsive disorder. *Journal of Anxiety Disorders*, *10*, 379.

Shapiro, F. (1991). Eye movement desensitization and reprocessing procedure: From EMD to EMD/R-A, and treatment model for anxiety and related trauma. *The Behavior Therapist*, *5*, 128–133.

Shapiro, F. (1995). *Eye movement desensitization and reprocessing (EMDR): Basic principles, protocols, and procedures.* New York: Guilford Press.

Sharp, D. M., Power, K. G., Simpson, R. J., Swanson, V., Moodie, E., Anstee, J. A., & Ashford, J. J. (1996). Fluvoxamine, placebo, and cognitive behaviour therapy used alone and in combination in the treatment of panic disorder and agoraphobia. *Journal of Anxiety Disorders, 10,* 219–242.

Sherman, J. J. (1998). Effects of psychotherapeutic treatments for PTSD: A meta-analysis of controlled clinical trials. *Journal of Traumatic Stress, 11,* 413–435.

Silverman, W. A. (1977). The lesson of retrolental fibroplasia. *Scientific American, 236,* 100–107.

Silverman, W. K., & Kurtines, W. M. (1996). Transfer of control: A psychosocial intervention model for internalizing disorders in youth. In E. D. Hibbs & P. S. Jensen (Eds.), *Psychosocial treatments for child and adolescent disorders: Empirically based strategies for clinical practice* (pp. 63–81). Washington, DC: American Psychological Association.

Simon, N. M., Connor, K. M., Lang, A. J., Rauch, S., Krulewisz, S., LeBeau, R. T., et al. (2008). Paroxetine CR augmentation for posttraumatic stress disorder refractory to prolonged exposure therapy. *Journal of Clinical Psychiatry, 69,* 400–405.

Sloan, T., & Telch, M. J. (2002). The effects of safety-seeking behavior and guided threat reappraisal on fear reduction during exposure: An experimental investigation. *Behaviour Research and Therapy, 40,* 235–251.

Smith, D., & Fitzpatrick, M. (1995). Patient–therapist boundary issues: An integrative review of theory and research. *Professional Psychology: Research and Practice, 26,* 499–506.

Soravia, L. M., Heinrichs, M., Aerni, A., Maroni, C., Schelling, G., Ehlert, U., et al. (2006). Glucocorticoids reduce phobic fear in humans. *Proceedings of the National Academy of Sciences, 103,* 5585–5590.

South, S. C., & Krueger, R. F. (2008). Marital quality moderates genetic and environmental influences on the internalizing spectrum. *Journal of Abnormal Psychology, 117*(4), 826–837.

Spiegel, D. A., & Bruce, T. J. (1997). Benzodiazepines and exposure-based cognitive behavior therapies for panic disorder: Conclusions from combined treatment trials. *American Journal of Psychiatry, 154,* 773–781.

Spielberger, C. D., Gorsuch, R. L., Lushene, R., Vagg, P. R., & Jacobs, G. A. (1983). *Manual for the State–Trait Anxiety Inventory.* Palo Alto, CA: Consulting Psychologists Press.

Stamm, B. H. (Ed.). (1999). *Secondary traumatic stress: Self-care issues for clinicians, researchers, and educators* (2nd ed.). Lutherville, MD: Sidran Press.

Stampfl, T. G. (1966). Implosive therapy: The theory. In S. G. Armitage (Ed.), *Behavior modification techniques in the treatment of emotional disorders* (pp. 22–37). Battle Creek, MI: V.A. Publication.

Stampfl, T. G., & Levis, D. J. (1967). Essentials of implosive therapy: A learning-theory-based psychodynamic behavioral therapy. *Journal of Abnormal Psychology, 72,* 496–503.

Stein, D., Hollander, E., & Rothbaum, B. O. (Eds.). (2010). *American Psychiatric*

Association textbook of anxiety disorders (2nd ed.). Washington, DC: American Psychiatric Association.

Stein, M. B., Sherbourne, C. D., Craske, M. G., Means-Christensen, A., Bystritsky, A., Katon, W., et al. (2004). Quality of care for primary care patients with anxiety disorders. *American Journal of Psychiatry, 161,* 2230–2237.

Steketee, G. (1993). Social support and treatment outcome of obsessive compulsive disorder at 9-month follow-up. *Behavioural Psychotherapy, 21*(2), 81–95.

Stewart, R. E., & Chambless, D. L. (2009). Cognitive-behavioral therapy for adult anxiety disorders in clinical practice: A meta-analysis of effectiveness studies. *Journal of Consulting and Clinical Psychology, 77,* 595–606.

Storch, E. A., Merlo, L. J., Bengtson, M., Murphy, T. K., Lewis, M. H., Yang, M. C., et al. (2007). D-cycloserine does not enhance exposure-response prevention therapy in obsessive–compulsive disorder. *International Clinical Psychopharmacology, 22,* 230–237.

Stravynski, A., & Amado, D. (2001). Social phobia as a deficit in social skills. In S. G. Hofmann & P. M. DiBartolo (Eds.), *From social anxiety to social phobia: Multiple perspectives* (pp. 107–129). Boston: Allyn & Bacon.

Summerfeldt, L. J. (2004). Understanding and treating incompleteness in obsessive–compulsive disorder. *Journal of Clinical Psychology, 60,* 1155–1168.

Summerfeldt, L. J. (2008). Symmetry, incompleteness, and ordering. In J. Abramowitz, D. McKay, & S. Taylor (Eds.), *Clinical handbook of obsessive–compulsive disorder and related problems* (pp. 44–60). Baltimore: Johns Hopkins University Press.

Swobota, H., Amering, M., Windhaber, J., & Katschnig, H. (2001). Long-term course of panic disorder: An 11 year follow-up. *Journal of Anxiety Disorders, 17,* 223–232.

Taylor, S. (1996). Meta-analysis of cognitive-behavioral treatments for social phobia. *Journal of Behavior Therapy and Experimental Psychiatry, 27,* 1–9.

Taylor, S. (Ed.). (1999). *Anxiety sensitivity: Theory, research, and treatment of the fear of anxiety.* Mahwah, NJ: Erlbaum.

Taylor, S. (2000). *Understanding and treating panic disorder.* New York: Wiley.

Taylor, S., & Asmundson, G. (2004). *Treating health anxiety: A cognitive-behavioral approach.* New York: Guilford Press.

Taylor, S., Asmundson, G. J. G., & Coons, M. J. (2005). Current directions in the treatment of hypochondriasis. *Journal of Cognitive Psychotherapy: An International Quarterly, 19,* 285–304.

Telch, M. J., Lucas, J. A., Schmidt, N. B., Hanna, H. H., LaNae, J. T., & Lucas, R. A. (1993). Group cognitive-behavioral treatment of panic disorder. *Behaviour Research and Therapy, 31,* 279–287.

Telch, M. J., Lucas, R. A., Smits, J. A. J., Powers, M. B., Heimberg, R., & Hart, T. (2004). Appraisal of social concerns: A cognitive assessment instrument for social phobia. *Depression and Anxiety, 19,* 217–224.

Thyer, B. A., & Sowers-Hoag, K. M. (1988). Behavior therapy for separation anxiety disorder. *Behavior Modification, 12,* 205–233.

Turk, D. C., & Salovey, P. (1985). Cognitive structures, cognitive processes, and cognitive-behavior modification: II. Judgments and inferences of the clinician. *Cognitive Therapy and Research, 9,* 19–33.

United Nations. (1987). United Nations convention against torture and other cruel, inhuman or degrading treatment or punishment. New York: Author.

Valderhaug, R., Gotestam, K. G., & Larsson, B. (2004). Clinicians' views on management of obsessive–compulsive disorders in children and adolescents. *Nordic Journal of Psychiatry, 58*(2), 125–132.

van Apeldoorn, F. J., van Hout, W. J., Mersch, P. P., Huisman, M., Slaap, B. R., Hale, W. W. 3rd, et al. (2008). Is a combined therapy more effective than either CBT or SSRI alone?: Results of a multicenter trial on panic disorder with or without agoraphobia. *Acta Psychiatrica Scandinavica, 117*, 260–270.

van Balkom, A. J. L. M., van Oppen, P., Vermeulen, A. W. A., van Dyck, R., Nauta, M. C. E., & Vorst, H. C. M. (1994). A meta-analysis on the treatment of obsessive–compulsive disorder: A comparison of antidepressants, behavior, and cognitive therapy. *Clinical Psychology Review, 14*, 359–381.

Van Etten, M., & Taylor, S. (1998). Comparative efficacy of treatments for posttraumatic stress disorder: A meta-analysis. *Clinical Psychology and Psychotherapy, 5*, 126–145.

Veronen, L., & Kilpatrick, D. (1983). Stress management for rape victims. In D. Meichenbaum & M. E. Jaremko (Eds.), *Stress reduction and prevention* (pp. 341–374). New York: Plenum Press.

Viana, A. G., Beidel, D. C., & Rabian, B. (2009). Selective mutism: A review and integration of the last 15 years. *Clinical Psychology Review, 29*(1), 57–67.

Walkup, J. T., Albano, A. M., Piacentini, J., Birmaher, B., Compton, S. N., Sherrill, J. T., et al. (2008). Cognitive behavioral therapy, sertraline, or a combination in childhood anxiety. *New England Journal of Medicine, 359*, 2753–2766.

Warwick, H. (1995). Assessment of hypochondriasis. *Behaviour Research and Therapy, 33*, 845–853.

Watson, H. J., & Rees, C. S. (2008). Meta-analysis of randomized, controlled treatment trials for pediatric obsessive–compulsive disorder. *Journal of Child Psychology and Psychiatry, 49*(5), 489–498.

Watson, J. B., & Rayner, R. (1920). Conditioned emotional reactions. *Journal of Experimental Psychology, 3*, 1–14.

Weissman, M. M. (1991). Panic disorder: Impact on quality of life. *Journal of Clinical Psychiatry, 52*(Suppl. 2), 6–8.

Wells, A., Clark, D. M., & Ahmad, S. (1998). How do I look with my mind's eye: Perspective taking in social phobic imagery. *Behaviour Research and Therapy, 36*, 631–634.

Weston, D., & Morrison, K. (2001). A multidimensional meta-analysis of treatments for depression, panic, and generalized anxiety disorder: An empirical examination of the status of empirically supported therapies. *Journal of Consulting and Clinical Psychology, 69*, 875–899.

Westra, H. A., & Dozois, D. J. A. (2006). Preparing clients for cognitive behavioral therapy: A randomized pilot study of motivational interviewing for anxiety. *Cognitive Therapy and Research, 30*(4), 481–498.

Whisman, M. A. (1999). Marital dissatisfaction and psychiatric disorders: Results from the National Comorbidity Survey. *Journal of Abnormal Psychology, 108*(4), 701–706.

Whitehead, W. E., Robinson, A., Blackwell, B., & Stutz, R. M. (1978). Flooding treatment of phobias: Does chronic diazepam increase effectiveness? *Behavior Therapy and Experimental Psychiatry, 9,* 219–225.

Whiteside, S. P., Brown, A. M., & Abramowitz, J. S. (2008). Five-day intensive treatment for adolescent OCD: A case series. *Journal of Anxiety Disorders, 22*(3), 495–504.

Widiger, T. A., & Miller, J. D. (2008). Psychological diagnosis. In D. Richard & S. Huprich (Eds.), *Clinical psychology, assessment, treatment, and research* (pp. 69–88). Oxford, UK: Elsevier.

Wilhelm, S., Buhlmann, U., Tolin, D. F., Meunier, S. A., Pearlson, G. D., Reese, H. E., et al. (2008). Augmentation of behavior therapy with D-cycloserine for obsessive–compulsive disorder. *American Journal of Psychiatry, 165,* 335–341.

Wilhelm, S., & Steketee, G. (2006). *Cognitive therapy for obsessive–compulsive disorder: A guide for professionals.* Oakland, CA: New Harbinger.

Wilson, J. K., & Rapee, R. M. (2005). The interpretation of negative social events in social phobia with versus without comorbid mood disorder. *Journal of Anxiety Disorders, 19,* 245–274.

Wolitzky-Taylor, K. B., Horowitz, J. D., Powers, M. B., & Telch, M. J. (2008). Psychological approaches in the treatment of specific phobia: A meta-analysis. *Clinical Psychology Review, 28,* 1021–1037.

Wolpe, J. (1958). *Psychotherapy by reciprocal inhibition.* Stanford, CA: Stanford University Press.

Zitrin, C. M., Klein, D., & Woerner, M. G. (1978). Behavior therapy, supportive psychotherapy, imipramine, and phobias. *Archives of General Psychiatry, 35,* 303–321.

Zitrin, C. M., Klein, D., Woerner, M. G., & Ross, D. C. (1983). Treatment of phobias: Comparison of imipramine hydrochloride and placebo. *Archives of General Psychiatry, 40,* 125–138.

Zur, O. (2001). Out-of-office experience: When crossing office boundaries and engaging in dual relationships are clinically beneficial and ethically sound. *The Independent Practitioner, 21,* 96–98.

Zur, O. (2005). The dumbing down of psychology: faulty beliefs about boundary crossings and dual relationships. In R. H. Wright & N. A. Cummings (Eds.), *Destructive trends in mental health: The well-intentioned path to harm* (pp. 252–282). New York: Taylor & Francis Group.

Zur, O. (2007). *Boundaries in psychotherapy: Ethical and clinical explorations.* Washington, DC: American Psychological Association.

Index

Page numbers followed by an *f*, *n*, or *t* indicate figures, notes, or tables.

385